Textbook of Pathophysiology

Textbook of
Pathophysiology

W. D. Snively, Jr., M.D., F.A.C.P.
Professor in the Life Sciences, School of Nursing,
University of Evansville, Evansville, Indiana;
Visiting Professor in Continuing Medical Education,
University of Alabama Medical Center, Birmingham, Alabama

and

Donna R. Beshear
Medical Writer; Research Associate

Illustrations by Robert Wiethop

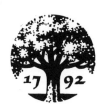

J. B. Lippincott Company

Philadelphia
Toronto

Copyright © 1972, by J. B. Lippincott Company

This book is fully protected by copyright, and,
with the exception of brief excerpts for review,
no part of it may be reproduced in any form, by
print, photoprint, microfilm, or by any other
means without the written permission of the publishers.

Distributed in Great Britain by
Blackwell Scientific Publications
Oxford, London and Edinburgh

ISBN-0-397-59051-2

Library of Congress Catalog Card Number: 70-175714

Printed in the United States of America

   3   4   2

Library of Congress Cataloging in Publication Data

Snively, William Daniel
   Textbook of pathophysiology.

   1. Physiology, Pathological. I. Beshear, Donna
R.,   joint author. II. Title.
RB113.S58 616.07 70-175714
ISBN 0-397-59051-2

acknowledgments

The authors gratefully acknowledge the generous assistance provided by the following individuals and institutions:

Audiovisual Department, Deaconess Hospital, Evansville, which provided numerous illustrations.

Department of Pathology, Henderson County Methodist Hospital, Henderson, Kentucky; and B. V. Cymbala, M.D., Director of the Department, who made his entire slide collection available to us.

Marjorie Fuller, Supervisor, Mead Johnson Research Center Library, and Rose Horn, Reprint Librarian, Mead Johnson Research Center, Evansville, who provided valued library research services.

Department of Pathology, Deaconess Hospital, Evansville, which provided slides of pathologic specimens.

Department of Radiology, St. Mary's Hospital, Evansville, which provided x-ray photographs.

Intensive Care Unit, St. Mary's Hospital, Evansville, which provided electrocardiographic strips.

Helen Smith, Ed.D., Dean, School of Nursing, University of Evansville, for valued counsel.

Ellen Lynch, R.N., B.S., M.S.N., Associate Director of Nursing, School of Nursing, Deaconess Hospital, Evansville, for valued counsel.

We are particularly indebted to David T. Miller, Vice President, J. B. Lippincott Company, for his valued counsel and guidance, and to Bernice Heller, Editor, Division of Higher Education, J. B. Lippincott Company, for her creative help and judicious guidance at every stage in the preparation and publication of this book.

preface

Pathologic physiology, or pathophysiology, is concerned with disruptions of normal physiology, with the processes that bring about these disruptions, and with the various ways in which the disruptions manifest themselves as symptoms, signs, physical findings, and laboratory findings. Plutarch said, "Medicine, to produce health, has to examine disease." Disease represents a change from the state of being in complete accord with one's external environment and in a state of internal equilibrium to a condition of dis-ease or discomfort. But we must, as William Boyd emphasizes, distinguish illness from disease. Disease refers to a specific state characterized by certain alterations in the body. These alterations presumably involve structure, even though that structure is microscopic or submicroscopic. Disease is caused by a process, known or unknown, and usually has certain symptoms, signs, and physical and laboratory findings. On the other hand, when we say a person is ill, we mean he is uncomfortable, is suffering from certain symptoms such as nausea, headache, abdominal cramps, or just plain fatigue that can't be explained on the basis of exertion. A patient can be diseased without being ill. Indeed, one may have a disease without recognizing it. For example, one may have arthritis of the bones of the neck yet have no symptoms whatever. The condition may be discovered in a routine x-ray examination. Later he may develop all sorts of unpleasant symptoms, such as pain in the arms, "dead" fingers, even paralysis and wasting of muscles. Then the patient is ill.

We must, however, beware of regarding disease as a static state, something that is found in the autopsy room. Disease is itself a process. Its manifestations change continually. It may end in the patient's recovery, or partial recovery or death. It may be as acute and explosive in its onset as a summer storm, or it may, like the falling of leaves in the autumn, represent the slow aging of tissues caused by the ravages of time. We should not ignore the importance of examining tissues after death. The Latin inscription in one autopsy room translates: "This is the place where death delights to serve the living." Wilens, in his *My Friends the Doctors*, says, "The old adage that dead men tell no tales does not hold true as far as the medical profession is concerned. Dead men have for centuries been telling doctors the story of *how* they got sick and *why* they died, and doctors have made use of this information very effectively in the treatment of other sick people."

Pathophysiology is concerned with the living sick, serving as an essential connecting link between the basic sciences of anatomy, physiology, and biochemistry on the one hand and medical and surgical therapy on the other. Its study is essential if one is to understand disease. Rudolph Virchow could well have been referring to pathophysiology rather than to pathology when he said, "Pathology has been released from the anomalous and isolated position which it has occupied for thousands of years. Through the application of its doctrines not only to diseases of man, but also to those of even the smallest and lowest animals, and to those of plants, it helps to deepen biological knowledge and to illuminate that region of the unknown which still envelops the intimate structure of living matter. It is no longer a matter of applied physiology—it has become physiology itself."

This book presents an integrated approach to human disease. It was designed for students in a variety of programs for health practitioners. It examines all that occurs when various disease-causing processes exert their effect on physiological function. First we shall examine what we regard as the basic pathophysiological processes that cause disease. In classifying these processes, our goal was to present a list that would be comprehensive, logical, and usable. We recognize that categories, no matter how logical they may appear to the human, are manmade rather than "natural." How nature's flaunting of categories frustrates man! Scientists are deeply concerned as to whether the euglena, that motile green creature that inhabits placid ponds, is plant or animal. Zoologists stay awake nights trying to decide whether the kangaroo is a mammal or an advanced reptile. These questions irk neither the euglena nor the hopping marsupial of Australia. But nature's refusal to be pigeonholed can cause enormous problems when one attempts to classify natural phenomena.

As will become clear in due course, few diseases result exclusively from one, or even two, pathophysiologic processes. Most are a commingling of many causes. Understanding the composite nature of disease leads toward, if not to, correct diagnosis and effective treatment. Understanding the roots of a given disorder is essential if one is to develop insight. It is similar to the necessity of mastering the fundamentals of football if one is to play a skillful game.

In preparing this text on pathophysiology, we are all too aware of the appalling glut of information—often called the information explosion—that confronts today's student. There has certainly been an enormous accumulation of knowledge within the past few decades. Still, as far back as any of us can remember, there always existed a larger body of clinically significant facts than any one person could master. Students may face a larger problem in their studies, but it is no new problem. And on the positive side, new tools are available for its solution.

How can today's student avoid becoming lost in the maze of facts? Obviously, he needs a key to unlock the door. That key may be the overused and abused term, *relevance*. If we focus on what is germane, we no longer face an insuperable obstacle. Students (and teachers as well) must develop a new sixth sense, a sense of the significant. They must use modern techniques to learn what is significant. In their minds must be the recognition that the march of science is as rapid as it is inexorable.

In this book, we have endeavored, then, to emphasize the relevant, to stress principles and concepts. We believe this approach leads to insight. Consider diseases affecting the kidney. The student who thoroughly understands the nephron, the anatomical and physiological unit of the kidney, is in the position of being able to predict with reasonable accuracy what kidney diseases will occur when certain pathophysiological processes involve the kidney. He will thoroughly understand the basis for such diseases as glomerulonephritis, pyelonephritis, and nephrosis, to name but three. On the other hand, should he merely learn to recite, parrot-fashion, the list of diseases affecting the kidney, including cause, symptoms, physical findings, laboratory findings, diagnosis, treatment, and prognosis, he will have no true understanding of disease of the kidney. Similarly, the student who understands the 16 basic imbalances in body fluids can predict which body fluid disturbances will occur in various disease states. He has a far deeper and more useful understanding of body fluid disturbances than if he merely memorized the changes occurring in these essential fluids in a host of diseases.

We have written this book so that it would be a simple matter to construct behavioral or instructional objectives based on the material it presents. For what we are trying to present is not a body of content to be driven into the mind of the student, but rather a text that will enable him to demonstrate his achievement in the field of pathophysiology in behavioral terms.

We have endeavored to enlist the visual senses to the fullest extent possible by the generous use of drawings, photographs, flow charts, and tables. Because the field of pathophysiology is subject enough for one book, we have assumed acquaintance with basic physiology and anatomy.

Although in this text we appear to focus on disease, let us always keep in mind the old French proverb, "There are no diseases, but only sick people."

contents

part one

Mechanisms and Models of Disease

introduction:
a unitary view of disease

Everyone concerned in any way with human health, be he Nobel laureate or ward aide, must come to grips with the question, What is disease? In the process of writing this book, we have been repeatedly reminded that man has made enormous progress toward answering this question—even though in many areas only the first few steps have been taken. Certainly one of the cardinal achievements of modern medical science has been an appreciation of disease as a disruption, or a dysfunction, of one or more normal physiological processes. In some instances the body recovers without help; but in many others, consequences of a more or less serious nature can be prevented only by successful treatment.

We term our view of disease and our approach to examining its varied manifestations *a unitary view of disease.* What do we mean by "a unitary view"? We mean a broad overview that regards disease as a dynamic process, not a static phenomenon. Such a view enables the health practitioner to avoid the shoals of fragmentation (in which only the immediate clinical ailment is recognized and treated) and keep to the deep channel of holism (in which the illness to be treated represents only one facet of the sick individual). As a result, the health practitioner views the patient as a sick *person* rather than as a "peptic ulcer" or a "fracture" or a "cerebrovascular accident." Such a view appears essential if one is to attain a true understanding of pathophysiology; he must be able to see the woods as well as the trees.

The unitary approach makes it clear that the hundreds of diseases encompassed by any disease nomenclature result from a small number of causative processes. If the student can clearly understand these basic processes he will have gained a vantage from which to view, with understanding, any disease.

No group of scientists would all agree as to just what these basic processes are. We have selected 12, as described in Part I. We have tested our list by analyzing a broad spectrum of diseases from the standpoint of their causation. We have found that virtually all could be explained on the basis of one or more of the 12 processes.

Today's student surpasses his predecessors in his appreciation of health care as a need—indeed, a right—of all mankind. He embarks on his chosen field of health practice with a clearer idea of his potential contributions to health improvement. The unitary view here encompassed should aid him in making his maximal contribution.

1

homeostasis and pathogenesis

Man is a tough and durable creature. By dint of amazing ingenuity and unflagging effort, spurred by a stubborn life-wish, he manages to inhabit almost every corner of the globe, no matter how inhospitable. He lives in the frozen tundra of the Arctic. He exists as a nomad in the deserts of northern Africa. He can eke out his days in the thin air of the Andes or on the inhospitable coast of Tierra del Fuego. He dwells in the sprawling, teeming towns on the humid coast of southern Asia. He rockets into outer space, even to the moon, and descends to the depths of the ocean. Throughout his long existence on this planet, a million years or more, he has been both hunted and hunter. He has survived countless struggles with viruses, bacteria, and other pathogenic microorganisms even though on at least one occasion, disease in the form of the bubonic plague threatened to extinguish his species.

Essential to man's survival is his own internal environment, the environment enclosed by his skin. The pervasive element of that internal environment is the body fluid that bathes the cells of his body and enabled him to leave his ancestral ocean. An internal environment could not exist without maintenance of temperature, composition, concentration, and volume within narrow bounds compatible with normal function. This is the goal of homeostasis, which is achieved through the activities of the widely distributed endocrine glands and the coordinating fibers of the nervous system.

As one reviews the history of medicine, he must be amazed by the tardiness of our recognition of homeostasis. This landmark physiological principle was not set out until 1857, when Claude Bernard introduced it at the Sorbonne in Paris. Said Bernard, "All the vital mechanisms, however varied they may be, have always but one end, that of preserving the constancy of the conditions of life in the internal environment." He thus set forth a fundamental concept which he named the *milieu intérieur* (internal environment), that increasingly guides medical thinking in its considerations of health and disease. The term *homeostasis,* which is the one generally used today, was coined by Walter Cannon, the great American physiologist, who introduced it in 1929. He pointed out

CONTRIBUTION OF CLAUDE BERNARD OF LANDMARK SIGNIFICANCE

that homeostatic processes are those that tend to restore the internal environment to a steady, or resting, state.

MECHANISM OF HOMEOSTASIS

Now, how does homeostasis operate? The cell, the basic unit of life, contains DNA (deoxyribonucleic acid), the transmitter of our genetic constitution which manufactures the myriad proteins required for cell function. Now, if the cell is to remain alive and to conduct its normal business, the composition of the bath water of the cells, the interstitial fluid (which comprises three-fourths of the extracellular fluid) must be precisely controlled. Experiment has shown that cells can stay alive when removed from the body if they are placed in a solution resembling interstitial fluid; but they die quickly in an isotonic solution of sodium chloride, whose composition differs greatly from that of interstitial fluid. Through such experiment is shown the ultimate function of all body organs and processes: to maintain constant the composition and concentration of the extracellular fluid and, via the cell wall, of the cellular fluid. Every body system, every organ, with the possible exception of the reproductive organs, is concerned with homeostasis. Par-

PRINCIPAL BODY HOMEOSTATIC MECHANISMS

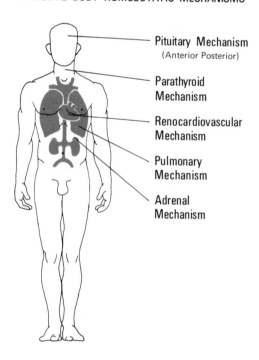

Pituitary Mechanism
(Anterior Posterior)

Parathyroid
Mechanism

Renocardiovascular
Mechanism

Pulmonary
Mechanism

Adrenal
Mechanism

ticularly involved are the renocardiovascular system, the parathyroid gland, the pituitary gland, the adrenal glands, and the lungs.

Acid–Base Balance

While recognizing that the several activities of the body have as their focus the maintenance of homeostasis, we might examine more closely how this is carried out. Let us take as our first example the maintenance of acid-base balance, to be discussed in detail in a later chapter. The acid-base balance of the body depends upon the hydrogen ion concentration in the extracellular and cellular fluid. Although hydrogen exists in these fluids in minute quantities, it is of incalculable im-

LABORATORY VALUES: NORMAL RANGES

Blood Formed Elements [*]

	Birth	3 mo.	1 yr.	5 yr.	12 yr.	Adults Women	Men
Hematocrit—% vol. of packed RBC/100 ml.	43–63	28–40	32–40	36–44	39–47	39–47	44–52
Hemoglobin— gm./100 ml.	14–20	9–13	11–12.5	12–14.7	13.4–15.8	13–16	15–18
RBC—million/ cu. mm.	4.1–5.7	3.1–4.7	3.9–4.7	4.0–4.8	4.3–5.1	4.2–5.0	4.8–6.0

Plasma Chemical Constituents

Plasma K^+	4.0–5.6	mEq /l.
Plasma Na^+	137–147	mEq /l.
Plasma Ca^{++}	4.5–5.8	mEq./l.
Plasma Protein	6–8	gm./100 ml.
Plasma Cl^-	98–106	mEq./l.
Plasma Cl^- plus Plasma HCO_3^-	123–135	mEq./l.
Plasma $HPO_4^=$	1.7–2.6	mEq./l.
Plasma pH	7.35–7.45	mEq./l.
Plasma HCO_3^-	25–29	mEq./l. (adults)
	20–25	mEq./l. (children)

Urine Values

Urine pH	4.5–8.2
Urine specific gravity	1.010–1.030

[*] In 94% of normal population.

portance. Its concentration depends largely upon the quantities of carbonic acid and base bicarbonate (by which we mean the bicarbonates of sodium, potassium, calcium, and magnesium) in the body fluids. The normal ratio of carbonic acid to bicarbonate is 1 to 20. As long as this ratio holds, the body is in acid–base balance. Should the ratio become disturbed, either because of a decrease or an increase in bicarbonate or because of a decrease or an increase in carbonic acid, the body slips over into an acid-base disturbance.

If we place carbonic acid on one side of a mythical balance and bicarbonate on the other side of the balance, we will achieve the conditions needed for acid-base balance as long as there is 1 part of carbonic acid to 20 parts of bicarbonate. Both the amounts of carbonic acid and of base bicarbonate can be doubled or halved, and the pH of the body fluid will remain within the narrow limits of normal, 7.35 to 7.45. But should either the carbonic acid or the base bicarbonate be increased or decreased without a corresponding change in the other, then an acid-base disturbance would occur and the homeostatic mechanisms would be called into play to maintain the balance level.

Acid–base disturbances due to metabolic disorders   Suppose that ketone bodies of diabetic acidosis neutralize base bicarbonate and cause a base bicarbonate deficit (as in metabolic acidosis). The body makes every effort to restore the balance to normal: the lungs blow off CO_2; the kidneys retain bicarbonate. These measures partially or completely restore the balance to normal.

ROLE OF THE KIDNEY AND THE LUNG

Now let us suppose that a patient with peptic ulcer takes excessive amounts of the alkali, sodium bicarbonate (baking soda)—so much, indeed, that the kidneys cannot excrete the excess. Bicarbonate excess (metabolic alkalosis) develops. Kidney excretion continues, to rid the system of the excess sodium bicarbonate. The rate and depth of respiration are decreased so that carbon dioxide is held back (carbon dioxide, when added to water, becomes carbonic acid, thus: $CO_2 + HOH = H_2CO_3$). The combined actions of kidney and lung will tilt the balance in the direction of normality, even if that state is not fully reached.

Acid–base disturbances due to respiratory disorders   Respiratory diseases also cause acid-base disturbances. Suppose the patient has pneumonia, his lungs being consolidated so that normal exchange of oxygen and carbon dioxide between blood and alveolar air stops. Carbon dioxide is retained in the blood. Carbonic acid excess (respiratory acidosis) occurs. Homeostatic mechanisms swing into action. The kidneys retain bicarbonate. The lungs cannot participate in the action since this is where the problem originated, but kidney retention of bicarbonate at least helps counteract the dysfunction.

Now let us suppose that because of hysteria, worry, or the early effects of salicylate intoxication, a person begins breathing deeply and rapidly, blowing off excessive quantities of carbon dioxide. A carbonic acid deficit (respiratory alkalosis) develops. The kidneys excrete bicarbonate to restore balance. The lungs do not participate because it was their dysfunction that initiated the imbalance.

You have noted that one effect of homeostatic controls is to increase or decrease the *bicarbonate* concentration—in order to promote normality of *hydrogen ion* concentration. Characteristically, homeostatic mechanisms are directed toward maintaining the important value at normal, so less important adjustments may suffer. The values shown in the table are maintained throughout most of the myriad activities of homeostasis.

Response to Stress Factors

We have still other examples showing how the body functions to achieve homeostasis. During periods of stress, the adrenal glands produce antistress, or anti-inflammatory, hormones, such as cortisol—an appropriate response to the challenge of stress which operates to maintain homeostasis. An endless number of examples of similar body activities could be cited.

Effects of cold   One of the most fascinating aspects of homeostasis concerns the differing sensitivities of body tissues to various levels of essential chemicals and of temperature. Sir Joseph Barcroft's laboratory in Cambridge, England, contained a small room wherein any known climate or altitude· could be duplicated. In a classic experiment, Sir Joseph once spent 14 days in an atmosphere equivalent to that of the highest slopes of Mount Everest. As a result of his studies, he emphasized that the *body* can tolerate wide alterations of acid-base balance and extreme cold. Then he pointed out that *mental processes* are far more sensitive than strictly somatic processes. A change in the hydrogen ion concentration of the body fluid for but a short time can cause an inability to concentrate that lasts for days. Cold sharply depresses the higher mental functions. A person starving and without adequate protection from cold would suffer from the acidosis that accompanies inadequate food intake and from the cold. Rational thinking would be crippled. These observations have an interesting application to primitive man. Until our forebears could so control their environment as to be kept reasonably warm and well nourished, they could make no real progress in the arts of civilization. Even today, of course, hungry people cannot be expected to think and plan properly. They are even less able to do so if they are also cold.

A poignant true story comes from the rugged mountains of northern California. A family of three made a forced landing in their small plane on a forested mountain slope in the dead of winter. The father wandered off through the deep snows in search of help, which he never found. The mother and daughter snuggled close in the fuselage. They had no food, and only the snow about the airplane for water. Although they had a supply of matches and were surrounded by a pine forest, they failed to start a signal fire with the gasoline in the airplane. They kept a sad diary, which indicated that they had lived for months before succumbing. But under those conditions, such prolonged life would have been impossible —obviously, they had mistaken hours for days and weeks for months. Their hunger and the deadening chill just wouldn't permit them to think creatively, or even clearly.

Factors That Tend Toward "Reverse Homeostasis"

FALLIBILITY OF
HOMEOSTASIS

We like to speak of the wisdom of the body, and we quite properly extol it; but we should not ignore the body's occasional lapses into quite stupid behavior, which often challenges the physician's best efforts and sometimes kills. Since homeostasis is a manifestation of the *human* organism—that frail structure—it cannot always operate in an infallible manner. What are some of these lapses?

Changes in temperature   When the temperature around us drops, perhaps to the point where we are in danger of freezing, body heat production accelerates and tends to offset the low environmental temperature. That is homeostasis at its best. But suppose one is wandering on the Arizona desert, where the temperature easily reaches 130° F. or higher. Does body heat production decrease, as one would expect? No, it does not. Heat production *increases,* in spite of the high environmental heat. Heat exhaustion and then heatstroke can quickly occur, partly due to this "reverse homeostasis."

Consider the matter of fever. Does it help combat infection? Scientists are not sure. But there remains no doubt that excessive fever, perhaps over 106° or 107° F., can be harmful and that extremely high fever, such as 110° F., cannot long be endured. Are the body homeostatic mechanisms "tricked" into "ordering" fever by bacterial toxins?

Stress   Another example of homeostasis gone awry: when stress assails one, the adrenal glands usually respond by producing appropriate amounts of the anti-inflammatory hormones, such as cortisol, or the "survival" hormones, such as aldosterone. Ideally, amounts produced balance each other. But in some circumstances homeostasis fails, and improper quantities of cortisol or of aldosterone are produced. Depending upon which imbalance occurs, disease may develop—rheumatoid arthritis if there is inadequate anti-inflammatory hormone, mineralocorticoid hypertension if there is excessive survival hormone. These diseases have been named *diseases of the general adaptation syndrome* by Hans Selye, who has greatly advanced our knowledge of the several effects of stress.

Antibody-antigen reactions   In other circumstances, too, homeostasis breaks down. The body possesses a complicated system of defenses against invading infectious organisms. Its antibodies vigorously attack proteins of the invaders so as to prevent disruption of homeostasis. But under certain circumstances—of which more later—these same antibodies attack the body's own proteins. The result may be serious disease of the thyroid, joints, eyes, or other body organs. Allergies, too, represent a sort of "homeostasis in reverse": as various mechanisms are called into play to counteract allergic irritants, disease far more serious than any damage due to the irritant may develop.

Genetic disorders   Diseases based on genetic factors provide another example of breakdown of homeostasis. For instance, in the case of PKU disease, the lack of a single cellular enzyme prevents normal metabolism of the amino acid phenylalanine. Cellular homeostasis is disrupted, with disastrous results to the individual.

Infection   Organisms of infectious diseases disturb homeostasis by producing exotoxins (harmful enzymes), by entering body cells and disrupting their integrity, by depleting the body of red cells, or by exerting other effects—all of which result in disturbed homeostasis. Diseases due to physical or chemical agents have similar outcomes. A serious burn destroys a great number of body cells, disturbing homeostasis in the process. Potassium from the destroyed cells is poured into the extracellular fluid. Dead cells provide a medium for multiplication of bacteria. A host of body fluid disturbances are encouraged. Chemical agents, too, can utterly disrupt the inner workings of the cells.

Neoplasia   Neoplasia (new growth) disturbs homeostasis in still other ways. Neoplastic cells seem to be more robust and certainly faster-growing than normal body cells, and so they appropriate available nutrients at the expense of the normal body cells. As tumors enlarge, they encroach on adjoining tissues, disturbing their homeostasis by pressure effects, ultimately causing necrosis. Malignant tumors spread through the lymphatics and the bloodstream to other parts of the body, where secondary tumors develop and create further disease.

Body fluids   We have already seen that it is through a delicate balance of water and electrolytes that the constancy of the internal environment is maintained. It follows that when there is a condition of sodium concentration deficit or excess, potassium concentration deficit or excess, calcium concentration deficit or excess, or, indeed, any one of many other conditions of imbalance, homeostasis suffers.

DYNAMIC
EQUILIBRIUM
THE "IDEAL"
STATE OF HEALTH

Nutritional disease   In diseases of malnutrition, whether the problem is one of too much food (as in obesity), too little food (as in kwashiorkor), or a lack of a nutritive substance (as in beriberi), the real sufferer is the cell. The aging process, too, disturbs homeostasis. It reflects the weakened efforts of aging cells to maintain homeostasis. When these efforts fail, degenerative diseases occur.

Endocrine disorders   The endocrine glands are of incalculable importance. Whether the disturbance occurs in the pituitary, in the adrenals, in the thyroid, in the thymus, or in one of the sex organs, the result is disturbance of homeostasis and the beginning of disease. As we shall see, the diseases of endocrine dysfunction constitute a long list.

Psychosomatic disturbances   Psychosomatic factors play a definite part also. The human organism, through the mind, reacts in a conscious, unconscious, or subconscious manner to external events, and these reactions may serve to benefit the total organism—or to harm it. When the external event causes a "storm" within, the autonomic nervous system sends appropriate distress signals to the glands, muscles, and visceral organs; the steady state is disrupted, sometimes violently—much in the manner of a tornado pursuing its deadly course through a pleasant countryside.

DISEASE AS IMBALANCE

Through the investigations of such scientists as Claude Bernard and Walter Cannon, our understanding of disease has advanced, and we view disease as an imbalance—a breakdown of the delicate steady state—rather than as merely the absence of good health. Our examination of the altered physiology that causes disease and of the ways in which it distorts homeostasis provides a splendid basis for our analysis of disease.

BIBLIOGRAPHY

Snively, W., and Sweeney, M.: Fluid Balance Handbook for Practitioners. Springfield, Illinois, Charles C Thomas, 1956.

Snively, W.: Body Fluid Disturbances. New York, Grune & Stratton, 1962.

The Merck Manual of Diagnosis and Therapy. Rahway, New Jersey, Merck Sharp & Dohme Research Laboratories, 1966.

Metheny, N., and Snively, W.: Nurses' Handbook of Fluid Balance. Philadelphia, J. B. Lippincott Co., 1967.

Sodeman, W., and Sodeman, W.: Pathologic Physiology. Philadelphia, W. B. Saunders Co., 1967.

Passmore, R., and Robson, J.: A Companion to Medical Studies. Philadelphia, F. A. Davis Company, 1969.

Snively, W., and Thuerbach, J.: Sea of Life. New York, David McKay Co., Inc., 1969.

Boyd, W.: A Textbook of Pathology. Philadelphia, Lea & Febiger, 1970.

2

genetics: diseases due to hereditary factors

Disorders of hereditary origin are assuming an ever-growing place in medical practice. Some 2,000 diseases either owe their entire cause to genetic factors or possess an important genetic component. Perhaps the increase in inheritable diseases stems from a gradual decline in childhood illnesses due to malnutrition and infection. Dr. Hymie Gordon, Consulting Physician to the Mayo Clinic Section on Medical Genetics, said, "In 1910, for example, there were six deaths from diarrheal diseases in infancy for every one owing to congenital malformations. But," Dr. Gordon pointed out, "a complete statistical turnabout occurred in little more than 50 years. In 1965, there was one diarrheal death for every six from congenital malformations." According to a recent estimate, 25 per cent of the country's medical problems can be traced in part to genetic factors. Some hereditary diseases occur with surprising frequency—Down's syndrome, or mongolism, for example, appearing about once in every 600 live births. One estimate of the incidence of genetic defects was placed at 5 per cent of all live births.

HISTORICAL BACKGROUND

The serious study of genetics dates back little more than a century. It was in 1866 that the Austrian monk, Gregor Mendel, crossed a red pea and a white pea in his monastery garden. In the second generation, four plants bore red flowers; but in the third generation, three were red and one was white. This led Mendel to propose the concept of a dominant character (in this case, red) and a recessive character (in this case, white). Although the factor for the recessive character was

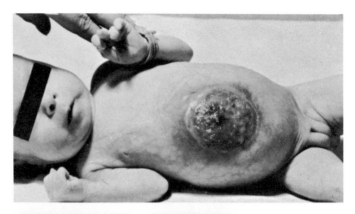

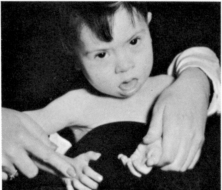

The child above was born with an emphalocele—a congenital anomaly in which the contents of the abdomen protrude through the wall and are covered with a thin membrane instead of skin. It is not an inherited disorder. An example of a condition that is both congenital and hereditary is Down's syndrome; the child (*left*) shows the characteristic facial features.

hidden in the second generation, it was, nevertheless, present. Unfortunately, Mendel's pioneer work attracted no attention at that time. The modern study of genetics dates from 1907, when T. H. Morgan began his work with the fruitfly, *Drosophila melanogaster*. Nevertheless, Mendel had laid a foundation, and his work and that of Morgan enabled modern scientists to move rapidly ahead.

TERMINOLOGY

In the field of medical genetics, as in virtually every other field of medicine, terminology is often confusing. The terms *familial* and *hereditary*, as applied to disease, have exactly the same meaning—that is, the transmission of a quality, character, or defect from one generation to another. On the other hand, a *congenital* defect, one present at birth, is not necessarily hereditary, or familial, since it may have been acquired in utero. Congenital syphilis, for example, used to be called, quite incorrectly, hereditary syphilis. Since it is transmitted to the unborn baby by the mother and not by the germ plasm, it is congenital but not hereditary. *Genetics,* itself, is the study of the mechanism of heredity.

HEREDITY VERSUS ENVIRONMENT

In recent years scientific investigation has shown that no illness results solely from inheritance or from environment; both hereditary and environmental influences play a role in the causation of all disease. Some diseases are overwhelmingly hereditary in their origin, whereas in others, environment plays the overwhelming role. In all diseases, however, both factors operate. Let us formulate a list of diseases, beginning with some that are almost entirely hereditary and ending with one or two that are almost entirely environmental. The list might start with hemophilia, almost entirely hereditary, and move on down through phenylketonuria (PKU), diabetes mellitus, schizophrenia, rheumatoid arthritis, essential hypertension, coronary artery disease, carcinoma of the breast, peptic ulcer, tuberculosis, and injury. As the hereditary importance of the causation of the diseases on the list decreases, the environmental importance increases. Even in trauma, heredity plays a role—for example, if the individual is, by his hereditary constitution, accident prone. Certainly heredity plays a role, however small, in the rapidity of the patient's recovery. Then too, such diseases as diabetes mellitus, schizophrenia, and hypertension are not solely hereditary. Nevertheless, hereditary factors play a role in each instance.

The list of disorders that are primarily hereditary includes the following:

hemophilia
mongolism
alkaptonuria
ochronosis
PKU disease
hyperaminoaciduria
hyperhistadinemia
the Fanconi syndrome
galactosemia
fructosuria
glycogen storage diseases
immunologic deficiency syndromes
porphyria
gout
methemoglobinemia
familial Mediterranean fever
hemochromatosis
Hurler's syndrome (gargoylism)
Wilson's disease (hepatolenticular degeneration)
albinism

ENVIRONMENTAL AGENTS AND HEREDITARY FACTORS BOTH CONTRIBUTORS TO DISEASE

HEREDITY RESIDES IN THE CELLS

The nucleus of the cell is the ultimate source of genetic information. Examination of the nucleus of a cell not ready to divide reveals dark-staining granules called *chromatin material,* arranged in loosely coiled strands known as *chromosomes.* The latter become clearly visible when they coil tightly just before mitotic cell division, by which somatic or body cells duplicate themselves and provide for the growth of the body. Each normal body cell, or somatic cell, has 46 chromosomes in its nucleus. Each chromosome bears thousands of genes strung along its threadlike structure, 100,000 genes for each cell. As Boyd has stated, the gene is the biochemical carrier of biological information from one generation to the next. In their totality, the genes determine what the human is in his totality.

The chromosomes and their passengers, the genes, consist of a remarkable and complex chemical, deoxyribonucleic acid, or DNA. DNA stores genetic information and puts it to practical use in the manufacture of proteins. The intriguing mystery of the structure of DNA was clarified in 1953 by Dr. James Watson and Dr. Francis Crick, who described the DNA molecule as a spiral ladder, a sort of *double helix.* Watson's book of this title makes the most fascinating of reading.

DNA, residing in its control center, the cell nucleus, governs the production of countless proteins. Without reviewing the somewhat complicated details, let us point out that DNA accomplishes its mission

DNA A DOUBLE HELIX

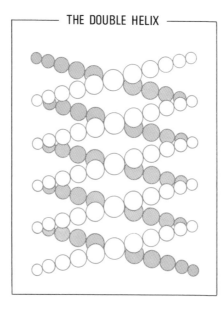

THE DOUBLE HELIX

The chemical structure of deoxyribonucleic acid (DNA) was a mystery until 1953, when Dr. James Watson and Dr. Francis Crick postulated the chemical configuration of DNA as a spiral ladder, or double helix (a helix is a spiral). The DNA molecule is enormously complex; the sides of the ladder are formed by alternating units of deoxyribose sugar and phosphate. Like a conventional ladder, the spiral ladder has rungs (not shown in the stylized illustration) formed by paired nitrogenous bases known as adenine, thymine, guanine, and cytosine. No one has clearly seen the minuscule DNA molecule under a microscope, but a shadowy image of its general form can be seen in *The Double Helix,* by James D. Watson.

with the assistance of two forms of ribonucleic acid, or RNA, which DNA splits off from its own substance. DNA has substance enough to produce these riboneucleic acid forms, since every nucleus contains about 3 feet of the exceedingly thin DNA molecule. Two sorts of RNA are thus produced: messenger RNA, or M-RNA, and transfer RNA, or T-RNA. Provided with chemical "code words," T-RNA proceeds to the cytoplasm of the cell, where it arranges the amino acids needed for construction of protein. These amino acids must be energized by adenosine triphosphate, or ATP, before leaving with T-RNA for their ultimate destination. M-RNA, also split off from DNA, incorporates in its molecule a pattern, or template, for the design of a specific protein. It takes millions of M-RNA molecules to provide the patterns for the proteins needed for a single cell.

FORMATION OF PROTEIN

Leaving the nucleus, M-RNA enters the cytoplasm and proceeds to a *ribosome,* a structural unit on which the actual synthesis of protein occurs. T-RNA, in the meantime, has been gathering amino acids. It goes to the M-RNA on the ribosome, where the amino acids become attached to the M-RNA protein template. After sufficient amino acids of the right kind have been brought to the M-RNA, the protein is completed. The completed protein is then available for utilization in the cell or elsewhere in the body. After the protein molecule has thus been made, the M-RNA disintegrates. DNA continues to form all the M-RNA needed, each molecule provided with the proper pattern for the fabrication of a specific protein, while the T-RNA molecules continue to bring amino acids to the M-RNA.

Through this mechanism are made the proteins of enzymes (thousands for this purpose alone), as well as the proteins that form skin, muscle, blood vessels, hormones, and all the organs of the body.

CONTRIBUTIONS OF DROSOPHILA MELANOGASTER

The investigations of chromosomes were greatly facilitated by study of the fruitfly, *Drosophila melanogaster.* Throughout the animal and plant kingdoms, most cells grow by dividing, and the chromosomes become visible as separate units under the microscope only during mitosis. A fortunate exception to such growth is seen in the larvae of *Drosophila melanogaster,* in which the salivary gland grows by enlargement of individual cells. A salivary gland cell can reach a size 1,000 times as large as most cells. This circumstance provided scientists with an invaluable opportunity to study chromosomes, their appearance, their duplication, and how they contribute to growth. The information and knowledge gained thereby could then be applied to the study of the chromosomes of man.

GENES AND CHROMOSOMES

In man the chromosomes number 46, of which 44 are somatic (body) and are known as *autosomes,* and two are sex chromosomes. The autosomes and the sex chromosomes are arranged in pairs; one member of each pair is maternal and one member is paternal. Thus there are 22 pairs of autosomes and one pair of sex chromosomes.

During the interphase of mitosis, when active cell division is not occurring, the chromosomes are extremely long and thin; it is during this period that the DNA content of the nucleus doubles. When the cell becomes ready to divide, the chromosomes condense by coiling up. Each now consists of two long, parallel strands, or *chromatids,* held together at a point of connection known as the *centromere.* When mitosis is complete, the chromosomes unwind and can no longer be seen. Nevertheless, they continue to participate actively in the metabolism of the cell.

Each chromosome is divided into two arms by the centromere; if the division is in the middle of the chromosome, the chromosome is X-shaped; if it is near the end, the chromosome is Y-shaped. For study purposes, scientists have arranged the 23 pairs of chromosomes into seven groups identified by the letters A to G, in order of decreasing length of the chromosomes. Such an arrangement is called a *karyotype.* Each normal female cell has an XX sex chromosome combination; each normal male

CHROMOSOMAL KARYOTYPE FOR FEMALE

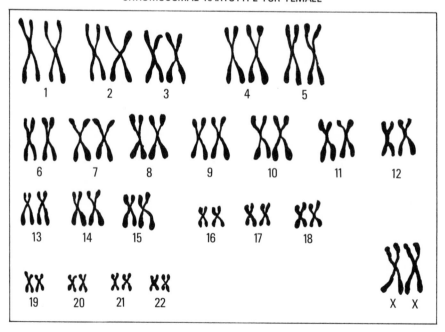

cell has an XY sex chromosome complex. When there are three chromosomes of one kind instead of only two, the condition is known as *trisomy*. Loss of an entire chromosome is known as *monosomy* and is nearly always fatal.

Genes vary in their power in a way that we shall shortly make clear. "Strong" genes are called *dominant*, "weak" genes, *recessive*. Although each somatic chromosome bears many genes, it has only one gene, and, therefore, half the genetic material, for any trait. The complementary gene is located in a corresponding site on the other chromosome of the pair. Both genes may be dominant, or both may be recessive. Or, one may be dominant and the other recessive. If the genes on a pair of chromosomes are the same, either dominant or recessive, a *homozygous* condition exists for those particular genes on that particular chromosome pair. When one of the genes is dominant and the other recessive, the condition is *heterozygous*. The characteristic corresponding to a dominant gene will always appear in the individual, regardless of whether the gene is paired with another dominant gene or with a recessive gene. A recessive gene, however, must be complemented by another recessive gene if the characteristic is to become apparent in the individual. If a recessive gene for an anomaly or disease is paired with a normal gene, the person with that gene will become merely a carrier, perhaps to pass on the recessive trait to his progeny.

KARYOTYPE—
A CHROMOSOMAL
"PORTRAIT"

CHROMOSOMAL KARYOTYPE FOR MALE

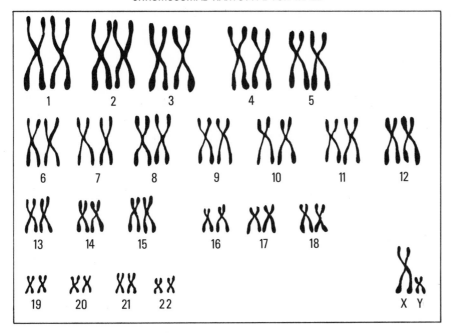

MECHANISMS OF DEVELOPMENT OF HEREDITARY DISEASE

Variation in the Number of Chromosomes

Among the abnormalities caused by variation in the number of chromosomes—in this case an extra sex chromosome—is Klinefelter's syndrome, or feminization of the male, which may be accompanied by mental retardation. A contrasting anomaly, in which there is a single sex chromosome, is Turner's syndrome, or masculinization of the female. Mongolism and certain other disorders in which mental deficiency is a component also stem from an abnormal number of chromosomes. In yet another abnormality, part of a short arm of a chromosome is missing. The result of this abnormality is the so-called cat cry syndrome, in which the infant is severely retarded and has a small head, widely spaced eyes, and a high-pitched, plaintive cry that sounds like a cat mewing.

Gene Malfunction

Any genetic defect will lead to faulty enzyme synthesis, since this is under control of the genes. The group of disorders so caused is known as *inborn errors of metabolism.* The metabolic block may affect protein, carbohydrate, lipid, nucleic acid, porphyrin, or pigment metabolism, but the primary abnormality is always in the genetic control of protein synthesis. Phenylketonuria (described later in this chapter), albinism, and galactosemia are included in this large group.

Mutation

The following passage by J. C. Kendrew lucidly illustrates the kinds of genetic accidents which can occur:

What kinds of mutation can we envisage? If we think of the hereditary information as a particular sequence of bases on the DNA, it can be compared to a message written in code, and a mutation would be rather like a misprint in the line of type. Here are a few examples, taken from newspaper articles, of the kinds of misprint which are liable to happen:

SAY IT WITH GLOWERS

We might call this sort of error a SUBSTITUTION; an incorrect letter has been substituted for the correct one.

THE PRIME MINISTER, WHO SPENT THE WEEKEND
IN SCOTLAND SHOOTING PEASANTS, . . .

In this example a letter has been left out, so we may call it a DELETION.

TREASURY CONTROL OF PUBLIC MONKEYS

Here, on the other hand, an extra letter has found its way into the type; it is an INSERTION.

PUT OUR TRUST IN THE UNTIED NATIONS

Here a section of type has been put in backwards; we may describe it as an INVERSION.

Finally, a sentence can sometimes suddenly turn into gibberish; this we simply call NONSENSE.

BBC SCIENCE PROGRAMMES ARE FRDOHMRF GPT YJR INOM

In fact, every one of these kinds of misprint is known to occur in the genetic material of living organisms, and the names I have given them are the names used by geneticists to describe the corresponding mutations.°

Since each gene consists of millions of atoms, rearrangement of the atoms can give the gene new properties. This type of change is a *mutation*, an abnormality in a gene which is acquired rather than inherited. The mutant genes bring about their effects through an alteration in biochemical function. Mutation is an essential mechanism of evolution, creating variations in living creatures. Some of the variations are favorable, some unfavorable. Nevertheless, life would never have evolved beyond its first primitive forms without mutations. Fortunately, most harmful mutations are recessive, producing no harm as long as the partner gene remains undamaged. LSD and tranquilizers such as chlorpromazine are believed to harm chromosomes by causing breaks in them. X-ray and ionizing radiation also can cause such breaks. Radiation may be natural, such as exists at high altitudes; it may be due to fallout, as occurs following the dropping of an atomic bomb; or it may result from medical procedures, e.g., x-rays and radium in diagnosis and therapy.

MUTATION AN INTEGRAL ELEMENT OF EVOLUTION

INHERITANCE OF TRAITS

Dominant Inheritance

Expression of a dominant trait indicates that the trait was present in a parent and a grandparent. The trait may be transmitted by either sex to a child of either sex. Should one parent possess the dominant gene, the chance of any child inheriting the gene is one in two. Any

---

° Kendrew, John C.: The Thread of Life, p. 80. London, Harvard University Press, G. Bell & Sons, 1968.

child who receives the dominant gene will express the trait. If two cousins with the dominant gene mate in the third generation, the chances are three in four that any child will inherit the trait. If either parent is homozygous dominant, it is inevitable. Such heredity is not sex-linked. Examples of dominant disease traits include short fingers and toes, multiple cartilaginous exostoses, Huntington's chorea, multiple polyposis of the colon and rectum, diabetes insipidus, and angioneurotic edema.

Recessive Inheritance

In recessive inheritance the defect appears only in an individual in whom both paired genes carry the defect. Persons who have only one recessive gene for the disease trait do not exhibit it but act as carriers. Such a condition may remain unsuspected for generations until a homozygous mating brings two recessive genes together. When two first cousins marry, or in isolated communities where closely related persons marry, the probability of homozygous individuals increases. The inhabitants of the tiny island of Tristan da Cunha, in the South Atlantic, all descended from seven men who landed there 150 years ago. The incidence of congenital defects in the population was 185 per 1,000 persons, whereas the incidence among the British is 25 per 1,000. Among the diseases manifested by the islanders were retinal lesions, with a high incidence of blindness. Examples of recessive inheritance are amaurotic family idiocy, in which blindness and idiocy are combined; retinitis pigmentosa, combining retinal sclerosis with pigmentation and atrophy; Friedreich's ataxia, a disease in which there is both spinal and cerebellar degeneration; alkaptonuria, a urinary abnormality; xeroderma pigmentosum, a skin disorder; and albinism.

Sex-Linked Inheritance

INHERITANCE
TRANSMITTED
BY X AND
Y CHROMOSOMES

Each of the 44 autosomes contributed by a male gamete, or sex cell, corresponds to an autosome provided by the female gamete. In addition, there are two chromosomes that determine the individual's sex, the X and the Y chromosomes. The female has two X chromosomes, XX, while the male has one X and one Y chromosome, XY. There are two types of spermatozoa. One has an X chromosome. When it unites with a female gamete, the offspring will be female. The other type of spermatozoa has a Y chromosome. When it unites with a female gamete, the offspring will be a male. A father, therefore, passes on to his sons the Y chromosome he received from his father. He passes on to each of his daughters the X chromosome received from his mother. Both of these sex chromosomes carry additional nonsexual genes known as *sex-linked* genes. Since the female has two X chromosomes, she will be merely a carrier if one of her X chromosomes carries a recessive sex-linked gene. But if a boy inherits such a recessive gene on his mother's X chromosome, he will express the trait or defect. Such a recessive gene can be passed from father to daughter and from mother to son, but only in the male will the trait represented by the gene become apparent. It will, however, be transmitted silently by the female, in whom the recessive gene is prevented from manifesting itself by the dominant normal gene of the other X chromosome.

Such transmission of the trait of a recessive gene occurs in hemophilia, a sex-linked disease in which the patient bleeds readily because his clotting ability is defective. As a rule, only males develop hemophilia, and only females transmit the disease. Most hemophilic boys die of hemorrhage before reaching maturity. Should it occur, however, that a hemophiliac reach maturity and marry a carrier female, then a daughter as well as a son may be hemophilic. In such an instance, the mother would contribute an X chromosome with a recessive gene for hemophilia and the father would contribute an X with a recessive gene for hemophilia. The female child would have two X chromosomes predisposing her to hemophilia.

Other examples of sex-linked inheritance of disease include color blindness, night blindness, progressive muscular dystrophy, and Leber's hereditary optic atrophy. Years ago, in testing Marine recruits in the hills of Kentucky for color blindness, one of the authors would now and then discover color blindness in one or more of the male members of a family but not in the female.

HEREDITARY DISEASES

The study of diseases due to genetic factors can be the work of a lifetime—or of several lifetimes. Obviously, in a book such as this one, it is not possible to do more than mention some of the mechanisms and a few of the disorders which are classified as hereditary. The interested reader will find detailed descriptions of these disorders in the appropriate textbooks, several of which are listed in the bibliography at the end of the chapter.

Blood Disorders

Included among the hereditary blood disorders are hemophilia, pernicious anemia, sickle cell anemia, and hemorrhagic telangiectasia. Blood groups follow the rules of human heredity. Certain substances in some of the groups (antibodies or agglutinins called *alpha* and *beta*) cause agglutination, or clotting, of substances (antibodies or agglutinable substances called A and B) in other groups. These agglutinating substances behave exactly like dominant genes. We shall study this subject in some detail in the chapter on diseases of the immune mechanism.

Metabolic Disorders

HEREDITARY
DISORDERS
HAVE
WIDESPREAD
MANIFESTATIONS

In inborn errors of metabolism, the error results from an enzymatic defect that may involve proteins, carbohydrates, lipids, or pigments. Perhaps the best known of such disorders is phenylketonuria, or PKU, a disorder of protein metabolism in which there is a deficiency of phenylalanine hydroxylase, a liver enzyme which normally changes phenylalanine to tyrosine. In PKU, severe mental retardation and several neurologic disturbances are observed. The defect is recessive.

Hereditary fructose intolerance involves abnormalities in the liver cells. Galactosemia stems from an enzymatic deficiency of the erythrocytes. In cystinuria, the enzyme system that normally regulates renal tubular transport is absent. The result may be excessive tubular reabsorption with accumulation of a catabolic substance in body fluids.

Skeletal Defects

A number of hereditary defects affect the skeleton. One is brachydactyly, or short fingers, with the fingers having only two phalanges, the second and third being fused. Another is multiple cartilaginous exostoses. Still another is fragilitas ossium, in which there are multiple fractures. It is usually dominant. In Marfan's syndrome (from which Abraham Lincoln may have suffered) the extremities are long and thin, the face is long and narrow, and the individual is "double jointed."

Neuromuscular Disorders

Among the neuromuscular disorders that are hereditary are progressive muscular atrophy, pseudohypertrophic muscular dystrophy, Friedreich's ataxia, peroneal atrophy, amyotonia congenita, and myotonia congenita.

Skin Diseases

Baldness, xeroderma pigmentosum, and von Recklinghausen's disease, or multiple neurofibromatosis, are included among the inherited skin disorders.

Eye Diseases

Among the numerous hereditary eye diseases are retinitis pigmentosa, hereditary optic atrophy, or Leber's disease, color blindness, and some forms of night blindness. The hereditary disease irideremia involves absence of the iris and blindness. Retinoblastoma, a neoplasm that is fatal unless removed early, is also hereditary.

Mental Diseases

Much evidence points to the possible hereditary nature of schizophrenia. Huntington's chorea appears to be hereditary. So do some forms of feeblemindedness, including amaurotic familial idiocy and mongolian idiocy.

Susceptibility to Infection

Heredity plays an outstanding role in susceptibility to infection. In general, exposure to an infectious disease over the centuries results in the survival of individuals who have been able to combat the infection, and they transmit this resistance to their descendants.

Our relative immunity to syphilis comes about because, over the centuries, our more susceptible ancestors all died of it. When syphilis first appeared in Europe, it was an acute infectious disease and was called the Great Pox. (Another unpleasant disease, by contrast, was named the smallpox.) Over the centuries, the survival of resistant humans has resulted in the conversion of syphilis to a nonexplosive chronic disease. It is, nevertheless, a relatively acute disease for those races that have never been previously exposed.

When Captain Cook visited some South Sea islands, his men transmitted the measles virus to the natives. The death rate was almost 100 per cent in those persons whose ancestors had never been exposed. Tuberculosis, a relatively mild, chronic disease among Caucasians, was highly fatal to American Indians.

Numerous examples could be given to illustrate the importance of heredity in susceptibility to infection. We all know robust individuals who never seem to "catch" anything, and others who seem to "catch" everything. Nutrition, hygiene, and other factors play a role, but perhaps heredity is the chief determinant.

Heredity in Cancer

There have been clear-cut examples of heredity involving certain neoplastic processes. One of these is polyposis of the rectum and colon, which has a pronounced tendency to become malignant. Neuroblastoma of the retina also shows a strong hereditary tendency.

Should both parents suffer from cancer, it appears probable that at least some of the children will do so. In one family, for example, both mother and father had cancer; their six children died of it; and a grandchild died of it—an entire family of nine, covering three generations. Although there is no "cancer gene," there is without a doubt some predisposition to develop cancer on a hereditary basis.

PROGRESS IN TREATMENT

EARLY STEPS BEING MADE IN CONTROL AND TREATMENT

Formerly, treatment of virtually all forms of hereditary disease appeared futile; presently, however, there is increasing reason for optimism. The depredations of at least one hereditary disease, PKU, can virtually be eliminated in certain favorable instances, although the treatment requires heroic effort and ingenuity. There are also other areas of excellent progress. Dr. Leon E. Rosenberg, of Yale University, has directed attention to a rapidly growing class of inborn metabolic errors that respond to large doses of vitamins, although the disorders do not represent vitamin deficiencies. The total number of vitamin-dependent forms of genetic disease is now about 12. Two of the entities respond to large doses of vitamin B_6. The incidence of one vitamin-dependent disease, homocystinuria, appears comparable to that of phenylketonuria. Dietary management of PKU has been beneficial, particularly when started in infancy.

An exciting new development has been the first clinical application of genetic engineering, in the case of two German sisters born with an unusual amino acid disturbance. The effort is being made to correct the inborn enzymatic defect in the two girls by infecting them with a virus, in the hope of altering their native DNA. The attempt is certainly experimental—but it may represent the shape of things to come.

Every effort should be made to diagnose hereditary disease. A detailed family history should be taken, with at least an hour set aside for an interview. The following information should be recorded regarding the patient's parents, brothers, sisters, and other close relatives: Name, year of birth and of death, and sex. Married and maiden names of female relatives should be noted. The health of each relative and the cause or circumstances of death should be investigated. Doctors' records, hospital notes, and death certificates should be studied. Abortions and neonatal deaths deserve special attention.

Especially helpful in the study of hereditary disease has been the investigation of twins. Identical twins, having developed from one fertilized ovum, provide a vehicle for studying the effects of heredity on disease. Frequently twins develop such diseases as the following more or less simultaneously: tumors; nervous and mental disease; noninfectious systemic disease, such as diabetes mellitus, and infections, such as tuberculosis.

DISEASE MODEL: PHENYLKETONURIA (PKU)

In addition to being an excellent model for a hereditary disease, phenylketonuria and its discovery are of some dramatic interest. In this disorder, an essential enzyme, phenylalanine hydroxylase, is deficient. Because this enzyme normally converts the amino acid phenylalanine to tyrosine, its lack results in an accumulation of phenylalanine in the blood and spinal fluid. One infant in every 10,000 to 20,000 births will be affected. If the infant is untreated, the result is brain damage and severe mental retardation. The patient acquires a peculiar, clinging odor like that of musty animal urine.

The discovery of PKU represents one of the great dramatic episodes in this century. It started in the spring of 1934, when a Norwegian dentist who suffered from chronic asthma informed a friend that he could not bear to remain in a closed room with his two young children because of their strange, penetrating odor. The children, 7 and 4 years old, were both mentally retarded, even though their parents were both of above average intelligence. Finally the dentist took the children to see Dr. Asbjorn Fölling, Professor of Nutritional Research at the University of Oslo School of Medicine.

Dr. Fölling, known personally to the senior author, is a generous, kind man and an inquisitive researcher. Dr. Fölling was not only sympathetic and curious when he saw the children, he was excited by the challenge. First he examined their urine to determine if they harbored a hidden infection; he found none. Then he tested a urine specimen for presence of diacetic acid. To perform the test, he used a chemical solution that turns the urine reddish-brown if it contains the acid. If the acid is absent, there is no change at all. To Dr. Fölling's bewilderment, the urine turned green. He tested again and again, but each time the urine turned green. He simply did not know why. Then he set to work relentlessly, and finally collected 20 quarts of urine from the children. Painstakingly and methodically, he began a systematic analysis of the urine designed to disclose the chemical that caused the urine to turn green. Organic compound after organic compound was ruled out as he applied the techniques of qualitative analysis. Finally, after a month of further work, he isolated crystals of the substance. Then, after 6 more weeks, he identified it as phenylpyruvic acid, a by-product of the metabolism of phenylalanine.

Next, he examined hundreds of mentally retarded persons in nursing homes and schools and found eight who suffered from the same symptoms as the children. Dr. Fölling's discovery of this disease, which was given the name *phenylketonuria,* was a tremendous contribution. Interest in the disease spread rapidly. Through the efforts of scores of investigators over the past 25 years, progress has been made in developing tests for its early detection; at present in the United States, 32 states require that every infant born in a hospital be tested and that immediate dietary treatment be started if the disease is discovered.

PKU ONE OF FIRST HEREDITARY DISORDERS TO YIELD TO MEDICAL MANAGEMENT

Only a generation ago, PKU was unknown. Today more than 30,000 mentally retarded persons all over the country are confined to institutions because their PKU was not diagnosed and treated when they were young. Treatment, though simple, is hard to control. The affected infant is put on an extremely low protein diet so as to decrease its intake of phenylalanine. A special formula extremely low in phenylalanine has been developed for the treatment of these children and has been distributed without cost to parents all over the world who could not afford this expensive food.

Failure to convert phenylalanine to tyrosine results in a decreased production of melanin, so that the patient has blond hair and fair skin. It is the excessive accumulation of phenylalanine or one of its products that harms the central nervous system, causing mental deficiency. Since the damage results from a failure to metabolize phenylalanine normally, it is rational to treat these patients with a low phenylalanine diet, which, started soon after birth, can be effective in preventing mental retardation.

PKU is transmitted as a recessive trait, so that a family in which the parents are normal and one child is affected has one in four chances of having another affected child with each successive pregnancy. Although the parents appear normal, each carries the gene for PKU. Until recently, there was no way of ascertaining whether an apparently normal person carried the gene or not, but it is now possible to detect most carriers by means of a PKU tolerance test similar to a glucose tolerance test. The heterozygous carrier demonstrates a curve in the blood phenylalanine level that is between the normal response and that of a patient with PKU. This indicates that the presence of one gene for the disease gives rise to a partial defect, insufficient to produce the disease.

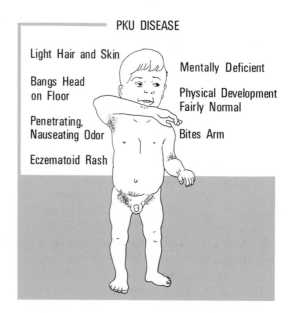

PKU DISEASE

Light Hair and Skin

Bangs Head on Floor

Penetrating, Nauseating Odor

Eczematoid Rash

Mentally Deficient

Physical Development Fairly Normal

Bites Arm

Another name for heterozygous carrier is *silent carrier*. In genetic constitution, the silent carrier bears a recessive gene for a specific disease but does not have the disease himself. Heterozygous carriers for several recessively inherited disorders can now be detected. In thalassemia, for example, which is an acute deficiency of red blood cells that is seen in southern climates, the heterozygous carrier does not manifest the disease in its full-blown state but may have a mild, symptom-free variation that can be discovered by examination of a blood smear.

CLINICAL CONSIDERATIONS

Knowledge of the existence and nature of hereditary diseases enables health scientists to be alert to the possible occurrence of such disorders and to refer patients or the parents of patients with these illnesses to genetic centers. A list of active genetic centers has been compiled by Dr. Henry T. Lynch, Assistant Professor and Chairman of the Department of Preventive Medicine and Public Health, Creighton University, Omaha. The 1969 edition of the *International Directory of Genetic Services* lists 427 genetic units in the United States and overseas, among which more than 150, located in a total of 44 states, offer genetic counseling.

As well as being aware of the nature of hereditary diseases, the health sciences student should develop a deep sympathy for the unfortunate persons afflicted by them. C. van Gastel said in 1970, "The salient fact about rare diseases is that they happen to people. There is another aspect to rare diseases: it is small consolation to a patient that his or her disease is very uncommon and therefore practically unknown. . . ."

TOPICS FOR DISCUSSION

1. In recent years there appears to be an increase in hereditary diseases. What, in your opinion, might account for this increase?

2. Discuss the various situations in which recessively inherited ailments become manifest.

3. What are the hazards presented by modern society that might well lead to gene mutations? What are the steps society must take to eliminate these hazards? If it appears impossible to eliminate them, how can they be reduced?

4. What circumstances would be required for hemophilia to become manifest in a female?

5. Was the fact that Gregor Mendel's basic discoveries went unnoticed for decades particularly unusual in the history of science?

6. What lessons can we learn from the discovery of PKU by Dr. Asbjorn Fölling?

7. How is DNA (deoxyribonucleic acid) involved in hereditary disease?

8. How does it happen that certain royal families seem extremely vulnerable to hereditary diseases? For example, porphyria is prominent in British royalty and hemophilia was notable in the Hapsburg line.

9. How are nutritional research and genetic disease linked?

10. What is the significance of genetic counseling in relation to hereditary disease?

BIBLIOGRAPHY

Books

Harrow, B., and Mazur, A.: Textbook of Biochemistry. Philadelphia, W. B. Saunders Co., 1966.

Beeson, P., and McDermott, W.: Textbook of Medicine. vols. I and II. Philadelphia, W. B. Saunders Co., 1967.

Gendel, B.: Genetics and Disease. pp. 37–55. In Sodeman, W., and Sodeman, W.: Pathologic Physiology. Philadelphia, W. B. Saunders Co., 1968.

Watson, J. D.: The Double Helix. Kingsport, Tennessee, Kingsport Press, Inc., 1968.

Chaffee, E., and Greisheimer, E.: Basic Physiology and Anatomy. pp. 14–56. Philadelphia, J. B. Lippincott Co., 1969.

Snively, W., and Thuerbach, J.: Sea of Life. New York, David McKay Co., Inc., 1969.

Boyd, W.: A Textbook of Pathology. pp. 493–519. Philadelphia, Lea & Febiger, 1970.

Articles

Voorhees, J., et al.: The XYY Chromosomal Complement and Nodulocystic Acne. Annals of Internal Medicine, 73:271, 1970.

van Gastel, C.: Rare disease and Uniqueness of the Patient. Annals of Internal Medicine, 73:474, 1970.

Bergsma, D., et al.: Birth Defects. Original Article Series, Vol. VI, No. 3. The National Foundation—March of Dimes, September, 1970.

Virus Is Used in a Genetic Therapy Test. Hospital Tribune, 4:1, 1970.

Vitamin-Response Type of Inborn Errors Rising. Hospital Tribune, 4:1, 16, 1970.

Medical News. JAMA, 213:2167, 1970.

Baker, D., et al.: Chromosome Errors in Men With Antisocial Behavior. JAMA, 214:869, 1970.

Danes, B.: Genetic Counseling. Medical World News, 11:34, 1970.

3

diseases due to hypersensitivity and autoimmunity

One frequently feels, as he studies the intricacies of body physiology, that he has been transported to a magic world far from everyday realities, viewing the sort of fantastic events described in *Alice's Adventures in Wonderland*. No phase of physiology or pathophysiology has a better claim to kinship with Lewis Carroll's masterpiece than does immunity and its pathologic variations, hypersensitivity and autoimmune disease. Immunity is fantastic in the best sense of the word. Hypersensitivity and autoimmune disease are bizarre in that word's worst sense —Alice would certainly have counted them among her bitter enemies. And while immunity deserves Cannon's words of praise when he proclaimed it "a manifestation of the wisdom of the body," hypersensitivity and autoimmune disease just as fully rate the censure of Boyd, who describes them as "revealing the stupidity of the body."

BASIC PRINCIPLES OF IMMUNITY

We shall do well to briefly review immunity before we discuss its pathologic variations. *Immunity* means, literally, not serving, or secure against. It may be viewed as a process by which the body, on the basis of past infections, learns to handle future infections more effectively. Immunity, then, represents a defensive action. Normally it is directed against foreign substances introduced into the body, usually via an infection. Since it stimulates a defensive reaction, usually carried out mainly by substances known as *antibodies,* the foreign substance is an *antigen,* or an *irritant*. Most antigens are proteins; some are complex carbohydrates. The essence of the immune process is body recognition that the antigen is chemically foreign—an alien, so to speak. By this means the body is able to destroy many invading organisms.

Immunity exists in several forms. *Natural immunity* is thought to occur

"LOCK AND KEY" MECHANISM

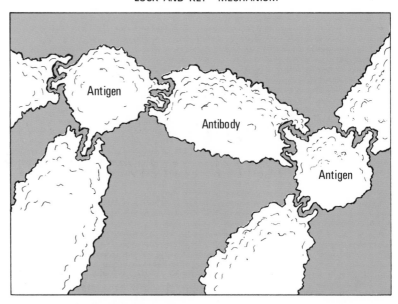

This illustration demonstrates how antibodies "lock" onto an antigen, effectively immobilizing and neutralizing the antigen and thereby preventing it from damaging body tissues.

as a result of a series of minor infections adequate to stimulate production of antibodies. *Acquired immunity* results from frank disease, as in some virus diseases, or from artificial immunization, as for diphtheria. Acquired immunity may be either *active* or *passive*. The active type is induced by inoculation with a suspension usually of dead or attenuated living bacteria or viruses. In passive immunity, the host receives protection although he plays no active role. When the serum of an immunized animal is injected into a human, the individual becomes immune to the infection. This type of immunity is short-lived since no change has occurred in the patient's cells. *Species immunity* is neither natural nor acquired, but is the immunity possessed by a species that is inherently unable to contract a given infection; there is no chemical affinity between the infecting agent and the animal's body cells. Tetanus toxin, for example, combines with human nerve cells and can kill a man, whereas it does no harm to the hen since it fails to combine with her cells.

THREE FORMS OF IMMUNITY KNOWN

Antibodies, the chief defensive agents in the human, are usually proteins, specifically gamma globulins, whose synthesis parallels the number of immature plasma cells in the tissues. Antibodies appear to be manufactured in the endoplasmic reticulum of the plasma cells. Antibodies remain in the blood long after the infection that stimulated their development has disappeared, and the plasma cells retain their ability to manufacture antibody to combat that infection.

The electron microscope has provided us with remarkable photographs of antigen-antibody complexes. When virus antigens and antibody are mixed and viewed under the microscope, one sees the virus particles

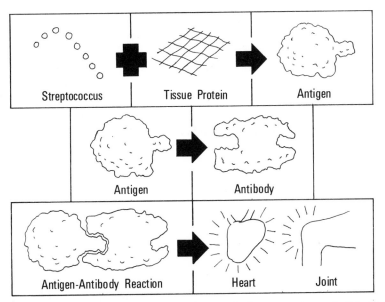

The series of events that may occur in rheumatic fever are shown in this series of illustrations. The individual first develops a streptococcal infection. The streptococcus combines with the individual's own tissue protein to form an antigen which stimulates production of an antibody. Antibodies attack antigens, and the resulting antigen-antibody reaction damages the heart muscle and the joints, frequently the knee and wrist.

clumped together, veiled over by a halo of fine filaments, the antibody molecules. The antibodies appear as long, rod-shaped molecules 200 to 250 angstroms in length (recall that an angstrom (Å) is but 1/10,000,000 mm.!).

The thymus gland is thought to play a key role in neonatal formation of antibodies and in the development of immunity. Here are produced most of the small lymphocytes that pass into the blood at birth and are then carried to the spleen and lymph nodes, where they multiply and, like the plasma cells, function in maintaining normal immunity.

Numerous specific antibodies are gamma globulins. (Persons who cannot synthesize gamma globulin cannot produce antibodies; their disorder, agammaglobulinemia, renders them extremely vulnerable to serious infections.) It should be kept in mind that not all antibodies are gamma globulins, nor are all gamma globulins antibodies. The essential point is that the cells "remember" the previous experience. This phenomenon is called an *anamnestic response,* and through it the individual's secondary defense mechanisms are instantaneously marshaled so that he may again combat the threatening microorganisms.

Other elements are involved in the body's defenses against infection. Important among them are the phagocytes, which ingest the foreign material, and the properdin system, in which the globulin properdin acts in conjunction with complement (a normal constituent of blood) and magnesium to destroy bacteria and neutralize viruses.

PRODUCTION
OF
ANTIBODIES
A NORMAL
MECHANISM

Antibodies are chiefly involved in the body's defense against bacteria and are less active against virus infections since they are produced late in the course of infection. Persons with a deficiency of gamma globulin, who develop little or no antibody, can recover normally from uncomplicated virus infection. Cellular resistance to viral infections appears to mount through production of *interferon,* a protein that is produced by cells that have reacted with a specific virus. The material is released into the intercellular fluids and acts on other host cells to obstruct the entrance of virus into these cells.

HYPERSENSITIVITY

Of the numerous classifications of hypersensitivity and allergy, William B. Sherman's impresses us as one of the clearest. We shall, in general, follow it in this section. Hypersensitivity and allergy are usually regarded as synonymous, but we shall see that allergy is but one expression of hypersensitivity. In 1906, von Pirquet introduced the term *allergy* to describe the reaction of organs and tissues following repeated contacts with irritants such as vaccine virus, tuberculin, and foreign serum. Allergy can reveal itself as an immediate reaction, occurring within a few minutes after exposure to an antigen, or a delayed reaction, occurring after 12 to 24 hours or longer. In *immediate hypersensitivity,* the plasma contains circulating antibodies capable of inducing sensitization in allergic persons. In *delayed allergy,* the plasma reveals no evidence of antibody activity, probably because this type of reaction occurs *inside* the lymphoid cells. William Boyd has contrasted the two types of hypersensitivity, using the term *anaphylactic* for the immediate reaction and *tuberculin* for the delayed type:

Anaphylactic Hypersensitivity (Immediate: early or humoral)	Tuberculin Hypersensitivity (Delayed: late or cellular)
Immediate reaction	Delayed reaction
Circulating antibody in serum	No circulating antibody
Passive transfer by serum possible	Transfer by cells
Not heritable	Heritable
Artificially induced	Naturally induced
Short duration	Long duration
Symptoms chiefly caused by smooth muscle spasm	Symptoms chiefly caused by edema
Desensitization easy	Desensitization difficult

The terms *hypersensitivity* and *allergy* include only reactions with a proved or probable immunologic mechanism; they do not cover individual idiosyncrasies independent of an immune mechanism.

Experimental Anaphylaxis

When 0.1 to 1 ml. of a nonpoisonous protein, such as egg white or horse serum, is injected into a normal guinea pig, no visible change is noted. But should a second injection be given 7 to 10 days later, there is an explosive reaction, manifested in restlessness, labored breathing, and convulsions, usually ending in death. Antibodies may appear in the serum. When this serum is administered to an animal of the same species or another species, it sensitizes the animal. Most of the symptoms seen in anaphylaxis result from the effects of pharmacologically active substances generated by the antigen-antibody reaction. Histamine heads the list of these chemicals, although serotonin, heparin, acetylcholine, and bradykinin have been involved in anaphylactic reactions in various species.

Human Anaphylaxis

Injection of a human with a protein such as equine antitoxin produces changes closely resembling those found in experimental anaphylaxis. Bovine serum globulin causes a similar reaction. Administered intravenously, it is metabolized similarly to the body's serum protein, but this process goes on only for a few days. Then, after 5 to 7 days, there is an explosive reaction to the foreign protein. The bovine protein disappears suddenly from the circulation. An antibody reacting specifically with the foreign protein becomes demonstrable in the recipient's serum. Serum sickness develops, with enlargement of the superficial lymph nodes, skin rashes, joint pain, and fever. The symptoms can be controlled clinically by use of such adrenal hormones as cortisone, but the recovered patient remains sensitized to the antigen that caused the illness. The laboratory test demonstrates that his plasma contains a gamma globulin antibody that forms a precipitate with the antigen in vitro. This plasma induces local and general anaphylaxis when it is injected into guinea pigs.

SIMILARITY BETWEEN EXPERIMENTAL ANAPHYLAXIS AND HUMAN ANAPHYLAXIS

As long as active sensitization exists, further injections of the same antigen will probably induce anaphylactic shock, with urticaria, asthma, and failure of the peripheral circulation. Such reactions can cause death within minutes.

Episodes resembling anaphylactic shock may follow penicillin injections or insect stings, and are most likely to develop in individuals with a personal or familial history of sensitization.

ATOPY

Many of the common allergic diseases of man—hay fever, bronchial asthma, infantile eczema, and atopic dermatitis—stem not from unusual exposure but rather from the everyday contacts of normal living.

Studies have repeatedly revealed that persons who have suffered from one disease of this group are more likely than the general population to develop others. Such sensitivity is called *atopy*. Heredity has an important role in its development. It is an inherited rather than an acquired condition.

Persons display sensitization to the antigens of pollens only with direct exposure to them. Perhaps previous exposure is essential to produce an atopic reaction to common food antigens, but this relationship cannot be proven, since these antigens can be transmitted from mother to child through the placenta or through human milk. The list of substances that may induce atopic sensitization includes pollens, mold spores, animal danders, vegetable dusts, and foods. Antigens have been identified as typical proteins or chemically similar substances of lower molecular weight. Sensitization has been traced to chemicals with simple structures, such as halazone and tannic acid, as well as to a wide variety of petroleum-related chemicals. Perhaps such substances act as haptenes, combining with body proteins to produce the antigens.

In atopic sensitization, an immediate wheal develops when minute quantities of the antigen are injected into the skin. The plasma of the sensitized person lacks precipitating antibodies (such as are found in acquired serum allergy); it does not cause local or general anaphylaxis when injected into the guinea pig.

The physician treats atopic sensitization by administering repeated injections of the specific antigens to which the patient is believed sensitive. The goal is to "desensitize" or "immunize" him. This treatment usually brings about a reduction in sensitivity. Early in the course of treatment the quantity of antibody increases but later decreases, until finally, virtually total desensitization may be achieved after 5 to 10 years.

SOURCES OF
ATOPIC
REACTIONS
FOUND
WIDELY
IN HUMAN
ENVIRONMENT

Pathophysiologic Response

In the affected individual, exposure to a specific antigen causes the smaller blood vessels to dilate as fluid moves from the plasma to the interstitial spaces. Small muscles undergo spasm. Mucous glands increase their secretion. Chemical mediators, chiefly histamine, freed by the antigen-antibody reaction appear to initiate these changes.

An atopic reaction may occur even when all connections with the cerebrospinal and autonomic nervous systems have been severed, as, for example, in paralysis. Although the reaction is basically immunologic, such factors as the emotional state, nonspecific irritants, and the physiologic activity of the involved organ have strong effects. Thus, a man who is overworked, who has family problems that worry him, or who is suffering from an infection is far more likely to react allergically to a pollen or to a food to which he is sensitive than if he did not labor under these stresses.

Eczema

The itching eczematoid lesion usually called *infantile eczema* in infants and *atopic dermatitis* in adults probably stems, in part at least, from atopic sensitization. Eighty-six per cent of adults treated for atopic dermatitis have had eczema during the first 5 years of life, and many eczematous infants develop atopic respiratory disease in later years. Skin testing contributes little to diagnosis in most instances. Elimination of foodstuffs that have induced pronounced reactions when administered intradermally may not affect the eczema. The disease may, in fact, persist after all conceivable antigens have been eliminated. As a rule, eczematous persons scratch the lesions, and this scratching may aggravate the condition.

INFANTILE
FORM MAY
BE FOLLOWED
BY ASSOCIATED
DISEASE IN
ADULTHOOD

Bacterial Antigens

In bronchial asthma, over half the patients demonstrate typical atopic sensitization to antigens; among the remainder, many have had hay fever or another atopic disease in the past. Generally a respiratory infection is present. Nevertheless, skin tests utilizing bacterial antigens have failed to induce the immediate wheal that is the hallmark of atopic sensitization.

DELAYED ALLERGIES

In both allergic contact dermatitis and delayed reactions to infective antigens, such as tuberculin, delayed sensitivity is demonstrated. The serum of the sensitized person contains no demonstrable antibodies, and the reaction must therefore take place inside lymphoid cells.

Allergic Contact Dermatitis

Dermatitis due to contact is attributed to many irritants, both organic and inorganic. The organic substance may have a simpler chemical structure and lower molecular weight than typical proteins. The antigens include salts of metals, such as nickel and mercury; simple organic compounds, such as formaldehyde; drugs; and poison ivy and other plants. These substances probably act as haptenes, combining with body proteins to produce antigens, which cause sensitization.

Delayed Sensitization to Infective Agents

A type of delayed sensitization has been observed in brucellosis, glanders, syphilis, coccidioidomycosis, and lymphopathia venereum. In these situations, hypersensitivity to the infecting agent converts the disease from a widespread infection with little inflammation to a localized one with severe inflammation.

Allergic Reactions to Drugs

Many persons experience an untoward effect from drugs at some time. These drugs are not intrinsic antigens, so that reactions to them are seldom on a purely immunologic basis. Use of drugs in skin tests may be undependable, dangerous, or both. Drugs that are usually innocuous may, in allergic persons, cause rhinitis, asthma, urticaria, and contact dermatitis; in extreme cases, these agents may induce fever, rash, a blood dyscrasia, and liver damage. Such effects do not follow exposure to natural antigens, such as ragweed, animal danders, and other sources found in man's normal environment.

Typically, there are no symptoms following the first dose of the drug, but, following a period of 7 to 14 days, fever or rash, or perhaps both, appear. These symptoms clear after the drug has been stopped and eliminated from the body, only to recur within a few hours should another dose be given.

Allergic reactions to certain nonprotein medicinal agents are puzzling. Penicillin, for example, is nontoxic to most individuals, even when given in very large doses (as in valvulitis). Yet, it can give rise to severe urticaria, which in a small number of cases may be followed by anaphylactic shock and death. Yet, penicillin is not an antigen, nor is it

PENICILLIN MAY BEHAVE AS AN ANTIGEN

capable of forming a stable chemical compound with protein that would cause it to behave like a haptene. The explanation may be that in the body, penicillin is degraded (reduced) to penicillanic acid and penicilloic acid, either of which *can* combine with protein and act as a haptene. Skin tests performed with penicillin are far from reliable in predicting reactions; worse, a minute quantity can initiate a fatal reaction. Allergy to the life-saving penicillins still presents a knotty problem to the healing professions.

DISEASE MODEL: URTICARIA

Urticaria, also known as hives, is a skin eruption characterized by sharp-edged, elevated, flat-topped wheals. It is usually of brief duration but causes intense itching that is nearly intolerable. The rash is sometimes accompanied by general symptoms.

Although urticaria can stem from various causes, most cases revolve about allergy, with that to food standing at the top of the list. Common food antigens include shellfish, nuts, and berries and other fruits, although if the circumstances are "right," any food can cause urticaria. Wheals may appear promptly after the particular food is eaten, or their appearance may be delayed for as long as 12 hours. There may be digestive and respiratory symptoms also.

As we have mentioned, drugs—notably penicillin—can cause urticaria. In some of these cases, the urticaria is a manifestation of a generalized reaction resembling serum sickness. The prodromal period may be as long as a week or more. The urticaria may persist for months even though no further penicillin is administered. Characteristically, it is agents containing protein molecules—of which antisera, insulin, and extracts of allergens are examples—that induce urticaria. Urticaria may develop after the allergic person has been in contact with silk, wool, or animal pelts. A chronic form may follow infection of the teeth, tonsils, sinuses, or other foci. Worm infestation and bites of insects such as lice, mosquitoes, the *Acarus scabiei,* and bedbugs may be associated. Then too, stress in the form of financial problems or emotional turmoil can contribute to an episode. An analogy might be drawn between the development of urticaria and blowing a fuse in an overloaded electrical circuit. For example, in a mildly sensitive person, eating strawberries might not cause wheals to appear. But strawberries plus fatigue plus an overdrawn bank account plus a throat infection might trigger an explosive attack that would force the victim to take to his bed.

ALLERGY THE MOST FREQUENT CAUSE OF URTICARIA

As the episode develops, there is cutaneous dilatation of small blood vessels, and transudation of fluid through the walls of capillaries. Evidence indicates that release of histamine is the initiating factor in producing the wheal (consequently, antihistamines in suitable dosage would tend to suppress the reaction). It is possible to produce such lesions in normal skin by injecting histamine or histamine liberators. Histamine release is apparently an outcome of an antigen-antibody reaction. Circulating antibodies are usually demonstrable. If antigen is injected, a wheal will develop. In some types of urticaria, notably those resulting from infection, protein-containing drugs, or delayed reactions to foods, it may be impossible to demonstrate antibody.

HISTAMINE LIBERATION INITIATES THE REACTION

In the typical case there are clusters of circular lesions from 1 to 4 cm. in diameter, with edges sharply raised above the skin surface. Both the wheal and the surrounding skin are reddened. The wheal blanches when the skin is gently stretched. The lesions usually fade in from 6 to 24 hours, when further crops appear in other skin areas. Wheals appearing on the eyelids, lips, or genitalia have less sharp definition. There is associated subcutaneous edema, producing a clinical picture that has been well described as giant urticaria. The unbearable itching may induce furious scratching, which, in turn, produces new elongated lesions. The palms, soles, and scalp are rarely involved.

One may find it difficult to distinguish urticaria from insect bites, since in allergic persons insect bites often induce typical urticarial wheals. Usually, however, a central puncture is seen following insect bites, and as the wheal fades, a small pruritic papule remains. As a rule, it is the exposed parts of the body that are bitten.

The physician employs ephedrine, antihistaminics, or epinephrine in treating urticaria; in a severe attack, prednisone or another cortisone derivative may be administered. A long-respected local remedy is calamine lotion with phenol. Sometimes penicillinase is administered if the urticaria was due to penicillin.

AUTOIMMUNE DISEASE

The essence of autoimmune disease is failure of the mechanism that normally suppresses the production of antibodies against one's own tissue. Antigenic substances formed within the body (therefore designated *autoantigens*) excite formation of antibodies, and the resulting antigen-antibody reaction causes tissue injury in one "target organ" or possibly in several. The term *autoimmune disease* poorly describes the illness. A better term might be *autoclastic*, which means self-destroying. This is precisely what occurs in autoimmune disease.

Normally, the body tolerates its own protein substances, reacting defensively (or immunologically) only against foreign protein substances. As Sir F. Macfarlane Burnet points out, it appears that the body labels its own tissues "self" and foreign tissues "not self." *When the body treats "self" as "not self," autoimmune disease occurs.*

SELF-NOT SELF PRINCIPLE OPERATES IN BLOOD TRANSFUSIONS

Blood groups provide an excellent example of the principle of self and not self, as will be described. Classification of blood types is based upon the following:

1. The presence or absence of the specific antigen A or B in the *red blood cells*. These are agglutinable substances, or *agglutinogens*.
2. The presence or absence of the specific antibody alpha or beta in the *plasma*.

The antigen content of blood determines the type designation, thus:

Blood Type	Antigen	Antibody
A	A	beta
B	B	alpha
AB	A and B	none
O	none	alpha and beta

Antibody alpha agglutinates (causes clumping) antigen A; antibody beta agglutinates antigen B. Type A donor blood should not be given to a recipient with type B or type O blood. Type B donor blood should not be given to a recipient with type A or type O blood. Type AB donor blood should not be given to a recipient with type A, B, or O blood. Should transfusion be carried out that violates the self-not self principle—as would occur if the precautions just described were not followed —the donor red blood cells would be agglutinated by the recipient plasma, and hemolysis (breaking down) into the plasma would follow. The end result would be a transfusion reaction with serious or even fatal results. Recipient red blood cells are not hemolyzed by donor plasma because donor plasma is greatly diluted by recipient plasma.

What is it that causes the body to violate the self-not self rule? The possibilities include somatic cell mutation, release of cloistered or inaccessible antigens into the bloodstream, cross-reactions between foreign and body antigens, and haptene formation. We shall discuss each of these.

Somatic Cell Mutation

Occasionally a random mutation takes place in a somatic cell by which the structure of the cell's hereditary material, DNA, is altered. The outcome may be that the mutant cell enters the circulation as an *immunocyte*, a cell capable of releasing antibodies that will react with body antigens. The antigen-antibody reaction is, as we have seen, destructive. The mutant cell continues to produce antibodies, as do its daughter cells.

The thymus gland (see Chap. 10) is believed to be crucial in respect to autoimmune disease, although its exact role is not known. Lymphoid cells are believed to act as carriers of antibodies made by the plasma cells. Inasmuch as the lymph cells are manufactured by the thymus, it appears reasonable to believe that the thymus might play an important part in somatic cell mutation. Note that in the case of somatic cell mutation it is release of foreign *antibodies* that causes the problem. In most instances of autoimmune disease, a foreign *antigen* is involved.

Inaccessible Antigens

Certain specialized body tissues carry out their functions in locations segregated from the body's general chemical laboratory. These cloistered tissues are the seat of chemical patterns that may, in certain circumstances, act as antigens, since the body has not "learned" to tolerate them. These are called *inaccessible antigens*. It may happen that through trauma or infection, these antigens are freed to enter the body's chemical reaction processes. If the body stamps them as intruders, as it is quite likely to do, autoimmune disease results. A good example of these remote substances is the lens protein of the eye. Antigen sequestered here does not normally reach the bloodstream in more than minute quantities; but should it be released into the bloodstream after injury to the eye, the body's immune mechanism would treat the protein as a foreign substance. In rapidly mounting numbers, antibodies specific for the antigen of lens protein would attack the uninjured eye. The disease that would be thus produced is sympathetic ophthalmia. In earlier years it was a frequent cause of blindness, and although with improved understanding and advanced techniques it has been brought under control, the physician must still remain alert to this possibility.

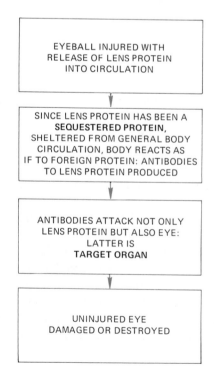

SEQUENCE OF EVENTS
IN SYMPATHETIC OPHTHALMIA

EYEBALL INJURED WITH
RELEASE OF LENS PROTEIN
INTO CIRCULATION

SINCE LENS PROTEIN HAS BEEN A
SEQUESTERED PROTEIN,
SHELTERED FROM GENERAL BODY
CIRCULATION, BODY REACTS AS
IF TO FOREIGN PROTEIN: ANTIBODIES
TO LENS PROTEIN PRODUCED

ANTIBODIES ATTACK NOT ONLY
LENS PROTEIN BUT ALSO EYE:
LATTER IS
TARGET ORGAN

UNINJURED EYE
DAMAGED OR DESTROYED

The thyroid gland, too, is vulnerable to autoimmune disease. It manu-factures the inaccessible protein thyroglobulin. All goes well as long as the thyroglobulin remains within the thyroid follicles. Should it escape, however, into the interstitial spaces of the thyroid, it would be treated as a foreign protein. This is precisely what occurs in Hashimoto's disease, which we shall examine later.

Cross-Reactions

In a cross-reaction, an antibody attacks a body substance closely related to but not identical with an invading antigen. Thus, a foreign antigen invades the body, which produces antibodies to repel it. But cer-

SEQUENCE OF EVENTS
IN RHEUMATIC FEVER

STREPTOCOCCUS
INFECTION

TOXINS FROM STREPTOCOCCUS
PROVIDE ANTIGEN
FOR HOST ANTIBODIES

BUT PROTEIN IN HEART
MUSCLE AND JOINTS
CROSS REACTS (CLOSELY
RESEMBLES) FOREIGN ANTIGEN

HOST ANTIBODIES ATTACK NOT
ONLY FOREIGN ANTIGEN BUT
HOST PROTEIN: ALSO ATTACKS
ORGANS (HEART AND JOINTS)
HARBORING HOST PROTEIN:
HEART AND JOINTS BECOME
TARGET ORGANS

HEART AND JOINTS
SEVERELY DAMAGED:
DAMAGE CONTINUES AFTER
INFECTION HAS DISAPPEARED:
A TRUE AUTOIMMUNE REACTION

SELF-NOT
SELF
PRINCIPLE
SEEN IN
RHEUMATIC
FEVER

tain body organs (thyroid gland, heart) sometimes contain a substance resembling the antigen. The antibodies react not only against the antigen but also against the body substance, just as if it were an antigen. The substance that resembles the antigen is designated an *antigenic determinant*. Rheumatic fever, which often follows streptococcal throat infections, is an example of autoimmune disease developing in this manner. Here, the antigens of the causative organisms, the hemolytic streptococci, resemble the antigens of the cardiac muscle. Antibodies formed to resist the bacterial antigens continue to react against the cardiac antigens long after the infection has cleared. This cross-reaction is the basis for severe damage to the heart muscle.

Varieties of Autoimmune Disease

The field of autoimmune diseases is a new one, and consequently the questions outweigh the answers by a great factor. No two diseases generally classified as autoimmune are alike: some are only questionably autoimmune, and few are universally accepted as autoimmune. The list of possible or probable autoimmune conditions includes:
  chronic glomerulonephritis
  sympathetic ophthalmia
  idiopathic myocarditis
  sarcoidosis
  acquired hemolytic anemia
  idiopathic hemorrhagic purpura
  Hashimoto's disease
  Addison's disease
  collagen diseases, including
      lupus erythematosus
      polyarteritis nodosa
      Wegener's granulomatosis
      rheumatoid arthritis
      rheumatic fever
Disorders less likely to be autoimmune are:
  ataxia-telangiectasia
  ulcerative colitis
  multiple sclerosis
  chronic hepatitis
Autoimmune diseases have several characteristics in common:

1. They often follow an infection.
2. Frequently they are familial, suggesting an inherited tendency to produce excessive antibodies.
3. The gamma globulin level is frequently elevated.
4. They often give rise to "false positive" tests for syphilis.
5. Administration of cortisone and ACTH frequently is beneficial.

Pertinent is William Boyd's warning: "It is dangerously, if not fatally, easy to be seduced by the concept of autoimmunity as an explanation for many so-called idiopathic diseases. . . . Autoimmune reactions are going to prove of great value in explaining a number of obscure conditions, but they will not provide a key to every mystery."

DISEASE MODEL: HASHIMOTO'S DISEASE

Hashimoto's disease, also called *struma, struma lymphomatosa,* and *Hashimoto's thyroiditis,* was described by Hashimoto in 1912. It is a chronic disorder involving the thyroid gland, with clinical symptoms including progressive enlargement of the gland, with or without symptoms of pressure. The parenchyma of the thyroid undergoes atrophy. Lymphocytes infiltrate the gland's substance, this infiltration perhaps representing delayed tissue hypersensitivity to a protein or proteins of the thyroid. It may be that thyroglobulin acts as a foreign substance to initiate Hashimoto's disease, as already described.

The disease chiefly affects women. Usually they consult their physician because of the mass in the neck or because of symptoms from pressure. Occasionally the disease appears to be associated with other

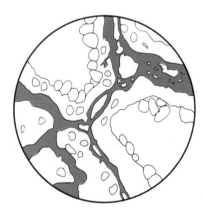 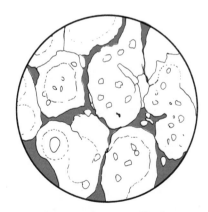

Normal Basement Membrane   Fragmented Basement Membrane

Hashimoto's Disease. In the normal individual, the important thyroid protein thyroglobulin is confined within the thyroid lobules by the basement membrane. The illustration on the left shows a normal basement membrane and portions of six thyroid follicles. In Hashimoto's disease, the basement membrane becomes fragmented for reasons unknown. The illustration on the right shows a fragmented basement membrane, portions of which surround fragments of thyroid follicles. This disruption of the normal structure of the thyroid gland permits thyroglobulin to escape into the interstitial tissues. Here it is treated exactly as if it were a foreign protein. Antibodies against thyroglobulin form, and these antibodies attack not only the escaped thyroglobulin but the thyroid gland itself.

conditions believed to be autoimmune in origin—rheumatoid arthritis, for example. The thyroid gland is not tender, and its configuration is firm and lobular. The pyramidal lobe almost invariably is thickened. Thyroid function usually is normal, although occasionally the radioactive iodine uptake and turnover are slightly elevated. The serum gamma globulin may be elevated. Antibodies in high titer against several thyroid compounds, especially thyroglobulin, may be found.

Slowly progressive enlargement of the gland usually necessitates its surgical removal. Hypothyroidism may appear in advanced Hashimoto's disease. Only when there are pressure symptoms or an unsightly swelling is surgical treatment imperative. Early in the disease, the condition may improve with administration of desiccated thyroid gland.

CLINICAL CONSIDERATIONS

A knowledge of the mechanisms of body immunity and the circumstances in which it may go awry is essential for all health workers. At a more practical level, we can extend far more sympathy to the sufferer from allergic disease if we know its basis. All too frequently allergic patients are suspected, and even accused, of being neurotics—especially by those who have never experienced the watery agonies of hay fever, the intolerable itching of hives, the splitting headache of food sensitivity, or the breathlessness of asthma.

Treatment of allergic disorders often develops into a prolonged ordeal, during which new allergies may be added to the old. Frequently the patient ends up learning to live with his allergies rather than obtaining a cure. Understanding that this may well happen helps both the patient and those involved in providing therapy.

Knowledge about hypersensitivity states, especially in relation to the administration of drugs, can help prevent needless tragedies or can enable one to better cope with emergency situations. Since autoimmune disease usually is manifested in the early stage as an infection, one should always consider this possibility when a patient who has suffered from an infection is not recuperating properly. Finally, autoimmune disease does not often develop; but, as has been well said, "The incidence of a rare disease is exactly 100 per cent if *you* have it."

TOPICS FOR DISCUSSION

1. Discuss the similarities between allergic disease and mild psychic disorders, such as the neuroses.

2. Why is *autoclastic* a more accurate term to describe autoimmune disease than *autoimmune?*

3. There is great variation from one autoimmune disease to another. What might account for this?

4. How do you explain the uncertainty of scientists in designating a specific disorder as an autoimmune disease?

5. Discuss the relationship between hypersensitivity and the adreno-cortical hormones.

6. What is the relationship between stress, as the concept was introduced by Dr. Hans Selye, and allergic disease?

7. Would you classify scientific knowledge in the field of allergy as at a primitive or at an advanced stage of development?

8. Corticosteroids such as cortisone are highly effective in the management of many allergic disorders. What hazards are involved in their use?

9. Discuss borderline "allergic" reactions, such as those caused by some drugs. Differentiate between sensitivity, or allergy, on the one hand and idiosyncrasy on the other.

10. The incidence of allergic diseases varies greatly from country to country. It appears to be much higher in the United States than in other countries. Can you explain this?

BIBLIOGRAPHY

Books

Beeson, P., and McDermott, W.: Textbook of Medicine. vols. I and II. Philadelphia, W. B. Saunders Co., 1967.

Douthwaite, A.: French's Index of Differential Diagnosis. Baltimore, The Williams & Wilkins Co., 1967.

Burnet, F.: Autoimmune Disease, pp. 15–30. In Sodeman, W., and Sodeman, W.: Pathologic Physiology. Philadelphia, W. B. Saunders Co., 1968.

Houston, J., et al.: A Short Textbook of Medicine. Philadelphia, J. B. Lippincott Co., 1968.

Sherman, W.: Allergy. pp. 216–223. In Sodeman, W., and Sodeman, W.: Pathologic Physiology. Philadelphia, W. B. Saunders Co., 1968.

Talso, P., and Remenchik, A.: Internal Medicine. St. Louis, The C. V. Mosby Co., 1968.

Boyd, W.: A Textbook of Pathology. pp. 142–185. Philadelphia, Lea & Febiger, 1970.

Passmore, R., and Robson, J.: A Companion to Medical Studies. vol. 2, pp. 1–13. Philadelphia, F. A. Davis Co., 1970.

Articles

Rebuilding the cell to cure disease. Medical World News, 11:23, (November 13) 1970.

4

infectious diseases

Almost as far back as written records go we find evidence that mankind has been afflicted by frequent recurrences of horrible epidemics. Periodically occurring without any apparent cause, each one has taken its toll of life and then departed as strangely as it came. They have halted social progress, determined the results of wars, and sometimes even threatened the existence of civilization itself.
—Ernest Caulfield [*]

We are sometimes too prone to believe that infection—overwhelmingly the leading cause of death in bygone years—no longer poses a formidable problem. Though disability and death stemming from infection have decreased dramatically in recent decades, infectious disease still constitutes an important threat to health. Many of the highly destructive infections of yesteryear have largely disappeared, yet, new ones have replaced them. Some of these were stimulated by the very antibiotic therapy that controlled or abolished their predecessors. With decimation of the normal flora by antibiotics, resistant variants and resistant strains of organisms can multiply and flourish. Although infection still occurs in the highly developed countries of the temperate zones, in the more heavily populated tropical and semitropical areas, infection is not an occasional event, but an ever present threat. Hundreds of thousands of persons are afflicted every year with infections such as leprosy, malaria, and Asiatic cholera, to name a few. Although the total impact of infectious disease on today's health may have decreased, the actual number of infections that must be diagnosed and treated is still great.

THE DISCOVERY OF THE INFECTIOUS NATURE OF CERTAIN DISEASES

During the Dark Ages, ignorance and superstition combined to prevent the discovery of infecting agents. Christians regarded disease as the result of sin, and according to this view afflicted persons were merely receiving their just deserts. Then, toward the end of the twelfth century,

---

[*] Caulfield, Ernest: The Throat Distemper of 1735–1740. New Haven, Conn., Yale Journal of Biology and Medicine, 1939.

the great Francis of Assisi founded the Franciscan Order, an important function of which was the establishment of hospices for care of the sick poor. Both religion and the biological sciences began to glimpse a new dawn. A long procession of great men helped to light the lamp of truth that was to reveal the infectious origin of much disease.

EARLY
STAGES IN
UNDERSTANDING
OF THE
INFECTIOUS
PROCESS

Girolamo Fracastoro (1484–1553), an Italian, stood out as a physician, poet, physicist, geologist, astronomer, and pathologist. His medical poem, *Syphilis sive Morbus Gallicus,* indicated the infectious origin of venereal disease. In 1546, he published *De Contagione,* which outlined the modern theory of infection and described epidemics of foot-and-mouth disease and of typhus fever. Fracastoro believed that disease was caused by a sort of gel that could be made to reproduce when placed in the proper medium.

An Italian Jesuit, Athanasius Kircher (1602–1680), stated that living organisms were a cause of disease. He was one of the first to use the microscope to investigate disease. Looking at the blood of plague victims with a microscope, he found that it vibrated with what he called "worms." The "worms" might have been white or red blood cells in rouleaux formation, or they might actually have been large bacteria.

The Dutchman Antony van Leeuwenhoek (1632–1723), called the "Father of Microbiology," saw the various types of bacteria under the microscope and sketched the rods, spheres, and spirals that his instrument revealed. He was the first to make such observations, which were so accurate that many of the forms he described are easily recognized. Unfortunately, the importance of Leeuwenhoek's discoveries was not understood at first, because at that time microorganisms were studied mainly to satisfy curiosity about their relationship to higher living forms, without awareness of their significance in fermentation and the production of disease. Such understanding had to await the coming of Louis Pasteur, who, with Robert Koch, founded bacteriology.

It had been thought by most people that bacteria arose spontaneously from soil, plants, or other unlike animals. This notion of *spontaneous generation* held sway until the latter part of the nineteenth century when Pasteur performed a series of experiments proving that microorganisms can originate only from organic matter. Pasteur also refined the process of fermentation to improve wine-making (an important industry in France), and it was later adapted to milk-processing (pasteurization). Pasteur isolated the organism that caused silkworm disease. He introduced the concept of *immunization,* or vaccination, and ultimately he successfully vaccinated a young boy who had been bitten by a rabid wolf. In so doing, he was applying the principle discovered by Edward Jenner, who about 50 years earlier had shown that material removed from a cowpox lesion could be used to inoculate against the far more serious disease of smallpox. Thus, in vaccination, attenuated (weakened) organisms do not produce disease, but instead stimulate the body to produce antibodies.

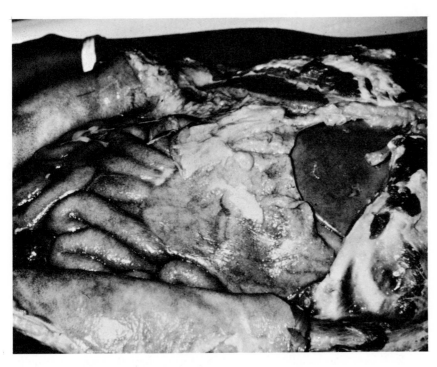

Purulent exudate covers bowel and omentum as
well as peritoneal wall.

Pasteur's companion genius, Robert Koch, described the complete life
history of the anthrax bacillus. He showed that anthrax can be transmitted to animals by use of cultures. Koch devised methods of fixing
and drying bacterial films on cover slips, of staining the films, and of
photographing the stained organisms. He listed six bacteria that cause
surgical infections, described the corresponding pathologic findings, and
cultured each organism through repeated generations in vitro and in vivo.
We still call the tubercle bacillus Koch's bacillus. Koch also discovered
the *Vibrio cholerae,* the causative organism of Asiatic cholera, which still
causes many human deaths.

Not one of these great medical pioneers escaped skepticism, ridicule,
scorn, and persecution. Yet they laid the foundation for the great advances in knowledge of infectious disease that were to arrive during the
mid-twentieth century. Discovery of the infectious nature of much disease
was agonizingly slow; in the meantime, untold millions suffered and
many died. Discovery of medical truths has ever been a long, slow
process. Infection was no exception.

PASTEUR
AND KOCH
THE
FOUNDERS OF
BACTERIOLOGY

CLASSIFICATION OF INFECTIOUS AGENTS

Infection is the invasion of the body by pathogenic organisms, whether or not detectable disease occurs. Obviously, infection is not the same as disease caused by infection. Disease can be other than infectious in origin, and infection can occur without disease. Human infection, with or without disease, can be caused by a virus, a rickettsial organism, a bacterium, a fungus, or an animal parasite. For an infection to be contagious, man-to-man or animal-to-man spread must take place. In some infections, this does not happen.

Under what circumstances, then, will an infection become a disease? This depends upon the invading organisms, the body responses they elicit, and the predisposing or defensive factors existing at the time of the infection.

Which invading organisms cause human infectious disease? The list is long. It includes:

1. Viruses: minute parasitic forms not visible under the light microscope, characterized by a lack of independent metabolism and by the ability to reproduce only within living host cells.
2. Rickettsiae: small rod-shaped to coccoid-shaped organisms usually placed between viruses and bacteria, transmitted by lice, fleas, ticks, and mites to man and other animals, and requiring living tissue to exist.
3. Bacteria: one-celled plants visible under the microscope. Organisms in the genera Bacillus and Clostridium are spore-forming.
   a. Bacilli (straight rods)
   b. Cocci (dot shaped)
      (1) Diplococci
      (2) Streptococci

| ANIMALS | PLANTS | | | |
Protozoa	Fungi	Bacteria	Rickettsiae	Viruses

(3) Staphylococci
  c. Curved rods
    (1) Vibrios (comma shaped)
    (2) Spirilla (wavy or corkscrew shaped)
    (3) Spirochetes (flexible, similar to spirilla)
4. Fungi: plant organisms of a low order of development, very few of which are pathogenic; includes mushrooms, toadstools, molds, yeasts, and related plants.
5. Animal parasites: organisms living on or within the bodies of animals or humans, obtaining an advantage without providing compensation. Includes a considerable range of organisms, some of which are by no means microscopic. Intestinal worms, for example, may be many feet in length.

Size

What is the size of infecting organisms? The variation is considerable. The smallest microorganisms, which measure about 20 mμ (mμ = millimicron = one thousandth of a micron), belong to the arbovirus group; the bacterium Staphylococcus measures about 1 mμ; and animal parasites, such as the beef or pork tapeworm, may be as long as 10 meters, or over 30 feet. So the largest organism that can infect man is 10 billion times as large as the smallest.

ORIGIN OF INFECTING ORGANISMS

Dormancy

Microorganisms may remain dormant in human tissue before they begin to reproduce and cause disease. For example, the virus of herpes simplex can persist for a long period without causing symptoms before it multiplies and produces a cold sore.

Normal Inhabitants

The mouth, upper respiratory tract, lower gastrointestinal tract, and skin are continuously inhabited by bacteria and fungi. These are regarded as normal, yet under certain circumstances they can cause disease. The conjunctiva of the eye, the distal part of the urethra, and the vagina also continuously support microorganisms, whereas the sinuses, terminal bronchi, upper respiratory tract, stomach, and upper intestine prove sterile on culture.

NUMEROUS SOURCES OF DISEASE FOUND IN THE NORMAL HUMAN ENVIRONMENT

Initial infection of the urinary tract can usually be traced to bacteria common in the lower gastrointestinal tract or on the perineum. Pharyngitis, sinusitis, and pneumonia can be traced to organisms common in the mouth in many instances. Infections of wounds or of the skin usually are brought about by organisms normally present on the skin.

Soil Organisms

Only a small number of the numerous microorganisms normally present in the soil cause disease. Soil contaminated by chicken or bird droppings contains *Histoplasma capsulatum*, the fungus that causes histoplasmosis. In certain areas of the midsouth of the United States, over 80 per cent of the population are infected with the organism, although most never manifest clinical disease. Dust in barracks or in hospitals can infect humans with a hemolytic Streptococcus. Man acquires infestation with hookworm by walking barefoot in soil infested with the embryos.

The Human Source

Man himself provides the source for many of the infections that afflict him. Tuberculosis is acquired after prolonged or intimate contact with a patient suffering from this infection. Syphilis is transmitted by contact with a syphilitic lesion in a person who has the disease. Ring-

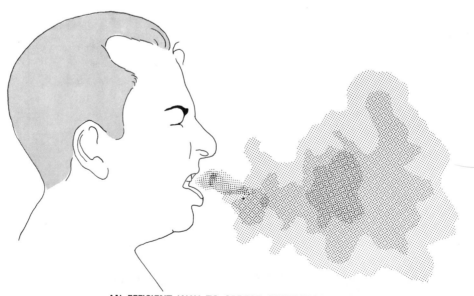

AN EFFICIENT WAY TO SPREAD MICROORGANISMS

worm spreads from person to person via contaminated clothing and structures such as floors. A considerable number of viral infections are transmitted from one person to another by direct contact and include measles, mumps, chickenpox, German measles, hepatitis, and poliomyelitis. Bacterial infections also may be transmitted directly, or in some instances indirectly. The person transmitting the infection may be a patient suffering from the disease, one convalescing from it, or a healthy carrier. One famous carrier of typhoid fever, Typhoid Mary, infected at least 50 persons over a 15 year period. The *carrier* harbors highly pathogenic organisms that communicate disease to others, yet he suffers no disease himself.

Water Supply

When sanitation breaks down, the water supply may be a source of infection, as in rural areas when shallow springs are used or in cities when fresh water is contaminated by broken sewer pipes. Disease that stems from contaminated water usually attacks the intestinal tract, as occurred in Chicago in 1933, when a large number of persons became infected with amebic dysentery because of faulty plumbing in the hotel they occupied. Asiatic cholera, endemic to many regions of the world, owes its spread to the drinking of water contaminated with sewage.

Milk

Milk is an excellent medium for the spread of infectious disease. Tuberculosis of the gastrointestinal tract and of bones can often be traced to the drinking of milk produced by infected cows. Brucellosis may result from drinking the milk of cows afflicted with this disease, and Q fever may be similarly acquired. Strangely enough, the animals may produce infected milk, yet remain asymptomatic themselves. Other diseases that may be spread by milk include typhoid fever, infectious hepatitis, and poliomyelitis.

Food

Infected food can spread disease in several ways. Gastroenteritis may result from eating food contaminated with any of several organisms. For example, food allowed to stand for some time, notably ham, custard, and salad dressing, acquires an enormous number of organisms, mainly staphylococci, that produce a powerful toxin. Infectious hepatitis may result from eating raw oysters or clams. Food that is improperly canned or bottled, usually in home processing, may be contaminated by a deadly bacterium, *Clostridium botulinum,* which produces a toxin that acts at multiple sites distant from the gastrointestinal tract. Humans can acquire liver abscesses from eating uncooked vegetables contaminated by the protozoon, *Entamoeba histolytica.* Ulcerative lesions develop in the cecum when the microorganism releases a destructive enzyme and actively moves into the bowel wall. When mesenteric vessels become eroded, the parasite is carried by the portal circulation to the liver, where it causes abscesses.

Animals

Animals can be counted among the most important sources of serious disease in humans. Tuberculosis, brucellosis, epidemic pharyngitis, and Q fever may be transmitted by cattle. Sheep and cattle with anthrax can transmit it to humans. Rabbits and other rodents carry tularemia, or rabbit fever, to humans. Birds can transmit a serious form of pneumonia. Rabies is transmitted to humans by the bites of rabid dogs, foxes, bats, and some other animals. Swine and cattle transmit tapeworm. The eating of insufficiently cooked pork may result in trichinosis, which causes muscle pain, edema of the eyes, fever, paralysis, and sometimes death. Monkeys may be a source of malaria. Animal contacts are of obvious importance in diagnosing infectious disease. The health scientist might ask several questions about disease transmission by animals. Has the patient been bitten, as in rabies? Has he eaten a meat containing a parasite, as in tapeworm? Has he handled an animal, as in tularemia? Has he been exposed to animal skin or fur, as in anthrax? Has he inhaled dust from bird droppings, as in psittacosis? Has he been bitten by an insect, as in malaria?

Insects

The widespread diseases of malaria and filariasis are caused by parasites that pass through the body of the mosquito, which then acts as the vector (carrier) by biting the human. During the fourteenth century, the common rat flea served as the carrier of bubonic plague, which killed 25,000,000 people—one fourth of the world's population. An important source of the germ that causes tularemia and Rocky Mountain spotted fever is the tick. Mosquitoes, ticks, and mice are reservoirs of human infection for St. Louis encephalitis, dengue fever, Rift Valley fever, and other illnesses. Flies can spread infection by contaminating food with microorganisms they have eaten or that they carry on their legs or bodies. The virus causing poliomyelitis has been recovered from flies.

Placenta

Even before birth, man is not free of the threat of infection. Congenital syphilis provides an example in which the embryo is invaded via the placenta. Often the infection kills the fetus, and an abortion or stillbirth takes place. Infection of the fetus with the virus of German measles may cause cataracts, deafness, and heart abnormalities if the mother is infected during the first 3 months of pregnancy.

Parenteral Transmission

Various infectious diseases, including serum hepatitis, syphilis, and malaria, may be spread by the intravenous or intramuscular route. With such a "main line" introduction into the bloodstream, the disease spreads rapidly and is soon manifest throughout the body.

Comment

For a disease to be contagious, the causative organism must be transmitted from one person to another by direct contact or through the air (airborne); examples of contagious disease are gonorrhea, typhoid fever, and the common cold. In noncontagious infections, the organism usually enters the host only by direct invasion; examples are tetanus (lockjaw) and botulism. The success of a disease-causing microbe in producing disease depends on the number of organisms and their virulence. That is, invasion by a small number of a certain organism might not cause illness, whereas invasion by a large number of that organism would certainly do so. Protective measures, such as inoculation, may be sufficient in the case of the former but would fail in the latter. Host resistance also plays a role.

Disease-causing microbes can enter the human body through the respiratory tract, the digestive tract, and the broken or unbroken skin. Respiratory microbes leave the body by way of the mouth in saliva or by way of the nose in lung exudates. Intestinal microbes leave in the feces or urine. Some microorganisms leave the host in the bodies of biting insects, such as the mosquito.

To transmit disease, microbes must survive sufficiently long outside the host. For example, *Salmonella typhosa,* which causes typhoid fever, is hardy, being able to live in water or ice for weeks, whereas *Treponema pallidum,* which causes syphilis, is fragile and dies quickly outside the body.

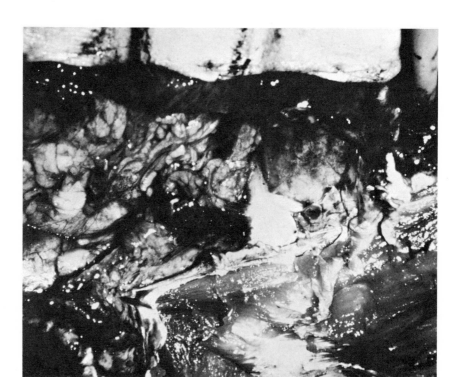

Tissues badly damaged by infection. Glairy exudate present. Failure of wound healing.

DAMAGING EFFECTS OF INFECTING ORGANISMS

Obstruction

Infectious agents may cause obstruction or exert pressure. The fish, beef, and pork tapeworms, enormous when compared to bacteria, can cause intestinal obstruction; the ascaris, minute in comparison to the tapeworm, produces the same effect by forming tiny globes in the intestine. The dracunculus, 1 meter long, causes a swelling under the skin, and *Loa loa* lodges beneath the conjunctiva. Filaria block the lymphatics and thus cause the deforming disease known as elephantiasis. *Tinea solium* forms a cyst in the brain, and the end result may be epilepsy.

Organisms need not be gigantic to cause pressure effects. Blindness, for example, can result from multiplication of *Loa loa* within the optic nerve, and *Bacillus anthracis*, the causative agent of anthrax, can cause death by obstructing blood vessels. Even in the severely infected patient, the mass of the patient dwarfs the total mass of the infecting organisms. Most microorganisms without a doubt cause disease by means that are not physical.

TOTAL
DAMAGE TO
THE HUMAN
ORGANISM
VARIES
ACCORDING TO
CHARACTERISTICS
OF INVADING
MICROORGANISM

Toxins

One of the chief mechanisms by which microorganisms damage the host is through release of a harmful chemical substance—a toxin. There are two types of toxins. *Endotoxins* are released by the disintegration of dead bacteria, and their toxicity is low. Only the endotoxins of gram-negative bacteria are regarded as of serious consequence in human disease. *Exotoxins*, liberated by gram-positive living bacteria during their metabolism, are far more powerful. Endotoxins produce generalized and diverse effects, whereas exotoxins attack the central nervous system, the heart muscle. and the adrenal glands. Some idea of the relative potency of endotoxins and exotoxins may be gained by the realization that 1 mg. of an endotoxin is lethal to ten mice (the laboratory animal usually used in such study), while 1 mg. of an exotoxin would be lethal to 31,000,000 mice.

Bacterial Enzymes

Bacterial enzymes, although not toxins, play a part in the production of infection by breaking down complex food materials (protein, carbohydrate, fat) into simpler substances that can be assimilated by the bacteria. One of these, hyaluronidase, hydrolyzes (splits) hyaluronic acid, an essential ingredient of the cellular ground substance of tissue, thus permitting the bacteria to spread more rapidly.

Another enzyme produced by bacteria is coagulase, which accelerates the formation of blood clots. This enzyme may lay down fibrin in the periphery of areas involved in infection, changing them to walled abscesses. In the center of the abscess, phagocytosis may be handicapped.

Certain bacteria produce the enzyme streptokinase, which liquefies clots through its action on a normal blood ingredient, plasminogen. Plasminogen then forms plasmin, which is an active protein destroying agent, and which inactivates complement, a circulating protein essential to normal defense against infection.

Another enzyme fabricated by bacteria is deoxyribonuclease, which can cause liquefaction of exudates such as pleural fluid. The viruses that cause influenza and mumps produce enzymes that release neuraminic acid, which helps the viruses attach to cells. Presence of the acid appears to promote infection.

Invasiveness

Invasiveness, or *penetrance,* refers to the ability of the infecting organism to penetrate tissue. Some microorganisms have minimal ability to invade tissue, but others make their entrance explosively. The diphtheria organism penetrates only the superficial cells of the upper respiratory tract, and causes its damage by manufacturing a powerful exotoxin. The tetanus organism likewise shows no tendency to spread, but it too manufactures an overwhelming toxin that passes to motor nerve endings in the spinal cord and interferes with motor function.

The common cold virus does not invade deep tissue, whereas other organisms are capable of doing so. Actinomyces produces an indolent but spreading infection under the skin, which can pass through such strong fibrous tissues as the diaphragm, pleura, chest cavity wall, and skin with destructive effects. The herpes virus penetrates tissue at the border between the mucous membranes and the skin of the mouth, causing the typical cold sore. This persistent virus is capable of causing further lesions some years after the initial infection, and other viruses may persist in tonsillar or adenoidal tissues for long periods.

Certain microbes, including the Staphylococcus, give rise to a lesion at the site of body entrance, then go on to invade the lymph vessels. Following initial invasion by the tubercle bacillus, there is invasion of lymph nodes and spread to chains of nodes. *T. pallidum* enters the lymphatics and passes to the regional lymph nodes; the virus of vaccinia spreads to the lymphatics that drain the site of vaccination; poliovirus spreads to the regional lymph nodes from its intestinal site of reproduction by way of the lymphatics.

Microbes may penetrate blood vessel walls, then spread via the bloodstream, as the gram-negative rod forms do. The Absidia, the fungi that cause sinusitis, rapidly invade vessel walls and spread via the bloodstream to remote organs. The mumps virus spreads through the bloodstream from the parotid glands to the testis and to the kidney. The viruses of infectious hepatitis and serum hepatitis may persist in the blood for over a year and can be transmitted in donor blood to a recipient during transfusion. Viruses also endure in the bloodstream in cases of dengue, yellow fever, and Colorado tick fever. Indeed, in malaria and filariasis, the microorganisms can be so numerous as to be visible in a single drop of blood when examined by the thick smear technique.

Virulence

Virulence means the intensity of disease caused by a given strain of a microorganism as shown by its power to produce toxic substances and its ability to establish itself within the host. We refer, therefore, to a *pathogenic,* or *disease-causing, species* and to a *virulent strain.* Scientists have been able to discover no specific enzymatic or biochemical distinctions that account for differences in virulence among strains of a species, and frequently the only detectable difference between strains is their ability to produce disease. For example, types I, II, and

III of the pneumonia organism are highly fatal; one strain of poliovirus is exceedingly virulent; the strain of influenza virus that caused the death of 20 million people between 1917 and 1919 was overwhelmingly virulent; but one strain of the tubercle bacillus is used in active immunization against the disease because of its low virulence.

Several bacteria and one fungus have protective polysaccharide *capsules* (a viscous substance that forms a covering layer around the cell) that inhibit phagocytosis and thereby increase the ability of the organism to produce disease. In one experiment, capsule material added to noncapsulated bacteria in animals caused increased virulence, since the capsule material dissolved in body fluids and neutralized circulating antibody. The capsule also causes a sort of immunologic paralysis by presenting such an enormous amount of antigen to the animal that it cannot produce antibody. The organisms that cause pneumonia and anthrax possess such capsules.

Organ Preference

Certain organisms appear to prefer certain organs—the reason for this being one of the mysteries of medicine. As an example, the virus that causes mumps attacks the parotid gland, testes, and ovaries. Other organisms invade the lungs. Conversely, some organs, such as the thymus, pancreas, and thyroid, produce specific chemical substances that combat the Streptococcus and other organisms.

THE CHANGING PICTURE OF INFECTION

Bacterial enzyme systems as they evolved over the ages have permitted certain strains of organisms to survive, so that when local environments have become hostile, bacterial mutations have brought latent enzyme systems to the fore. Unfortunately for mankind, the excessive use of antibiotics has encouraged such mutations, by reducing the numbers of the normal flora in certain areas and allowing foreign flora to proliferate. Bacteria which are harmless in their normal habitat may cause serious infection in the new environment. Thus, excessive use of antibiotics has promoted a shift from streptococcal infections to those caused by gram-negative bacilli, resistant staphylococci, viruses, and fungi. Moreover, viruses have shown a pronounced ability to attack bacteria and drastically increase their virulence through *transduction,* in which the genetic makeup of a bacterial cell is actually altered.

MUTATION PROMOTES TRANSDUCTION

SUPERINFECTION

Early in the history of penicillin therapy, physicians began to observe the phenomenon of *superinfection*, thus: antibiotic therapy, by eliminating nonresistant pathogens, can provide the opportunity for a normally harmless bacterium, resistant to the antibiotic, to multiply and to cause disease because of the increased nutrients made available to it. This increase in nutrients results from suppression of growth of other microorganisms and disruption of the body's normal bacterial flora. Sometimes, indeed, an antibiotic appears to directly stimulate growth of a microorganism. For example: chloramphenicol can directly inhibit antibody production; the antianabolic effect of tetracycline can cause suppression of the body's immune responses.

FACTORS PREDISPOSING TO INFECTION

Age

Age is important among the factors predisposing to infection. Infections occur more commonly and are more severe during infancy and old age, bacterial pneumonia and tuberculosis being especially significant during these periods. Mumps, measles, poliomyelitis, varicella, and infectious hepatitis strike adults more severely than children, while viral respiratory disease is less common in the elderly than in the young. Disseminated histoplasmosis occurs more often in infants, cryptococcosis in the middle-aged, and blastomycosis in the older persons. It may be that the young have more frequent infections because they lack antibodies. These crucial defenders against infection are transferred from the mother to the fetus before birth, gradually decreasing during the first 6 months of life, as the child begins to manufacture his own antibodies. In older age groups, production of antibodies in response to antigens decreases, yet the reasons for this are not always clear. Middle-aged persons are increasingly exposed as a result of certain occupational activities, but this is not the whole explanation. Perhaps the stresses and worries of middle life provide a clue.

Occupation

Occupation may increase one's exposure to infecting organisms. Brucellosis shows an increased incidence in stockyard workers, sporotrichosis in gardeners, tularemia in hunters, anthrax in wool workers. Miners and stone cutters are afflicted by certain lung diseases such as tuberculosis, but in this instance, increased susceptibility stems from increased exposure to silica rather than from increased exposure to the tubercle bacillus.

Sex Differences

Occupation does not account for the high risk of severe poliomyelitis in women of childbearing age. Infections of the urinary tract occur ten times as frequently in the female as in the male, probably because the ureters may be obstructed by a pregnant uterus, because urethral trauma may occur during intercourse, or because the female urethra is shorter. Meningitis and septicemia occur almost twice as frequently in males as in females. Osteomyelitis, tuberculosis, and cryptococcosis are seen in males more frequently.

Race

Tuberculosis afflicts Negroes more often than Caucasians. Coccidioidomycosis in disseminated form occurs three times as often in Mexicans, 15 times as often in Negroes, and five times as often in Filipinos compared to the incidence in Caucasians. Such factors as housing, exposure to dust, crowded living quarters, availability of medical care, and ability to purchase drugs may outweigh racial differences.

Nutrition

One would expect that good nutrition would protect against infectious disease, particularly since the formation of blood globulins—the source of antibodies—depends upon adequate protein intake. This is generally the case, but there are a few rare exceptions. Experimentally, rats and rabbits with protein deficiency have a lowered resistance to pneumonia, yet vitamin B deficient mice show lower susceptibility to poliovirus. During World War II, thousands of concentration camp inhabitants died of starvation and infection. Among the underdeveloped countries of the world, infection is a very common cause of death among starving populations.

Fatigue

Although experimental evidence is not available to support the opinion that fatigue predisposes to infection, many—perhaps most—physicians believe that fatigue increases susceptibility to pneumonia, the common cold, tuberculosis, and poliomyelitis. The reasons for this are not clear as yet.

Temperature Effects

Cold appears to predispose to infection. While decreased temperature decreases bacterial multiplication, it suppresses antibody formation, and also decreases the ciliary motion of the tracheal mucosa. Higher temperatures, on the other hand, increase bacterial reproduction, but also increase antibody response to antigen.

Secondary Disease

Patients who have decreased gamma globulin or abnormal globulins are susceptible to repeated bacterial infections, although they do not show increased susceptibility to viral disease. Persons with diabetes mellitus are particularly susceptible to infection; as an example, tuberculosis strikes diabetics four times as often as it does normals. Diabetics are likewise more susceptible to the fungus disease phycomycosis, pyelonephritis due to gram-negative bacteria, and certain skin infections. Perhaps the high levels of glucose in the urine and blood may predispose diabetics to infection, or it may be that the acidosis that develops in poorly controlled diabetes is responsible. There is certainly a delay in the migration of defensive cells to sites of infection in acidosis.

A secondary disease, or an intercurrent (superimposed) infection, often kills a patient with a serious primary disorder, such as rheumatoid arthritis. Why are these secondary infections so deadly? In emphysema and bronchiectasis, for example, the cause may be bronchial obstruction and inadequate drainage, while in chronic lymphatic leukemia and Hodgkin's disease, decreased antibody production may be responsible for increased frequency of infection. Viral influenza may be followed by bacterial pneumonia.

Increased Susceptibility Due to Radiation

Ionizing radiation is known to increase susceptibility to infection. Persons exposed to effects of the atom bombs dropped on Hiroshima and Nagasaki developed infections 2 to 3 days after exposure. These may have resulted because of damage to cells, particularly lymphocytes, which are essential to host defense and among the most radiosensitive of cells. Extensive cell necrosis, edema, hemorrhage, and sloughing appear to remove barriers to microbial invasion and spread. Destruction of plasma cells impairs antibody synthesis.

Drug Effects

Many extrinsic factors predispose man to infection. Although therapy with corticosteroids such as cortisone has been effective in arthritis and allergies, it has many undesirable consequences, including suppression of the normal inflammatory response to infection and injury, and impairment of antibody formation. In this way corticosteroids may cause a reactivation of tuberculosis, a fatal outcome in chickenpox (usually a mild disease), and an increase in the frequency of such illnesses as pneumococcal pneumonia and septicemia. In fact, these steroids affect unfavorably almost every weapon for host defense.

A second group of drugs, including 6-mercaptopurine, dactinomycin, and azathioprine, have been employed to suppress host rejection of organ transplants, with similar unfavorable results. Death from infection occurred in as many as a third of such patients in some series.

FACTORS TENDING TO COMBAT INFECTIOUS DISEASE

Skin Protection

Many organisms, including various species of the Staphylococcus, continuously reside on the skin, representative of the horde of microbes ever present in the air. Such factors as drying, loss of surface skin cells, and acid pH have a bearing on the development of skin bacteria. Indeed, natural mechanisms may be more effective than energetic washing. A few years ago some hospitals tried the approach of not washing newborns for the first few days. It appeared that these unwashed babies had a greater resistance to infection than babies bathed according to usual practice. Although the newer approach was not widely followed, results suggested that the skin of the normal newborn does secrete protective substances.

THE NORMAL INDIVIDUAL POSSESSES MANY INTRINSIC DEFENDERS

Respiratory Defenses

A large number of microorganisms have contact with the respiratory tract. Most of those striking the mucosal surface are entrapped by mucin, which is secreted in the amount of 1 liter a day by the glands of the upper respiratory tract, and which possesses both antiviral and antibacterial activity. Then phagocytes remove most bacteria that finally reach the terminal bronchioles of the lung, alveolar ducts, and alveoli. Contained in the nasal secretions are antibodies to many viruses.

Digestive Defenses

Mucin and ciliary action aid in the defense against infection in the upper digestive tract. Saliva kills some bacteria, as does gastric juice. Bile, being alkaline, neutralizes the antibacterial action of stomach acids, thus aiding bacterial growth, and by the time food and intestinal secretions have reached the lower small intestine and colon, the bacterial population has increased a millionfold. This population of essentially normal bowel bacteria may well prevent invasion of deep tissues by potential pathogens by depriving them of nutrients or by exerting an antibiotic effect.

Flushing

Both the flow of urine and urine acidity help prevent infection of the urethra. Included among the other protectors of the genitourinary tract are a mucoprotein capable of inhibiting certain viruses, minute amounts of antibody, gamma globulin, and other antibacterial and anti-mycobacterial substances.

Normal Flora That Assist in Defense

The vagina is enabled to resist the effects of pathogens by means of microorganisms that are normally present. Thus, estrogen secreted by the ovaries favors deposit of glycogen, which supports growth of lactic acid-producing bacteria, and lactic acid in turn depresses growth of certain vaginal pathogens.

Systemic Defenses

Among the body's systemic defenses are antibodies, which circulate even in the newborn infant's blood (see Chap. 3). Antibodies are proteins so modified by the presence of an antigen that they react specifically with the antigen. Antigens are proteins or polysaccharides (complex carbohydrates), usually fragments of cells of plants, animals, or microbes or derived from such fragments. Antibodies aid in preventing disease or assist in recovery by attacking the microorganisms, which they either destroy or dissolve. They promote phagocytosis, destroy microbial debris, and neutralize toxins. Various techniques are available by which antibodies can be demonstrated in the laboratory, including agglutination or precipitation of the products of microorganisms, neutralization of toxins, and induction of anaphylactic reactions in sensitized animals. Because of their specificity, antigen-antibody reactions are useful in diagnosis of disease, by identifying bacteria isolated from the patient or detecting antibodies in the patient's serum.

Antibodies against the Pneumococcus promote swelling of the pneumococcal capsule. Antibodies against the Asiatic cholera organism destroy the microbe. Other antibodies inactivate toxins. Opsonins, also present in the blood, are antibodies that render bacteria more attractive to the phagocytic leukocytes by uniting directly with the bacteria, thus changing their external electrical charge. A simple analogy might be useful. Examine a drop of milk under the microscope. You will notice that the tiny fat globules remain discrete or separate. Normally, fat globules coalesce. Why do they not do so in milk? The reason is that they are coated with protein bearing an electrical charge that repels the other protein-coated fat globules. If the protein membrane is removed, the fat globules coalesce. In viral infections, an additional protective material, the protein interferon, is freed from infected cells to protect them and cells not yet infected (see Chap. 3).

Other blood substances possess antimicrobic activity. These include complement, a heat-labile component of normal serum; certain lipid fractions that neutralize viruses; a heat-stable substance, leukin, released by leukocytes and bactericidal for a few species of bacteria. Properdin, a globulin which does not require antigen, exerts antibacterial activity when magnesium and complement are present.

Polymorphonuclear leukocytes serve well in preventing infection, indeed, these active, phagocytic, mobile cells may spell the difference between life and death. Other cells found in the reticuloendothelial organs, such as the liver and spleen, destroy circulating microorganisms.

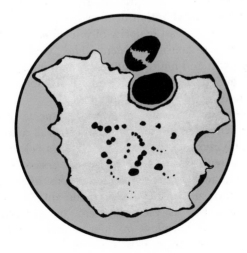

A neutrophilic leukocyte engulfing two bacteria. First, the leukocyte approaches the bacterium. When it comes in contact, the great arms, or pseudopods (false feet) project from the cytoplasm of the leukocyte, surround the bacterium, and engulf it. Within the leukocyte, the bacterium is digested and rendered harmless.

General Measures

The patient's medical attendants can do much to aid in the defense against infection. Nonspecific therapeutic measures include rest, diet, replacement of water and electrolytes, sedation, and treatment of symptoms. The appropriate vaccine (e.g., tetanus, poliomyelitis, pertussis, diphtheria, measles, rabies) may be employed (see p. 30). These provide active protection since the body is stimulated to develop its own antibodies.

Passive Protection

Antiserums, which are produced in animals by giving them vaccines, help modify or even prevent disease. The antitoxins against diphtheria and botulism were eminently successful. Hyperimmune gamma globulin given immediately after exposure prevents infection or lessens its severity in various diseases; but such protection is passive since the patient plays no role himself in combating the illness. The immunity lasts no longer than a month.

Therapeutic Agents

The introduction of chemotherapeutic agents, including antibiotics, during the thirties greatly changed the picture of infectious disease. As a result, many infections that formerly had high morbidity and mortality rates now cause little trouble. These agents reduce the severity of symptoms, the duration of illness, the frequency of sequelae, and the fatality rate in the vast majority of infections. A chemotherapeutic agent that kills the organism is *bactericidal*, while one that merely suppresses the growth and multiplication of the microbe is *bacteriostatic*. Because of their activity against a wide range of bacteria, many of these agents are known as *broad-spectrum antibiotics*.

There are both beneficial and unfavorable aspects of chemotherapy. For example: penicillin acts on the bacterial cell wall when the bacterium is multiplying; polymyxin acts on the bacterium's cell membrane; tetracycline interferes with its protein synthesis; griseofulvin inhibits the organism's nucleic acid synthesis; sulfonamides affect the organism's intermediary metabolism. In such fashion, the antibiotics act to destroy the microorganisms. But as the pathogenic microorganisms are suppressed, other bacteria—harmless in their normal habitat—are allowed to proliferate and thus cause new illnesses (see p. 60). Hence the success of chemotherapy still depends on intact host defenses; treatment may fail when resistance is depressed. A further consideration is that the use of chemotherapeutic agents is often accompanied by side effects, some due to individual sensitivity.

HOST RESPONSE TO INFECTION

In many infections, host response is entirely absent. Perhaps 80 per cent of the population of the western United States has been infected by the fungus *Histoplasma capsulatum*, but few people sickened. Mumps virus may cause illness in only some members of a family, the others being infected (as shown by persisting immunity or a rise in antibody titer) but not developing signs of illness.

On the other hand, inflammation can occur without infection. Inflammation has been defined as a reaction to damage in which there are multiple microscopic, functional, chemical, and clinically apparent changes. The traditional signs of inflammation include calor, or fever; dolor, or pain; rubor, or redness; tumor, or swelling; and loss of function.

HOST
RESPONSE
USUALLY
GENERALIZED

Temperature Regulation

The elevated temperature that frequently accompanies infection may be a defensive mechanism. Normal body temperature is usually cited as 37° C., or 98.6° F.; no doubt there is a normal range, perhaps from 97° F. to 100.4° F. Fever results from increased production of heat with decreased loss, or from decreased loss with normal production of

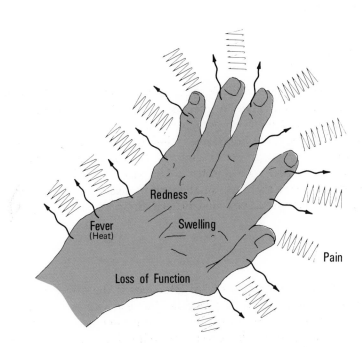

Redness

Swelling

Fever
(Heat)

Pain

Loss of Function

SIGNS OF INFLAMMATION

heat. The patient with fever feels that his body is warm and may notice that his face is flushed.

A chill frequently precedes fever. The patient feels cold and puts on additional coverings or clothes. He begins to shake. He may sit huddled in a chair or lie in bed with his knees drawn up to his chest. His teeth chatter and his face muscles twitch, so that he may have difficulty in speaking. His skin pales, or may even become blue, and looks like "goose flesh." The duration of the chill may range from 10 to 60 minutes.

Sweating often accompanies fever. Although generalized, it is most profuse in the axillary and genital areas. Interestingly enough, the palms and soles do not sweat during fever, but the skin and hair become wet. As the patient becomes warm, he may throw off his bedclothes. He may become intensely thirsty, yet when he drinks water he loses sodium, and may have fatigue, nausea, weakness, and muscle cramps.

Loss of Appetite

Infection constitutes a threat to the well-being, perhaps the life, of the host. It would be expected that an infectious process would, therefore, be challenged by mobilization of all body defenses, including activation of the sympathetic nervous system. One of the effects of such activation is decreased gastrointestinal activity. Thus loss of appetite may represent a defensive action on the part of the body. It certainly is a common symptom.

Skin Reactions

A few examples will illustrate how accurately the skin reflects generalized infection. Jaundice occurs in infectious hepatitis, Weil's disease, malaria, yellow fever, pneumococcal pneumonia, typhoid fever, and other disorders. Some infections, including scarlet fever and measles, cause dilatation of the blood vessels of the skin. In typhoid fever, meningococcemia, and endocarditis, skin lesions may be produced as multiplication of bacteria blocks small blood vessels. Vesicular skin lesions occur in chickenpox, smallpox, and rickettsialpox.

Malaise

Almost invariable in severe infections is the symptom malaise, which means feeling bad, feeling terrible, just not with it, not up to par, and so on. On some occasions, however, a person can feel well even though he is dangerously ill. A sense of well-being may be part of the disease, as in advanced tuberculosis, in which the patient shows *spes phthisica*, or the feeling of hope and cheerfulness about recovery. Malaise cannot be measured quantitatively. The mechanisms producing it are not understood, and it is not known whether malaise definitely helps combat infection.

General Symptoms

Most patients respond to infection with loss of interest and lack of enthusiasm toward their usual relationships and activities, and generalized weakness. They may become fatigued readily so that they cannot carry on their usual work, and they may take to bed. Contributing to such symptoms may be high fever, drenching sweat, sodium deficit, potassium deficit, water deficit, or deficit of extracellular fluid. These reactions may represent protective actions on the part of the body to limit inflammation and prevent further harm to body tissues, although in infectious mononucleosis and brucellosis the weariness and fatigue seem to be unduly severe.

DISEASE MODEL: LOBAR PNEUMONIA

As the model disease for the infectious disease group, we might do well to choose pneumococcal pneumonia, caused by the pneumococci. Since the infection usually involves one or more lobes, it is designated lobar pneumonia.

Development of Clinical Disease

Pneumococci reach the lungs through the respiratory tract and finally lodge in the alveoli, where they multiply. The products of their metabolism set up inflammation, first shown by outpouring of protein-rich edema fluid into the alveolar spaces. The fluid then serves as a culture medium for the pneumococci and also as a transport vehicle from one alveolus to another, from lobule to lobule, and from lobe to lobe.

The first 12 to 16 hours of pneumonia has been called the *stage of red hepatization* because the consolidated lung appears red and livery. This red color is caused by widespread dilatation of pulmonary blood vessels, which is characteristic of early pneumonia. A few hours after the initial dilatation of the lung capillaries and of the outpouring of edema fluid into the alveoli, polymorphonuclear leukocytes enter the alveolar spaces. They rapidly become so numerous that they form most of the bulk of the consolidated lung, although they are scarce in the zone of edema fluid where the pneumonic lesion is progressing. Some of these leukocytes are

PHAGOCYTOSIS ESSENTIAL TO RESOLUTION OF THE PNEUMONIC PROCESS actively phagocytic, taking up pneumococci by surface phagocytosis, which does not require the help of opsonins. Surface phagocytosis occurs when the leukocytes trap the bacteria against the wall of an alveolus or against another leukocyte. The more leukocytes in the alveolar space, the more active the surface phagocytosis. In tissue sections, pneumococci are scanty, but in the solid portion of the lung, they are plentiful in the advancing margin of the lesion, where edema fluid is more abundant and leukocytes are fewer.

At the time of spontaneous recovery, the *macrophage reaction* takes place, i.e., large mononuclear cells enter the alveoli, engulf any pneumococci still present, and phagocytize the polymorphonuclear leukocytes. This process continues until resolution is complete, when the lungs become clear to x-ray and physical examination.

The disease is frequently preceded by an upper respiratory infection. The symptoms and signs usually appear suddenly. There is usually a shaking chill, sharp pain in the involved chest, and cough, with the early production of a pinkish sputum that later becomes rusty. Fever and headache occur. Commonly, all these symptoms appear, although one or more may be absent. If rusty sputum is present, this virtually makes the diagnosis. There is shortness of breath, with the respiration at a rate of 25 to 45 per minute, and breathing is often painful because of the pleuritic involvement. There is a peculiar expiratory grunt. Delirium is common, especially in alcoholic patients. In children, onset of the disease may be announced by a convulsion. The patient sweats profusely and he may be cyanotic. His temperature rises rapidly to 101° F. to 105° F. The pulse speeds up to 100 to 130. Soon fine rales are audible over the involved area. Breath sounds are suppressed. A little later, consolidation of part of a lobe or of several lobes takes place. A pleural friction rub is often heard in the early stages. At this time there is a dry, hacking cough, except when bronchitis has preceded the pneumonia, in which case cough is productive of purulent sputum. The paroxysms of coughing may be extremely painful, but in the later stages, cough is more productive and usually painless. As the disease progresses, the sputum changes from pinkish to blood-flecked to rusty at the height of the illness, and finally to yellow and purulent when the disease resolves. Gastrointestinal symptoms are often noted, including abdominal swelling, jaundice, and diarrhea. Nausea and vomiting sometimes usher in the disease.

In right-sided pneumonias that involve the middle and lower lobes, right upper quadrant tenderness and rigidity may suggest the diagnosis of gallbladder disease, appendicitis, or peritonitis. Herpes, usually of the face and lips, is often present.

One should suspect pneumococcal pneumonia in any patient who has had an acute illness with fever associated with chill, pain in the chest, and cough, especially if he has been expectorating a thick, rusty sputum. Upon physical examination, one finds rapid heart rate, rapid breathing, cyanosis, and signs of solidification of part of the lung, confirming the

UPPER
RESPIRATORY
INFECTION
PREDISPOSES
TO PNEUMONIA

diagnosis. X-ray examination provides further confirmation or may show consolidation before physical examination does. Usually, but not always, the white blood count is elevated. Sputum smears and cultures reveal the pneumococcus, as do blood cultures in bacteremic patients.

Prognosis

Ninety-five per cent of patients with lobar pneumonia who receive adequate treatment now survive, although before the advent of modern forms of therapy the death rate was often 30 per cent or more. Patients treated during the first 3 days of illness are more likely to recover than those treated later. The outlook is usually better for those under age 50. The following factors make the outlook less favorable and convalescence more prolonged: a positive blood culture; involvement of two or more lobes; white blood count over 5,000; blood urea nitrogen over 70 mg. per 100 ml.; and the presence of any chronic disease, meningitis, or endocarditis.

Treatment

Supportive measures should be instituted at once. These include complete bed rest, administration of fluids, and administration of oxygen and analgesics when they are needed. Sputum and blood are collected for culture. Specific therapy should be started as soon as possible, the therapeutic agent being chosen on the basis of the history, results of the physical examination, and the gram-stain of the sputum. After blood and sputum have been cultured, antibacterial therapy can be changed if need be. When pneumococcal pneumonia is suspected, penicillin may be the antibiotic of choice, although the tetracyclines or erythromycin might in some instances serve well. If antibiotics are unavailable, sulfonamides can be used. Finally, antimicrobial therapy should continue until the patient has been afebrile for 48 hours.

CLINICAL CONSIDERATIONS

Observation and Diagnosis

Close observation can prove life-saving for the patient with an acute fulminating infection; it is only slightly less important to the patient with infection of moderate intensity. One should pay close attention to the vital signs, especially their changes from hour to hour and day to day. The "whole" patient should be kept in focus—his color, his energy, his demeanor, his attitude. Naturally, such events as vomiting, diarrhea, excessive sweating, chills, and convulsions demand prompt action.

TOTAL
PATIENT
CARE
NECESSARY
FOR
OPTIMAL
RECOVERY

Support

The patient should receive—and eat—a proper diet. What he eats, not what he is served, should be recorded. Some patients with infectious disease will require special supplements: more protein for the patient who does not eat his meat, eggs, cheese, fish, and dairy products in proper quantities; a vitamin B complex supplement, perhaps one of magnesium, for the alcoholic; supplemental vitamin C for the patient with an aversion to vegetables and greens. The body fluids should be maintained in a balanced state; to accomplish this, one looks for signs of imbalances of the body fluids and sees that accurate and complete intake-output records are maintained. Early imbalances are reported so prompt action can be taken.

Conservation of the patient's energy rates a high priority, particularly in severe infection. The patient should never be disturbed unnecessarily, even when hospital routine appears to demand it. He is permitted all possible sleep; he is not forced to sit in a wheelchair for a long period while awaiting an x-ray examination, for example.

The sicker the patient, the more he needs psychological support. One can help the patient see the bright side by chatting with him and buoying his flagging spirits. Especially is this essential in such stressful conditions as an infected burn. An optimistic outlook gives the patient the will to live and speeds recovery. Should the patient be isolated for bacteriologic reasons, the situation should be explained to him. At the same time, he should not be allowed to feel isolated from friendly, interested attention.

Symptomatic Therapy

Although treatment directed toward symptoms may be looked upon as secondary in importance to primary therapy, it may be decisive. Fever probably helps counteract infection; nevertheless, it should be reduced, if possible, when it reaches 104° F. Relief of headache or other pain, measures to help the patient sleep, and provision of a needed decongestant all help speed clinical progress.

Primary Treatment Modalities

The optimal primary or specific therapy can be chosen only on the basis of thorough understanding of antibacterial therapy, so that optimal dosage is employed. For example, when one is aware that penicillin kills only dividing microbes, he will see that the medication is given at the exact time and intervals specified. This permits the penicillin blood level to fluctuate and allows the bacteria to divide so they can be more readily killed. The informed person knows that such anti-biotics as the tetracyclines are bacteriostatic. The blood level of such drugs should be maintained at a constant concentration so as to keep the organisms from multiplying.

Familiarity with the occasional but real hazard of "allergy" to the peni-cillins and related antibiotics is essential, as is knowledge of the toxic effects of such agents as chloramphenicol. Only if one has such knowl-edge is it possible to recognize an untoward reaction early and to in-stitute indicated treatment.

TOPICS FOR DISCUSSION

1. How can one account for an infection occurring without disease?
2. Contrast the infectious diseases of the Middle Ages with those of today. Contrast the relative impact on the people of both periods.
3. Contrast the infectious diseases of a century ago with those of today.
4. Were health scientists more concerned with infectious disease a century ago than they are today?
5. What are some of the special problems in relation to infectious dis-ease posed by our modern civilization? In answering this question, con-sider such matters as jet airplane travel, the highly sophisticated diag-nostic facilities available, and the plethora of antibiotics.
6. Discuss superinfection as a problem in the modern day management of infectious disease.
7. Prior to 1900, which segment of our population (children, adults, or elderly) were most victimized by infectious disease?
8. What symptoms and findings of infectious disease can be regarded as aiding the host?
9. Consider the divergent roles of microorganisms found in man's normal environment.

BIBLIOGRAPHY

Books

Haggard, H.: Devils, Drugs, and Doctors. New York, Harper & Bros., 1929.
Caulfield, E.: The Throat Distemper. New Haven, Connecticut, Pub-lished for the Beaumont Medical Club by the Yale Journal of Biology and Medicine, 1939.
Selye, H.: The Stress of Life. New York, McGraw-Hill Book Co., 1956.
Schmidt, J.: Medical Discoveries. Springfield, Ill., Charles C Thomas, 1959.

Stewart, G.: The Penicillin Group of Drugs. New York, Elsevier Publishing Company, 1965.

Carpenter, P.: Microbiology. pp. 385–435. Philadelphia, W. B. Saunders Co., 1967.

Roueche, B.: Annals of Epidemiology. London, J. & A. Churchill, Ltd., 1967.

Garrod, L., and O'Grady, F.: Antibiotic and Chemotherapy. Baltimore, The Williams & Wilkins Co., 1968.

Utz, J.: Role of the Invading Organism and Other Topics. pp. 193–213. In Sodeman, W., and Sodeman, W.: Pathologic Physiology. Philadelphia, W. B. Saunders Co., 1968.

Boyd, W.: A Textbook of Pathology. pp. 309–439. Philadelphia, Lea & Febiger, 1970.

Articles

Neva, F., et al.: Malaria: host-defense mechanisms and complications. Annals of Internal Medicine, 73:295, 1970.

5

diseases due to physical agents

It is almost self-evident that population control, environmental quality, resource conservation, and the quality of life are all facets of a single central problem which has become a central concern of governments. This may well be "the hinge of history" when man's long-term future may be decided.

Rather than condemnation of the past, be grateful that the environmental movement is now sufficiently strong to provide opportunity to rectify our errors and chart a new course for the future while there is time. And there is yet time.
—Philip Handler *

Since man appeared on the planet Earth, physical agents have taken their place along with infection as causes of disability and death. They have appeared in countless forms: a club, an arrow, a high-velocity bullet, an auto collision—to mention but a few. Nor should we neglect natural disasters, such as earthquakes, floods, hurricanes, tornados, avalanches, and forest fires. We have chosen representative examples of disorders caused by physical agents from an almost endless list. We shall see that while injuries due to physical agents have much in common, certain agents exert specific effects.

TRAUMA

BOTH LOCAL AND SYSTEMIC EFFECTS PRODUCED BY TRAUMA

Trauma is the leading cause of death in persons between the ages of 1 and 37 years, and in all age groups it ranks fourth as the cause of death and first as the cause of disability. Trauma—that is, mechanical injury, or wound—occurs when a physical agent acts on the body so as to damage tissues. Trauma can injure any tissue and thus affect any body function; the initial damage can set in motion a chain reaction leading to additional problems. We shall use the classification of Fallis in our discussion: †

---

* Handler, Philip: Can Man Shape His Future? Perspectives in Biology and Medicine, Winter, 1971. The University of Chicago Press. © 1971 by the University of Chicago. All rights reserved.
† Fallis, B.: Textbook of Pathology. New York, McGraw-Hill, 1964.

1. Abrasion: denuding of the outer skin layer by friction. There is slight bleeding.
2. Contusion: also called a *bruise*. Blood is released within a tissue or organ but there is no surface bleeding. The finer blood vessels, particularly the capillaries, are disrupted by blunt force.
3. Laceration: a tear occurring when an external crushing, stretching force rips tissues apart.
4. Incised wound: a cut produced by an instrument with a sharp edge. The wound margins are smooth and tissue destruction is minimal.
5. Puncture wound: also called a *penetrating* wound. It is caused by a slender, pointed object such as a glass sliver, a pointed knife, or a hatpin.
6. Fracture: a break in a bone. A simple fracture occurs when the broken bone ends do not penetrate the skin; a compound fracture involves penetration of the skin by the broken bone ends; a comminuted fracture causes shattering of bone; and a pathologic fracture is one occurring in an area of bone already diseased, as by a tumor.

TYPES OF TISSUE INJURY

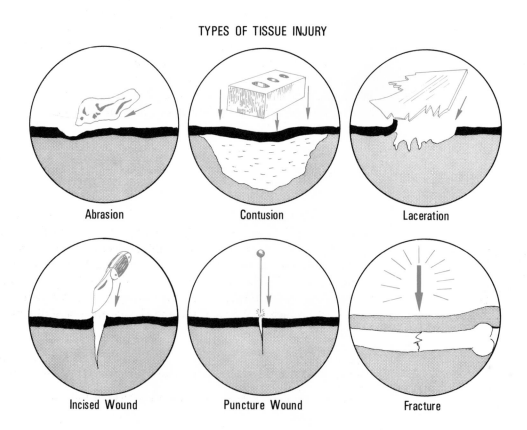

Abrasion   Contusion   Laceration

Incised Wound   Puncture Wound   Fracture

Trauma can produce pain; bleeding; loss of function; embolism consisting of blood clot, fat particles, or air; and infection. Inflammation, caused by the freeing of histamine by the injured tissues, usually accompanies severe tissue injury. Visceral organs, including the spleen, the liver, and the intestine, may be ruptured. Severe internal injuries can occur without bruising of the skin; e.g., the spleen may be ruptured in an auto accident. The injury may cause inflammatory and gangrenous changes in the fat cells of the subcutaneous tissues.

Shock

An effect of trauma that may of itself cause death is shock. As William Boyd has pointed out, the victim of shock lies quietly, oblivious of his environment. His face is ashen. Sweat drips from his eyebrows. His deep-sunk, weary eyes are lackluster. His cheeks are hollow, his brow is creased and his skin is cold. The vital processes reflect the patient's desperate condition: the temperature is below normal; the pulse is feeble, thready, and irregular; breathing is shallow; the blood pressure is low or unobtainable. Tubular damage in the kidney may cause the organ to fail (shock kidney). Naturally, every effort is made to prevent shock from reaching the extreme stage.

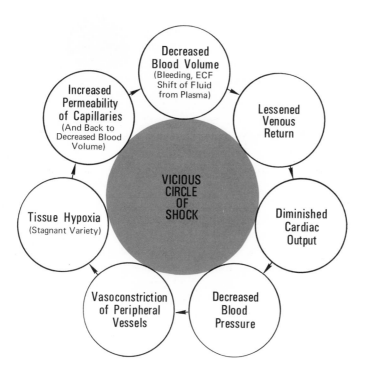

SHOCK SYNDROME
DUE TO MULTIPLE
CAUSES

Shock is a state of collapse of the circulation, often associated with inadequate return of blood to the heart. The blood vessels are depleted of blood. Shock may result from trauma, and it may also follow surgery, massive bleeding, body fluid disturbances, bleeding into the heart muscle, severe infections, poisoning, and drug reactions.

When shock results from deficient blood volume, as from blood loss, return of blood to the heart slackens. This type is *hypovolemic* shock. Heart output decreases and arterial blood pressure falls; the bodily response to this is constriction of blood vessels and an increase in the heart rate. The output of hormones, including aldosterone, antidiuretic (water conserving) hormone, and epinephrine, is increased. These defenses suffice until about 20 per cent of the blood volume has been lost.

In some cases, shock results from laking or pooling of blood in the dilated blood vessels. This is *normovolemic* shock. Sometimes this laking is the initial response to trauma; then it is called *primary shock*. Unlike the situation in shock due to decreased blood volume, the heart slows rather than accelerating—*bradycardia* occurs. This, along with the dilatation of blood vessels, causes a sharp reduction in cerebral blood flow. Fainting characterizes this type of shock. (Placing the patient in the horizontal position usually brings prompt relief, in contrast to the major measures often required for management of shock due to decreased blood volume.)

Systemic Effects

Consider what happens following extensive surgery or a compound fracture of the humerus. First, there are significant changes in body metabolism, most of which appear to hinder rather than help recovery. These include the following:

1. Loss of protein (usually measured as nitrogen excretion) from the skeletal muscles. Serious protein depletion can result. The cause of the phenomenon is not known; it has been called the *toxic destruction of protein*.
2. Transfer of substances needed for protein synthesis from other parts of the body to the wound area. New tissue grows in the wound site while tissue destruction goes on elsewhere in the body.
3. Under the stimulus of epinephrine and norepinephrine, the liver frees carbohydrate. These hormones of the adrenal medulla are secreted in greater than normal quantities in response to the individual's fear and apprehension resulting from the shock state.
4. Sodium retention as a result of greater renal tubular reabsorption stimulated by increased production of the adrenocortical hormone, aldosterone.
5. Pronounced retention of water resulting from the action of antidiuretic hormone on the renal tubules.

A number of hormones carry the message of injury to the tissues and organs of the body: adrenocortical hormones, including cortisone-like hormones and aldosterone; the adrenal medullary hormones epinephrine and norepinephrine; and antidiuretic hormone.

ELECTRICITY

An electrical current surging through the body may cause burns or death. The charge enters the body at one point and leaves it at another, and both locations usually appear to be burned. Sometimes tissues at the point of exit are torn. Often the point of exit is on the victim's feet, because the charge travels toward the ground. An electrical burn often *appears* to be mild. At first it is dry and bloodless; within 36 hours, however, the burn assumes a rosy color, swelling develops, tissues disintegrate, and an ulcer forms. Such a burn may require two or three times as long to heal as would a nonelectrical burn of similar magnitude.

An electrical burn produces the same general effects as does any severe burn. Rapid death from electrical shock is probably due to respiratory failure: sometimes the unconscious apneic shocked patient can be resuscitated by prolonged artificial respiration. An electric current may severely injure the nerve cells. Blood vessels, which are excellent electrical conductors, may also undergo serious damage.

Lightning has the same general effects as other forms of electric shock. A characteristic feature is the *current markings*, or *lightning figures*—tree-like red lines on the skin, which are probably produced by the splitting up of the current within the body.

IONIZING RADIATION

Of all physical agents, perhaps ionizing radiation causes the most damage in that it injures not only organs and cells, but the very molecules and atoms of protoplasm. Exposure to radiation causes a change, either a loss or a gain, in electrons, the negatively charged electric particles that are a part of the atoms that go to make up the human body. The free electron may become attached to some other atom, which then loses its electrical neutrality and becomes charged, or ionized. This loss or gain in electrons can cause alterations in the behavior of the affected molecules. Obviously, such alterations—affecting as they do the very stuff of which we are made—can have dire consequences. The tissue changes and the clinical symptoms and signs vary with the dose of radiation and the time after exposure. In addition to the effects observable within days, there may be later effects of a very serious nature, including malignant neoplastic change, which may not be manifest until years later.

ELECTRON CHANGES THE BASIS OF RADIATION DAMAGE

Tissues vary in their sensitivity to radiation. The following grouping grades tissue sensitivity from least to most sensitive: muscle and connective tissue, bone cells, nerve cells, lining cells of pleura and peritoneum, kidney epithelial cells, epithelium of the lung alveoli and biliary passages, liver cells, epidermis, epithelium of the intestine, proliferating cells of the bone marrow, gonads, lymphoid cells.

TISSUE
DEGENERATION
IS PRINCIPAL
EFFECT OF
IONIZING
RADIATION

Formerly, sources of radiation harmful to man were limited to high energy x-rays employed in diagnosis and therapy, and radium and related radioactive materials. Today the source list has grown to include nuclear reactors, cyclotrons, linear accelerators, and similar types of equipment, as well as cobalt and cesium bombs. Radiation exposure in industry represents a real hazard as a cause of injury and death. The development of power reactors increases the potential for accidents. Nuclear weapons testing and the nuclear power industry have increased the radioactivity normally present in the earth and the atmosphere.

Acute radiation sickness may follow therapeutic radiation, particularly of the abdomen, with symptoms of nausea, vomiting, diarrhea, anorexia, headache, malaise, and tachycardia. These symptoms subside within a few hours. There are also delayed effects of radiation. Prolonged or repeated exposures at low dose rates can produce cessation of menstruation, decrease in fertility in both sexes, decrease in libido in the female, anemia, leukopenia, thrombopenia, and cataracts. More severe exposure causes numerous effects: loss of hair, atrophy and ulceration of skin, keratosis, and possibly skin carcinoma. If radium has been employed, osteosarcoma may develop. Organs that may be damaged by still greater doses are the kidneys, muscles, and lungs. Chronic ulceration, fibrosis, and perforation of segments of the intestine have been reported.

Both somatic (body) and germ cells may be affected by exposure to radiation: if body cells, cancer, cataracts, degenerative disorders, or premature aging may ensue; if germ cells, the number of mutations increases, and those perpetuated by matings of affected individuals will result in an increasing number of persons with inherited disease.

Avoidance of overexposure is the only sure preventive of radiation injury. Once injury has been incurred, treatment is complex and generally unsatisfactory.

COLD

Extreme cold causes frostbite on exposed body parts, particularly when there is accompanying high wind, which causes rapid heat loss. In mild frostbite, the body part is first white and bloodless, then becomes red, swollen, and painful while thawing. Necrosis of the outer skin layer may occur. In severe frostbite, gangrene of the entire part may develop. Should the cold be severe enough to crystallize the fluid of the cells, the ice crystals would tear the cells apart. Gangrene results from loss of circulation due to extreme contraction of the blood vessels and damage to the capillaries.

In exposure to severe cold, blood is driven from the surface into the interior of the body. The temperature of the body falls, metabolism slows, and finally the victim succumbs to an irresistible desire to sleep. When body temperature reaches 70° F., the heart stops beating. (The dreadful effects of cold are described in the fascinating documentary, *Abandoned*, by A. L. Todd, listed among the references.)

LIGHT

Light waves consist of a very small band of *electromagnetic radiation*—that is, energy waves ranging from very long wave lengths, such as radio waves, to those of very short length, such as the cosmic rays. Like other forms of energy, light waves can cause injury. The shorter the wave length, the less the penetrating power. The energy of the short waves is dissipated in the skin, causing irritation. Waves shorter than the short wave end of the visible spectrum—the ultraviolet rays—cause the most irritation. Those beyond the long wave end—the infrared rays—penetrate most deeply and irritate least.

Ultraviolet light produces sunburn. Sunburn occurs independently of heat production, for climbers on high snowy peaks may be badly sunburned, and indeed, severe burns can occur at high altitudes in thick mist because of the high concentration of ultraviolet rays and the absence of protective atmosphere. Blondes burn more readily than do brunettes.

Sunburn represents a first-degree burn in most instances. The blood vessels of the burned area are congested; there is swelling, and white blood cells may migrate to the area. Blisters may appear. Pronounced peeling takes place as the burned area undergoes healing.

Persons such as farmers or sailors exposed for long periods to bright sunshine often develop thickened patches, or *keratoses*, on the skin of the face and back of the hands. Skin carcinoma may develop in these keratoses.

Certain individuals may manifest hypersensitivity to light, as in the metabolic disease, congenital porphyria. In such persons, sensitization to light follows experimental injection of hematoporphyrin. Animals so injected may be burned by light from which ultraviolet rays have been excluded.

Ultraviolet rays exert a photochemical action on the lipids of the skin by activating skin cholesterol and converting it to vitamin D. The lack of this vitamin is one cause of rickets; thus sunlight or ultraviolet light from a mercury vapor lamp can be used in treatment and is as effective as cod liver oil.

ALTERATIONS IN ATMOSPHERIC PRESSURE

A sudden increase in environmental pressure can cause caisson disease, also known as *diver's palsy* and *decompression sickness*. A caisson is a watertight cylinder containing air under high pressure that is used for sinking bridge piers. Caisson workers, workers in tunnels under rivers, and divers are subjected to high air pressures, and should they be returned to normal atmospheric pressures too rapidly, they would develop headache, dizziness, shortness of breath, general body pains (the "bends"), and sometimes paralysis. Under these high pressures, a large amount of air is dissolved in the blood plasma. The oxygen is absorbed, but the nitrogen may form bubbles of air emboli in the small arteries to the brain. Tissue destruction results, and there may be temporary or permanent paralysis. This problem does not occur if proper precautions are taken to reduce the pressure gradually.

Decreased pressure, as may be experienced when one travels in an unpressurized plane flying at extremely high altitudes, causes expansion of gases in body cavities such as the intestine, with results similar to those described above.

HEAT

Several systemic disorders may result from exposure to high environmental heat, of which by far the most serious is heat stroke, or paralysis of the heat-regulating mechanism. The temperature required to cause heat stroke varies with the humidity and the individual. When the air is completely saturated with water vapor and the environmental temperature is above 90° F., body temperature rises and loss of body heat by radiation ceases since radiation causes heat to flow from higher to lower temperatures; then temperature control depends entirely on vaporization of sweat. Should the sweating mechanism fail, then body temperature soars and heat stroke ensues.

HEAT STROKE, HEAT EXHAUSTION, AND SUNSTROKE HAVE SAME CAUSATION

Body temperature may rise to as high as 117° F. in heat stroke. Rectal temperature may be much higher than oral or axillary temperature. Heat stroke resulting from direct sun exposure is termed *sunstroke*, but it is identical with heat stroke. Sometimes death occurs suddenly with the onset of heat stroke. Or, the patient may fall unconscious, as soldiers on forced marches in tropical countries have so often done. The skin is hot and dry; the patient appears unable to perspire.

The chief pathologic findings after death from heat stroke include hemorrhages in the skin and mucous membranes, congestion or hemorrhages in the brain, edema of the brain and lungs, enlargement of the spleen, and cloudy swelling of the liver, kidneys, and heart.

Heat exhaustion is a milder form of response to heat stress. The distinction between heat exhaustion and heat stroke may not always be

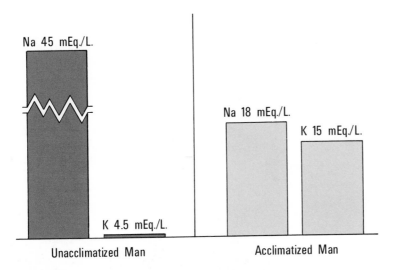

Na 45 mEq./L.

K 4.5 mEq./L.

Unacclimatized Man

Na 18 mEq./L.

K 15 mEq./L.

Acclimatized Man

The unacclimatized man loses in his sweat much sodium and little potassium. Under acclimatization, he produces increased amounts of aldosterone, which causes the sweat to contain little sodium and much potassium. Thus, persons exercising heavily in hot climates need to add potassium to their diets.

clear-cut. In heat exhaustion, the heat regulating mechanism is severely strained; in heat stroke, it is overwhelmed. The difference between heat exhaustion and heat stroke may therefore be merely one of degree.

Body potassium deficit may contribute to the development of illness due to heat stress. Gardner reported a striking correlation between potassium deficit and heat exhaustion during a prolonged heat wave in the Mississippi Valley in 1966. Many of the patients had been taking potassium-depleting diuretics. Toor and others found that during the torrid Israeli summer, when temperatures reach 117° F., healthy persons complained of weakness and lassitude. Toor found that subclinical potassium deficit had developed in many of these individuals, who previously had been in normal health. This finding appeared to be associated with kidney impairment in several such persons.

Curiously, potassium deficit appears to occur in some well-acclimatized persons exposed to prolonged heat. With acclimatization, sodium is conserved but potassium is lost, especially in the sweat. Increased production of the sodium-conserving, potassium-wasting aldosterone may be responsible. Clearly, potassium should not be omitted from mineral preparations designed to prevent heat stress disease.

DISEASE MODEL: SEVERE BURN

Burns are among the most frequent of all injuries caused by physical agents. Locally, a burn causes pain, which in some cases is great. The immediate threat to life in a newly burned patient, however, involves body fluids. Later, infection becomes an important threat to survival. Be-

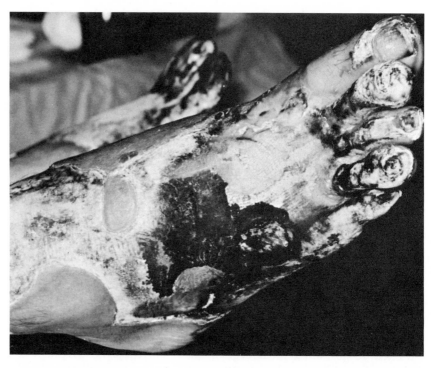

Burned foot, showing second- and third-degree burns. Portions burned to the second degree are light colored or white. Third-degree burn areas are blackened.

cause burns offer so many complex problems and because of their enormous present-day role as a cause of disability and death, we have chosen severe burn as our disease model for this chapter.

The depth of the burn affects both the volume and the composition of fluid lost from the circulation. In a first-degree burn, dilatation of blood vessels with slight reddening of skin is the significant change. A second-degree burn involves more severe damage with injury to deep tissues and formation of blisters containing fluid rich in protein. This fluid may accumulate beneath the surface of the burn before swelling appears. In a burn of the third degree, the entire thickness of skin is destroyed. Capillaries close to the surface of the wound are blocked with blood. No exchange of water and electrolytes takes place in the surface of a third-degree burn, while underneath the surface, great quantities of water and electrolytes accumulate.

Effects on the Body Fluids

Four major hazards mark the course of the severely burned patient during the first few days following the burn, all involving body fluids. They might be termed the Four Horsemen of Disaster:

INTERRUPTION TO NORMAL TISSUE CONTINUITY CAUSES DERANGEMENT OF ALL HOMEOSTATIC MECHANISMS

1. Losses of body fluids. Plasma, interstitial fluid, and blood (essentially a suspension of red cells in plasma) are lost following a burn. First, water and electrolytes shift from plasma to interstitial fluid in the region of the burn. Edema fluid appears; its volume may equal one-half the volume of extracellular fluid. Second, a protein-rich fluid is lost through leakage from the burned surface. The fluid consists of plasma and interstitial fluid in approximately equal quantities. Such losses occur chiefly in second-degree burns. A third source of fluid loss is leakage of blood from the capillaries and small blood vessels of the burned surface. Some is lost in dressing changes. Finally, the burned patient has fluid losses independent of the burn. Water lost as insensible (not perceptible to the senses) perspiration and urine equals about 1,500 ml. per square meter of body surface per day.
2. Shock. The danger of shock is present during the critical first 2 or 3 postburn days. It may be caused by pain, fear, or a decrease in plasma volume.
3. Renal depression. Kidney function is depressed in severe burns. The usual cause is decreased plasma volume and it is therefore temporary. Such renal depression must be distinguished from that due to organic damage. If the burn has injured the kidney to the point where its regulatory function is badly impaired, the patient's chances of survival are slim indeed.

ALL ELECTROLYTES
DEPLETED IN
SEVERE BURN

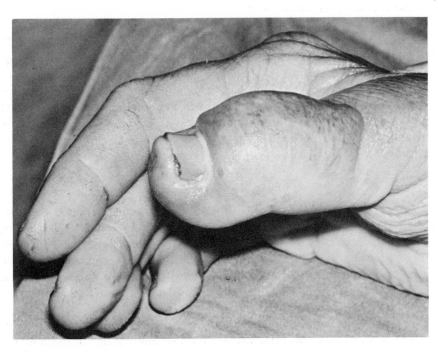

Deep burn, apparently of second degree, of right thumb and thenar eminence. Swelling caused by plasma-to-interstitial fluid shift.

4. Remobilization of edema fluid. This term refers to a shift of water and electrolytes from interstitial fluid to plasma. Remobilization begins on the third, fourth, or fifth day after burning. It is accompanied by diuresis and usually lasts 3 days or more. The volume of edema fluid in a burn may exceed the total normal plasma volume. As this fluid shifts back into the plasma, fatal acute pulmonary edema may ensue, because the heart and kidneys cannot handle the volume of water and electrolytes forced upon the vascular system. This dire event usually takes place only when the patient has been given excessive fluids during the first 2 or 3 postburn days.

Clinical Gauges of Fluid Deficits

Thirst is an early symptom following a burn. A patient permitted to drink unlimited amounts of water may develop a sodium deficit. Its clinical symptoms were perhaps mistaken for "early toxemia" in earlier years.

Vomiting may be a sign of circulatory collapse, acute gastric dilatation, or paralysis of the intestines. It is a common occurrence in severe burns.

Disturbances of the central nervous system include restlessness, disorientation, and maniacal behavior—signs of lack of oxygen in the brain and the need for more fluids.

Urinary output, measured hourly, is an excellent index of the patient's fluid state. A urinary flow of 30 to 50 ml. per hour is adequate for an adult.

Pulmonary edema may be caused by excessive fluid therapy, damage to the respiratory tract by the burn, remobilization of edema fluid, or invasive infection. The signs and symptoms of infection should be kept in mind in the treatment of burns, since these findings can be confused with those of fluid imbalances. In infection, the rectal temperature usually ranges from 104° F. to 107° F.

Metabolic Effects

The severely burned patient experiences an increased outpouring of protein, yet is restricted in food intake. Protein deficit is therefore likely to develop. Protein malnutrition has baleful effects, including impaired wound healing and decreased resistance to infection. Negative protein balance can become irreversible if permitted to last too long. Blocker, in a personal communication, has called this passing of the point of no return *burn decompensation.*

There is a marked increase in adrenal cortical activity, as is always seen in stress reactions—and a severe burn certainly is one of the supreme forms of stress. The protein metabolism is disturbed, as a result, and the increased catabolism contributes to the development of osteoporosis. Then too, the immobilization that is necessary in the treatment of severe burn contributes further to osteoporosis.

Excessive losses of calcium and phosphorus are universal in severely burned patients, yet replacement of the minerals in large amounts does not counteract the imbalances and may cause a dangerously high urinary content of calcium and phosphorus. Kidney stones can result.

During the first 2 or 3 postburn days, large amounts of potassium are excreted in the urine. Plasma potassium levels are normal, or even high, since potassium is leaving the cells; hence, potassium should not be given during the first 48 hours after the burn. Beginning about the fourth or fifth day, potassium begins to be retained, and the body requires additional potassium to compensate for the earlier losses.

Extraordinarily large fat losses often follow a burn. The early fat loss can average as much as 600 grams per day in a severely burned patient. This amount of fat is equivalent to more than a pound of butter! In addition, increased tissue demands for ascorbic acid (vitamin C) may occur after a burn.

The characteristic *alarm reaction* as described by Selye often appears in the burned patient. There is enlargement of the adrenal glands, shrinkage of the lymph glands, and acute ulceration in the gastrointestinal tract. Menstruation often ceases after a burn and does not reappear until late in convalescence. Mild testicular atrophy is quite common.

Psychological Effects

The severely burned patient not only suffers agonizing physical pain but is highly vulnerable to emotional disturbances. He faces a threat to survival, a fear of disfigurement, prolonged physical discomfort, frequent anesthesia, many surgical procedures, and a tedious convalescence. Moreover, he is separated from his loved ones and home. Such multiple, severe psychological threats may actually weight the balance against recovery.

All in all, a severe burn constitutes a supreme insult to the body. An understanding of the body's response to such an injury throws much light on the pathophysiology of disease caused by physical agents.

CLINICAL CONSIDERATIONS

Most of the injuries caused by physical agents will be encountered, at one time or another, in the hospital emergency room. When a patient so injured appears, one should first focus on his general condition. Thus, heart and lung status should receive first attention. Shock, whether incipient or advanced, should receive immediate treatment. If pain is prominent, it should be relieved, though oversedation can be hazardous.

Proper cleansing of the wound may be as important as skilled surgical repair. The wound should be cleaned gently, with as much time as is required being taken to obtain a truly clean wound. No tissue that appears viable should be harmed. The same precaution holds for surgical repair.

In the management of a patient with this type of disorder, one should devote attention to the patient *as a whole* and on his body systems *individually*—otherwise, secondary effects of the primary injury will be missed. Certainly the psychological effects of a serious wound deserve full attention. One prominent surgeon visits all patients on his burn ward every day they are in the hospital. He would not think of doing otherwise!

Since diseases due to physical agents are in large measure preventable, every health caretaker should manifest an active interest in their prevention.

ANALYSIS OF SEVERITY OF BURNS *

CRITICAL BURNS

Second-degree burns covering over 30% of body
Third-degree burns of face, hands, or feet or over 10% of body
Electrical burns
Burns complicated by
   Injury to lungs or air passages
   Extensive injury of soft tissues
   Fractures
Disposition required: General hospital; care by burn team

MODERATE BURNS

Second-degree burns of from 15 to 30% of body
Third-degree burns of less than 10% of body, not including face, hands, or feet
Disposition required: Community hospital

MINOR BURNS

Second-degree burns of less than 15% of body
Third-degree burns of less than 2% of body
Disposition required: Ambulatory treatment

TOPICS FOR DISCUSSION

1. Why are disorders caused by physical agents so widespread in today's society?

2. What occupational groups are particularly exposed to injuries caused by physical agents?

---

* Adapted from Artz, Curtis P. and Moncrief, John A.: The Treatment of Burns. Philadelphia, W. B. Saunders Co., 1969.

3. Why is the accident rate on farms considerably higher than that in factories?

4. Why are diseases due to physical agents uniquely preventable?

5. At what school level should safety education begin?

6. How prevalent are accidents in the home?

7. What are some of the practical steps one can take to prevent accidents in the home?

8. What arrangements should be made for emergency handling of accidents caused by physical agents in the rural community?

9. Name some harmful physical agents not covered in this chapter.

10. Since auto accidents are the greatest single cause of disability and death in the United States, what steps would you recommend to reduce the toll?

11. Discuss the relationship between the use of drugs, including alcohol, and disorders caused by physical agents.

12. What civic, social, and professional groups in your city might show leadership in preventing disease due to physical agents?

BIBLIOGRAPHY

Books

Selye, H.: The Stress of Life. New York, McGraw-Hill Book Co., 1956.

Todd, A.: Abandoned. New York, McGraw-Hill Book Co., 1961.

Fallis, B.: Textbook of Pathology. New York, McGraw-Hill Book Co., 1964.

Merck Manual of Diagnosis and Therapy. ed. 11. Rahway, N.J., Merck Sharp & Dohme Research Laboratories, 1966.

Snively, W., and Thuerbach, J.: Sea of Life. New York, David McKay, Co., Inc., 1969.

Boyd, W.: A Textbook of Pathology. Philadelphia, Lea & Febiger, 1970.

Articles

Snively, W.: The body's response to burning. GP, *20*:131, 1959.

Schamadan, J., et al.: Preliminary communication: evaluation of potassium-rich electrolyte solutions as oral prophylaxis for heat stress disease. Industrial Medicine and Surgery, *37*:677, 1968.

Bockel, J.: The tragedy of trauma. Science News, *98*:82, 1970.

Shires, G., and Jones, R.: Initial management of the severely injured patient, JAMA, *213*:1872, 1970.

Sliney, D.: Evaluating health hazards from military lasers. JAMA, *214*:1047, 1970.

6

diseases due to chemical agents

Any substance that injures health or destroys life when it is introduced into or absorbed by a living organism is a poison, or toxin. We are exposed every day to countless potentially hazardous substances. They exist in the food we eat, in the liquids we drink, and even in the air we breathe. Numerous substances commonly found in the home, such as cleaning fluid, detergents, and insecticides, contain toxic chemicals. Factory workers are frequently exposed to toxic agents, as are miners and farmers. Some chemicals are so toxic as to cause immediate death when taken into the body even in tiny amounts. Others pose no immediate threat to health when absorbed in minute quantities but are quite toxic when absorbed in large amounts or when exposure to them has been prolonged. Thus, poisoning may be either *acute* or *chronic*. Acute poisoning is likely to have a suicidal or homicidal basis, whereas chronic poisoning is usually on an occupational or environmental basis.

Chemical agents injure cells by disturbing biochemical activities associated with the minute-to-minute survival of cells. For example, carbon monoxide and cyanide combine with hemoglobin and block the transport of oxygen, thereby causing cell hypoxia. Aniline and other aromatic compounds cause oxidation of hemoglobin to methemoglobin; the resultant cyanosis may be fatal. Widespread cellular injury may cause such severe structural damage that death is inevitable. If, however, structural damage is slight or absent, the effects of the poison are usually quickly reversed, and recovery is often complete.

Since tissues are composed of several kinds of cells, it follows that cells differ in their susceptibility to chemical injury. This individual cell susceptibility accounts in great measure for the morphologic changes that take place in chemical poisoning.

Chemical poisons enter the body by (1) being inhaled (lungs), (2) being ingested (gastrointestinal tract), and (3) through contact (skin and mucous membranes). Their action takes place in (1) the site of entry, (2) the site of excretion, or (3) a sensitive tissue having affinity for the specific poison.

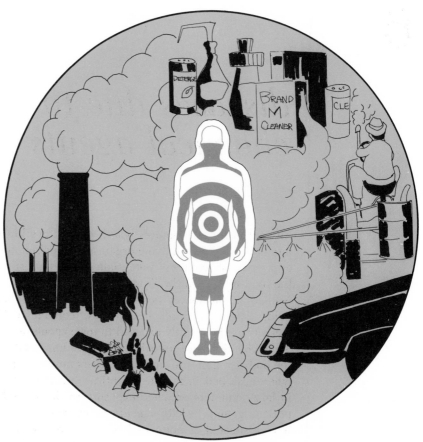

MODERN MAN IS THE TARGET FOR NUMEROUS CHEMICAL POISONS

Chemical poisons may be *exogenous* or *endogenous*. Exogenous poisoning is due to an outside cause. Endogenous poisoning may be caused by either of two situations. In one, a substance normally present in the body in fairly large amount (e.g., calcium, bilirubin), in certain illnesses becomes increased in concentration (e.g., hypercalcemia in lung carcinoma, hyperbilirubinemia in jaundice). Endogenous poisoning may result from a substance normally present in the body in such small amount that its presence is not detectable by usual analysis (e.g., sulfate). Normally such products of catabolism are excreted very rapidly (e.g., by kidney or liver), but in an illness involving the target organ, the organ's capacity to excrete or to detoxify the substance becomes greatly impaired or fails altogether. Then too, an exogenous poison may have such profound effects as to lead to endogenous poisoning. In this chapter, we shall discuss all these factors in some detail.

CUMULATIVE AND CHRONIC POISONING

A chemical agent that is not *acutely* poisonous even in a large amount may have deleterious effects if taken in small amounts over a long period. For example, an adult can safely ingest 180 mg. of iron a day for prolonged periods. But under certain circumstances (e.g., chronic liver disease, hereditary tendency to absorb excessive iron), iron may accumulate in his body leading to a serious disease of the liver, pancreas, lymph nodes, and heart muscle known as hemochromatosis. Ingestion of no more than 3 to 5 mg. of iron per day may be involved.

One of several things happens when a poison is absorbed by tissue in amounts that are not immediately and obviously injurious. If the agent is freely soluble in water, it is excreted unchanged in the urine. Lipid-soluble toxins, however, are not so readily excreted; they are first converted to water-soluble substances through reactions that take place in the liver and in the cells of the intestine and kidney, then excreted in urine or feces. Provided the chemical is never present in amounts sufficient to damage tissue, the excretory mechanisms are able to deal with it just as efficiently as they do tissue metabolites and unneeded substances in foods.

NORMAL EXCRETORY MECHANISM ADEQUATE TO DEAL WITH MANY POISONS

Poisons that cannot be excreted rapidly or rendered readily water-soluble accumulate in tissue. Mercury, for example, accumulates in kidney tubules if excretion cannot keep pace with absorption. When lead taken in by mouth exceeds the amount that can be adequately excreted, the excess is laid down in bone. Some lead can be laid down and retained in bones indefinitely without producing toxic effects, but when a critical level has been reached, maturation of red blood cells and hemoglobin formation are disrupted. Rapid mobilization of the accumulated lead, as occurs in acute intercurrent disease, raises the blood level and produces systemic toxicity.

The respiratory tract possesses an efficient mechanism for excreting irritant substances, and this protects the body from the cumulative toxic effects of polluting particulates. In normal circumstances, the mechanism is adequate; but should the environment be loaded with pollutants, the mechanism would fail and the lungs would be damaged.

Chronic effects may follow structural damage due to a single dose, or to repeated doses. Probably the most dreaded consequence is the possibility of cancer. Chemical carcinogenesis is described in Chapter 7.

STRUCTURAL DAMAGE

Numerous poisons and drugs have a selective action on certain organs, chiefly lung, brain, liver, and kidney, and on bone marrow. Poisons absorbed from the intestine by the portal system primarily affect the liver. The kidneys are heavily exposed to poisons excreted in urine. Highly irritating gases, such as sulfur dioxide, nitrous fumes, and phosgene, first attack the lungs and upper respiratory tract, where they may cause so much damage that they do not reach the bloodstream. Apparently, the respiratory epithelial cells are so damaged by these highly reactive substances that the normal communication between cells and bloodstream is blocked. On the other hand, chloroform absorbed through the lungs during anesthesia may not harm them but may damage the liver.

SITE OF ACTION A CRITICAL FACTOR IN EXTENT OF DAMAGE

As mentioned earlier, the site of action has a bearing on the effects of the toxin. Brain cells, for example, do not regenerate, so damage to the brain is likely to have more serious consequences than damage to the liver, which is often restored to a nearly normal state even after widespread cell destruction. Damage to the renal glomeruli is irreversible, whereas damage to the tubules is not necessarily so.

Damage to the Lung

The problem of air pollution—smog—has in recent years been recognized as an important cause of lung injury due to chemical agents. There are two known types of smog. The first is the wet and heavy atmosphere found in areas where fog is prevalent. In this type, the air contains sulfur dioxide, soluble fluorides and chlorides, and unknown substances. This type has caused many deaths. The second type occurs on sunny days with little wind and is caused by the combination of sunlight and pollutants emanating from high-temperature combustion processes and hydrocarbons from automobile exhaust. Open burning of trash contributes to this type of pollution also. Transportation fuels alone create over 90 million tons of pollutants each year, including carbon monoxide, oxidants, nitrogen compounds, lead, hydrocarbons, and particulate matter.

While pollution levels vary from day to day and from area to area, nearly everyone is exposed to air pollution all the time. Even at low levels it is harmful. Elderly persons with cardiovascular or pulmonary disease, asthmatics, and children are especially vulnerable. There is a definite cause-and-effect relationship between high pollution levels, as measured by the sulfur dioxide content of the air, and death from respiratory illness in individuals with chronic bronchopulmonary disease. The number of acute respiratory disorders increases sharply during episodes of high air pollution (see Chap. 17). There also may be a direct relationship with such problems as cough, dyspnea, and purulent sputum. Latent allergies to airborne antigens, such as dust, molds, and pollens, may become activated and cause clinical symptoms when the pollution level is high.

Some pollutants, including sulfur dioxide, nitrogen compounds, and ozone, apparently interfere with the clearing mechanism of the bronchi

CARBON MONOXIDE HARMS RABBITS; HOW ABOUT MAN?

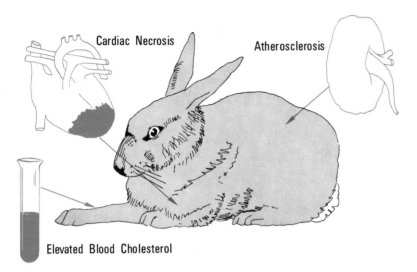

Cardiac Necrosis

Atherosclerosis

Elevated Blood Cholesterol

so that there is paralysis or destruction of the ciliary apparatus and increased production of mucus. There may be bronchospasm and acute inflammatory changes in the bronchial wall. Carbon monoxide combines with hemoglobin to form carboxyhemoglobin, thereby removing 5 to 10 per cent of the hemoglobin from the circulation. The oxygen tension is decreased so that less oxygen is available to tissue. Because of the greater oxygen needs of the myocardium as compared to other tissues, carbon monoxide is a possible pathogenic agent in death due to cardiac disease. It also may have a long-term effect, as suggested by studies such as one in which high blood cholesterol levels, atherosclerosis, and cardiac necrosis developed in rabbits exposed to high levels of carbon monoxide.

Tobacco smoking, cigarette smoking especially, also increases the risk of lung disease. James I of England described smoking as "a custom loathsome to the eye, hateful to the nose, harmful to the brain, dangerous to the lungs, and in the black stinking fume thereof nearest resembling the horrible Stygian smoke of the pit that is bottomless." There appears to be a direct relationship between smoking and the epidemic rise of chronic bronchopulmonary disease and bronchogenic carcinoma. (There is also overwhelming evidence that smoking is an important factor in development of coronary artery disease.) Some 16 substances capable of initiating cancer in experimental animals have been identified in tobacco smoke.

Some chemical poisons that affect the lungs are particulate and only slightly soluble, and thus exert their main effect in the immediate area of localization. Inhalation of silica, for example, leads to nodular areas of chronic inflammatory reaction within the lung. This is seen very often in coal miners and others whose occupation exposes them to silica dust (see Chap. 17).

Damage to the Brain

Carbon disulfide, widely used in the manufacture of rayon, causes irreversible changes in the central nervous system, giving rise to dementia and premature senility. Methyl and ethyl mercury salts, used extensively in fungicides, damage portions of the cerebral and cerebellar cortices. While the victim may show no adverse mental effects, he suffers gross ataxia, blindness, dysarthria, and other effects. Methanol, also called methyl alcohol, causes permanent blindness by destroying the retina. Exposure to manganese, as occurs in manganese mining, may have deleterious effects on the nuclei of basal cells, and thus produce a syndrome resembling Parkinson's disease. The liver may be damaged also.

Damage to the Liver

Because of its diverse functions, the liver is particularly vulnerable to damage by toxic agents. Carbon tetrachloride, a common ingredient of stain-removing solvents, causes acute hepatic necrosis and fatty change when toxic amounts are inhaled, ingested accidentally or with suicidal intent, or injected into experimental animals. This agent is not a powerful liver poison; rather, it causes renal tubular necrosis, which leads to acute renal failure. Thus the damage to liver cells is indirect. Tetrachloroethane, a widely used industrial solvent, causes necrosis of liver cells. This is why, incidentally, the user of these substances is always warned not to work in poorly ventilated quarters.

The fungus *Amanita phalloides,* sometimes mistaken for an edible mushroom, causes total liver necrosis, followed by death, within a few days. Yellow phosphorus, present in some rat poisons, also produces liver cell necrosis, as does ferrous sulfate in large quantities. Other drugs known to cause liver cell necrosis include cinchophen, acetaminophen, chloroform, tetracyclines when given intravenously in large doses, and some monoamine oxidase inhibitors. Phenothiazine derivatives and certain steroids are occasional causes of intrahepatic biliary obstruction and jaundice.

The liver possesses an amazing ability to regenerate, so that recovery is usually complete if the victim survives. Scar tissue may, however, interfere with regeneration, with resultant cirrhosis. This is particularly likely with repeated exposure to toxins, as in alcoholism.

Damage to the Kidney

Because renal blood flow and oxygen consumption are high, the kidneys are particularly susceptible to damage from poisons that induce cellular hypoxia. The excretory role of the kidneys is important, too, since absorbed poisons leave the body mainly by this route. The renal tubule cells thus are exposed in many instances to a chemical concentration many times that in the systemic blood. Sulfonamides, streptomycin, kanamycin, polymyxin, and amphotericin B are nephrotoxic. In mercury poisoning, the mercury is distributed throughout the tissues, but is concentrated in the kidneys, where it induces proximal tubular cell degeneration and necrosis leading to renal failure. Gold and arsenic, once widely used in medical therapy, are other causes, as is poisoning due to organic mercurial diuretics. Repeated exposure to lead, phenacetin, and perhaps aspirin may cause chronic renal failure. Carbon tetrachloride (in solvents), chlorates (in weedkillers), tetrachloroethylene (in solvents), and ethylene glycol (antifreeze) may produce renal tubular necrosis.

Damage to Bone Marrow

The action of poisons on bone marrow is not well understood. In some persons, perhaps because of an inherent defect in drug detoxification capacity or in marrow metabolism, exposure to drugs that are safe for most persons depresses organ function and causes marrow aplasia. Unfortunately, these incidents cannot be anticipated—only after many such instances over a period of months or years is a specific drug so identified. Tests on laboratory animals are of no avail, since drugs known to cause marrow aplasia and aplastic anemia in susceptible humans do not produce the same effects in laboratory animals. In many instances chloramphenicol is the cause of bone marrow depression. Troxidone, the sulfonamides, hydantoin anticonvulsants, phenylbutazone, gold, and perchlorates are other such agents.

Benzene in large quantities damages bone marrow in both man and animals. Alkylating agents may have similar effects on dividing cells. This has been demonstrated in laboratory animals, which ultimately die from bone marrow damage if they survive the intestinal injury caused by the drug. These agents in suitable amounts induce sterility in male insects, rats, and mice, and great amounts may destroy the germinal layer of the testis.

Aplastic anemia, which is depression of all the cellular constituents of marrow, is occasionally a disastrous consequence of treatment with alkylating agents; a much more common development is granulocytopenia, a fall in the total white count. Thrombocytopenia, with bleeding into the skin and other organs, may follow therapy with alkylating agents.

A number of drugs, including antihistamines, organic arsenic compounds, phenacetin, amphetamines, and mephenesin, induce hemolysis by an unknown mechanism that is not associated with hypersensitivity. Methyl chloride and naphthalene, used in some air conditioning systems, may also induce hemolytic reactions.

EFFECTS OF SOME COMMON POISONS

Corrosive Acids

NUMEROUS
CHEMICALS
WIDELY USED
IN INDUSTRY
MAY CAUSE
SEVERE
DAMAGE IF
HANDLED
CARELESSLY

The mineral acids, i.e., nitric, hydrochloric, and sulfuric, are corrosive, rapidly destroying or decomposing tissues that they contact. Thus they can produce burns of the lips, mouth, pharynx, esophagus, and stomach. The intense irritation causes the stomach to contract and lie in folds. Scattered patches of necrosis appear over the folds. If the patient survives, these necrotic patches slough, leaving a raw surface. All corrosive acids induce similar changes, but the color of the burns varies. Hydrochloric acid burns are white, those due to nitric acid are yellow, and sulfuric acid burns are brownish-red or black. The acid dissolves epithelium and connective tissue, and causes water to move out of the cells. Microscopically, the tissue appears necrotic on the surface with intense inflammation of surrounding tissues. Corrosive acids are often used in suicide attempts.

Accidental poisoning is a frequent occurrence in munitions works, where smokeless powder is made from nitrocellulose, which is obtained by treating cotton with nitric acid. There is severe inflammation of the larynx and trachea when these fumes are inhaled.

Caustic Alkalis

Strong alkalis, such as lime, caustic soda, and caustic potash, are corrosive. They convert tissue protein to alkaline proteinase and convert fat to soaps. With tissue breakdown, some of the bound alkali is released, extending the area of destruction. Commercial lye is the most common cause of alkali poisoning. A child may ingest it accidentally, and it is used in many suicide attempts. The lesions are similar to those produced by corrosive acids. There is severe burning, acute inflammation, and softening of tissue of the lips, mouth, throat, esophagus, and stomach. If the patient recovers, scar tissue will form which will cause esophageal and pyloric stricture.

Phenol

Poisoning by phenol (carbolic acid) differs in several ways from poisoning by other strong acids. Burns over the lips, mouth, esophagus, and stomach have a peculiar opaque, dead-white appearance. As with poisoning by other acids, the stomach contracts, and necrotic patches appear on the summits of the folds. Phenol causes immediate coagulation of the mucosa of the upper alimentary tract, followed by sloughing necrosis of tissue if the patient lives for some time. Dilute phenol causes an intense hemorrhagic inflammation rather than coagulation. The characteristic odor of phenol is recognized when the stomach is opened at autopsy.

Bichloride of Mercury

A concentrated solution of bichloride of mercury coagulates tissue similarly to phenol. Grayish-white patches of coagulation necrosis are seen, and surrounding tissue is inflamed.

Bichloride of mercury in tablet form produces severe local necrosis with deep ulceration in the stomach. After a few days, gastrointestinal and renal symptoms develop, since whatever the mode of entry, whether via skin and mucous membrane as in vaginal douche, or by mouth, mercury is excreted via the colon and the kidney. There is intense hemorrhagic colitis, and the renal convoluted tubules are extensively necrosed. Within 24 hours there is oliguria, often followed by anuria. Within 1 week, calcium salts are deposited in the necrotic tissue masses, many of which lie free in the lumen of the tubules. Just what causes this acute calcification is not understood.

Arsenic

Arsenic is a strong poison that can have either acute or chronic effects. In acute arsenic poisoning there is severe hemorrhagic inflammation along the entire gastrointestinal tract, including enteritis and colitis. At autopsy, Paris green or arsenic crystals may be seen in the folds of the stomach. Chronic arsenic poisoning chiefly affects the skin and nervous system. Cutaneous manifestations include pigmentation and marked keratinization. Weight loss, diarrhea or constipation, anorexia, fatigue, peripheral neuropathy, headache, and confusion are other effects. The disastrous effects on the central nervous system may result in mental disorders, peripheral nerve paralysis, and blindness. Before penicillin became available, arsenic was employed in the treatment of syphilis, and there were many instances of acute, sometimes fatal, poisoning.

Alkaloids

Poisonous alkaloids include strychnine, atropine, cocaine, and opium (morphine). These substances do not produce characteristic postmortem changes, and chemical analysis is the only means of detecting their presence in the body.

Methyl Alcohol

Methyl alcohol is absorbed by ingestion, or by inhalation of the fumes from liquid alcohol used in industry. It is a common ingredient of bootleg liquor. Methyl alcohol oxidizes to formaldehyde and formic acid, both of which are highly toxic. Autopsy findings include edema and hemorrhage in the brain, and small hemorrhages in the gastric mucosa. Those who survive acute intoxication may suffer optic atrophy and blindness.

Ethyl Alcohol

Ethyl alcohol, the principal ingredient of all popular "cocktail hour" drinks, deserves special mention because, unlike the other poisonous substances we have been talking about, it is ingested deliberately and often chronically by millions of persons. As a social lubricant, it occupies a unique place in modern life. It is estimated that some 7 million Americans are alcoholics, i.e., dependent upon alcohol in their day-to-day functioning. In France, where alcohol is taken as wine with meals, the rate of addiction is the world's highest.

A sufficient quantity of alcohol, i.e., a blood level of 600 mg. per 100 ml. or higher, usually is fatal. This fortunately is a rare occurrence, because the victim is likely to become stuporous before ingesting a lethal amount. What is far more likely is a state of chronic alcoholism. As the addict often "drinks his calories," he may suffer from various nutritional deficiencies. More serious even than these are hepatic cirrhosis and pneumonia, which develop rather frequently in alcoholics. Then there are disastrous psychic consequences due to the physical dependence on alcohol, ranging from hallucinations, to "rum fits," to delirium tremens. But probably the most devastating effect of alcoholism is the social cost—in disrupted family life, time lost from work, and automobile accidents due to drunken driving.

Chlorinated Hydrocarbons

Chloroform, carbon tetrachloride, dichloromethane, and tetrachloroethane are chlorinated hydrocarbons that are widely used as cleaning solvents in the dry cleaning of clothing and certain household furnishings and in the cleaning of electrical and electronic equipment. These agents are poisonous if swallowed, inhaled, or allowed to contaminate the skin. The vapor is extremely irritating to the eyes, nose, throat, and lungs. Their acute effects were described earlier in this chapter.

Carbon Monoxide

Carbon monoxide is nonirritating, colorless, tasteless, and odorless, so—unlike the chlorinated hydrocarbons—it gives no warning of its presence. Poisoning is by inhalation from car exhausts, sewers, some manufacturing processes, and faulty gas refrigerators and heaters fueled by gas, coal, oil or kerosene in poorly ventilated areas. As described earlier, carbon monoxide combines with hemoglobin to block the transport of oxygen and thus cause cell hypoxia. The brain, being the tissue most dependent on a continuous supply of oxygen, is primarily affected. If the victim does not die of asphyxia he may recover completely, or he may suffer residual disability, depending on the degree of cerebral damage that was sustained.

In chronic carbon monoxide poisoning, which is due to prolonged inhalation of low levels of the gas, there are many symptoms, including headache, dizziness, weakness and nausea. In concentrated form carbon monoxide is rapidly fatal. The victim loses consciousness suddenly and may die within minutes. Carboxyhemoglobin is of a bright color, so that the face, blood, and viscera become cherry-red. This, plus abnormally fluid blood, are the chief findings at autopsy.

Cyanides

Cyanides are among the most lethal poisons known. They are used industrially in cadmium plating, metal cleaning and polishing, coal tar distillation, electroplating, and in rat extermination. Cyanides are absorbed through the skin and act with such speed that even a few minutes' exposure may be fatal. Cyanides give off a smell of bitter almonds. Symptoms include flushing and headache. A characteristic peach-kernel odor is often noted when the stomach is opened at autopsy; the gastric mucosa is a bright chestnut-brown color.

Hydrogen sulfide gas is given off in coal pits, gas wells, and sewer gas, and is as rapidly fatal as hydrogen cyanide. The gas causes respiratory failure within a few seconds and death quickly follows. Autopsy findings include greenish cyanosis and greenish discoloration of the blood and viscera.

Barbiturates

Most cases of barbiturate poisoning result from ingestion with suicidal intent. In fact, barbiturate overdosage is the leading cause of drug-induced deaths. The barbiturates are relatively safe sedative-hypnotic drugs and, when taken on a physician's order, are usually harmless, but as little as five to 10 times the hypnotic dose can be extremely dangerous. The victim becomes comatose, and his respiration is severely depressed. As a result, inspissated mucus collects in the bronchial passages. The systemic anoxia may lead to vascular collapse and death. The barbiturates are commonly taken with alcohol to enhance the state of euphoria produced by each of them singly, and this can lead to rapid central nervous system depression ending in death. It should be noted that the barbiturates, unlike many of the other poisonous substances we have described, cause damage because of the central nervous system depression, and are relatively free of toxic reactions involving injury to vital organs.

Salicylates

Salicylates are an important cause of death in young children, who often have easy access to them. Excessive intake (not enough to cause death) causes gastric irritation, dizziness, nausea, fever, and diarrhea. Severe fluid and electrolyte imbalance results from acute intoxication, and there is an increase in the metabolic rate and production of carbon dioxide. The blood sugar level is raised and ketone bodies are formed—the picture is rather similar to diabetic acidosis. Salicylate overdose is an occasional cause of suicidal death.

Poisonous Plants

Poisonous plants are found in abundant numbers throughout the United States, the most common ones being chokeberry, jimson weed, stinkweed, and meadow saffron. Ergot, which may grow as a fungus on grains, is a source of potential poison. In North America, most cases of acute mushroom poisoning are due to members of the genus Amanita, which contain five toxins so potent that ingestion of only two or three mushrooms may be fatal. There is hepatic necrosis and renal degeneration and necrosis. The heart and brain also show degenerative changes.

Venomous Animals

In this category are included the venenating arthropods, such as scorpions, spiders, bees, wasps, and ants; the venomous reptiles, such as the Gila monster, the coral snake, and the rattlesnake; and the venomous marine animals, such as the jellyfish, marine snails of the genus Conus, and stinging corals.

Spiders and scorpions are common in most areas of the world. Their venom is neurotoxic, and usually the symptoms include pain and local inflammation, nausea, vomiting, headache, rapid respiration, and weakened pulse. There may be paralysis of the involved area. The stings of bees, wasps, and ants usually cause only local inflammation and pain, although in allergic persons a violent reaction ending in death can occur.

The only characteristic common to all species of venomous reptiles is the presence of maxillary fangs. This makes recognition of venomous reptiles difficult. In the United States the most common ones are the North American copperhead, the cottonmouth moccasin, and the rattlesnake. These bites cause severe pain, edema, nausea, vomiting, thirst, sweating, and fever. The prognosis is favorable if no further symptoms develop, but the bite may be serious or even fatal if such symptoms as numbness and tingling of the face, muscle spasms, and a sharp fall in blood pressure develop.

With the growing popularity of aquatic sports and increased investigation of marine sources of food, the medical importance of marine venoms is increasing quite rapidly. In most cases the sting causes intense burning pain, muscle cramps, dyspnea, and nausea. In severe cases there may be numbness, paralysis, and finally vascular collapse.

DISEASE MODEL: LEAD POISONING (PLUMBISM)

There are many industrial uses of lead and consequently many opportunities for exposure. Any procedure that produces lead vapor or mist, or lead dust exposes workers to inhalation and absorption of lead. Lead may be inhaled as dust or fumes, it may be absorbed through the skin, or it may be ingested. It is dissolved and absorbed from the digestive tract, deposited in the liver, and released into the circulation. The kidneys excrete some of the lead; but if intake outruns renal excretory ability, the excess is laid down in bone. With accumulation of toxic amounts in bone, there is severe anemia, weakness, insomnia, headache, and irritability. If the patient is careless about oral hygiene, lead sulfide is deposited along the gingival margins and produces a blue-black "lead line."

An early sign is pigment deposition in the retina. Constipation is common. Painful colic (often called "painter's colic" or "lead colic") may occur. Inflammation of the peripheral nerves, particularly the musculospinal and peroneal, may result in drop wrist and drop foot. In later stages, there may be depression, convulsions, delirium, and mental changes. With degeneration of the cerebral cortex, general paralysis may develop.

Lead poisoning in children is extremely serious, yet frequently goes

HOW LEAD POISONING AFFECTS MAN

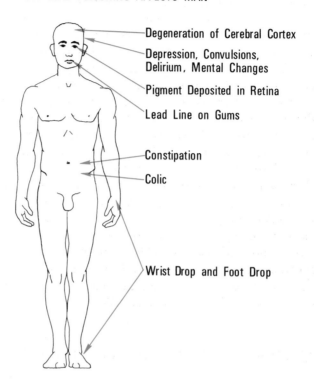

Degeneration of Cerebral Cortex

Depression, Convulsions, Delirium, Mental Changes

Pigment Deposited in Retina

Lead Line on Gums

Constipation

Colic

Wrist Drop and Foot Drop

LEAD POISONING IN CHILDREN A DISEASE OF POOR LIVING CONDITIONS

unrecognized at first. It is most likely to occur in areas where housing is poor or old and lead paint had been used in interior painting. (Today all children's toys and furniture must be painted with lead-free paint by the manufacturer.) The child may ingest lead paint scales from his crib or other furniture or may eat chips of lead paint from the walls (pica— perverted appetite). Drinking water that has passed through lead pipes is another source.

The child develops pronounced anemia and gastrointestinal symptoms of constipation, colic, and vomiting, but the most striking symptoms are those of lead encephalitis, and include visual disturbances and change in mental state. Convulsions and coma may follow if treatment is not begun quickly. The blood pressure may be elevated. Choked disc and separation of the cranial sutures may be seen. The symptoms result from the rapid increase in intracranial pressure due to pronounced cerebral edema. The pressure of the cerebrospinal fluid is greatly increased. In-flammation of peripheral nerves is rare. Seldom does a child exhibit the "lead line" on the gums, although roentgenograms will demonstrate a lead line in bone. The growing ends of long bones show increased density in areas where lead is deposited. This line is nearly always present, even in mild cases.

TREATMENT OF ACUTE POISONING

Several steps should be carried out promptly. The first is to evacuate the bulk of the poison from the stomach and intestine via gastric lavage, emetics, or cathartics. Next, an antidote must be administered to inactivate the poison that was not removed by gastric lavage. If a stomach tube has been used, the antidote and other needed liquids can be instilled before the tube is removed. Occasionally, it may be necessary to administer an antidote parenterally.

The next step is to eliminate the poison that has already been absorbed. This may be done by forcing fluids, either by mouth or parenterally. Dextrose in saline solution is generally used for this purpose. Venesection followed by blood transfusion may become necessary to remove all absorbed poison. Finally, symptomatic treatment is given as indicated.

CLINICAL CONSIDERATIONS

Potentially hazardous chemical agents abound in today's world, and the victims of such damage can be seen every day in almost all hospitals. The victim's life may depend on the knowledge of those caring for him. Early recognition of symptoms associated with chronic or cumulative poisoning may prevent severe damage.

In acute poisoning, prompt diagnosis is of utmost importance. The history, related circumstances, and significant objects found near the patient at the time the incident was discovered are of vital importance in making the diagnosis. Bits of food, as well as drinking glasses, bottles, or other containers may provide a clue as to the type of poison. All relevant information should be recorded.

Knowledge of treatment procedures and the proper antidotes for the various classes of poisons is essential. Information on emergency measures may be relayed via telephone to relatives of the victim. It may well mean the difference between life and death. For example, if induction of vomiting is not contraindicated, the victim or a relative can be told how to induce vomiting by placing a finger in the throat or by administering such easily prepared solutions as mustard in water or salt in warm water. If evacuation of the poison can be accomplished at home, less poison will be absorbed before the patient receives medical attention.

Death by poisoning may assume great medicolegal importance. Therefore, those who may be called upon to perform or assist at an autopsy should be familiar with the probable pathologic findings and with precautions to be observed in collecting tissue samples for chemical analysis. All postmortem findings should be recorded; no details should be left to memory.

Undoubtedly, among our modern blessings are the pharmaceutical agents that have in such large measure reduced the morbidity and mortality from disease. That these advances do not represent unmixed blessings does not detract from their inestimable worth. We have come a long way since the 1860's when the physician-poet Oliver Wendell Holmes said: "Excluding opium, which the creator, Himself, seems to prescribe, and excluding wine, which is a food, and excluding the vapors which produce the miracle of anesthesia, I firmly believe that if the whole materia medica, as now used, could be sunk to the bottom of the sea, it would be all the better for mankind and all the worse for the fishes." *

Almost any medication possesses potential for harm if used carelessly. In this sense we may regard medications as potential poisons. We read in Shakespeare that antidotes are poisons. This applies especially to potent drugs, however effective and lifesaving they may be. A recent category of illness has come to be recognized: iatrogenic disease, that is, disease resulting from drug therapy. Unfortunately, such disease can occur when drugs are used with great care and forethought. Today, thoughtful physicians emphasize the advantages of using a minimal number of drugs for a given patient, and then only when definitely indicated.

TOPICS FOR DISCUSSION

1. List the potentially harmful chemical agents to which you have been exposed today.

2. To what harmful chemical agents might the average person be exposed during the course of a week and what precautions might he take?

3. What precautions should be observed in the home to keep toxic agents out of the reach of children?

4. What steps might local or federal government take to help reduce environmental exposure to chemical toxins?

5. Did you recall, in discussing the preceding question, that the federal government recently established the Environmental Protection Agency? What are this agency's responsibilities concerning chemical poisons? What legal means are at its disposal?

6. List the forms of pollution you would encounter in a large city such as Los Angeles.

7. List the forms of pollution you would encounter in the country.

8. Why are Eskimos advised not to eat snow?

---

* Address to the Massachusetts Medical Society, May 30, 1860.

BIBLIOGRAPHY

Books

The Merck Manual of Diagnosis and Therapy. ed. 11. Rahway, New Jersey, Merck Sharp & Dohme Research Laboratories, 1966.

Boyd, W.: A Textbook of Pathology. pp. 489–492. Philadelphia, Lea & Febiger, 1970.

Passmore, R., and Robson, J.: A Companion to Medical Studies. vol. 2. Philadelphia, F. A. Davis Co., 1970.

Articles

Bean, W.: Vitamania, polypharmacy, and witchcraft. Editorial, Archives of Internal Medicine, 96:137, 1955.

Snively, W., and Becker, B.: Illinois medicine—a century ago. Illinois Medical Journal, 134:157, 1968.

Segal, M.: Air pollution and the physician's responsibility. Health Science Review, 1:2, 1970.

Pollution levels linked to daily mortality rates. Modern Medicine, 38:75, 1970.

Brass, A.: Tobacco and health. JAMA, 213:1879, 1970.

Thromboembolism, oral contraceptives, and cigarettes. Annals of Internal Medicine, 73:486, 1970.

Air pollution. Science News, 99:80, 1971.

Carnow, B.: Air pollution and physician responsibility. Archives of Internal Medicine, 127:91, 1971.

7

neoplasia

A cancer cell seems to be simply a cell that has
gone several steps beyond the average number of steps of modification:
"several" steps, because it takes one step to become sufficiently emancipated
from its neighbors to step out of bounds; another step, to emigrate
and lodge in a new environment, as does a metastatic cell; a third step, to
be able to conceal its alien nature to its new neighbors; a fourth step, to be
fit to thrive in the new community and to be nurtured there instead of
expelled; a fifth step, to proliferate in the new location; and a sixth step, to
prey on its neighbors and crowd them out. In principle, these steps are
perhaps no different in kind from the ones that transform an early
embryonic cell stepwise into a muscle cell, or a pancreas cell, or a thyroid cell,
or make an embryonic cell degenerate, as many do.
—Paul A. Weiss *

During the course of normal wear and tear, cells continuously proliferate
to replace the worn-out tissue. Following injury or disease, cell proliferation increases to repair and regenerate the damaged tissue, then slows
to normal when it has served its purpose. Sometimes, however, cell proliferation begins and continues indefinitely at a rate faster than normal.
Such accelerated activity, which has no apparent relationship to growth
and maintenance of body tissues, leads to development of a tumor mass.
This process is *neoplasia* (new growth).

In this chapter, we shall see that some neoplasms are not clinically
significant and that others are deadly; that tumors differ not only in their
clinical effects, but in numerous other ways as well; and that several
factors can cause or predispose to tumor growth and that these agents
frequently work together. With this background, we can then discuss the
various ways in which neoplasia causes disease. Our disease model, carcinoma of the stomach, will help illustrate just how cancer goes about its
deadly work. Finally, we shall see why a good understanding of neoplasia
is essential for anyone who is caring for a patient with a tumor.

---

* Weiss, Paul A.: A Cell Is Not an Island. Chicago, Ill., Perspectives in Biology and
Medicine, Winter 1971. The University of Chicago Press. © 1971 by the University
of Chicago. All rights reserved.

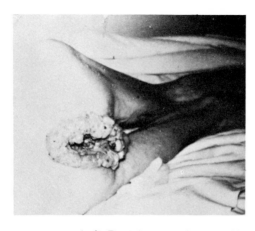 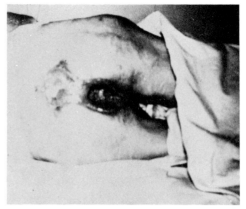

Left, Rectal cancer has proliferated into a large external lesion; the disease is making the patient cachectic as well. *Right,* The malignant tissue has been removed and the wound is healing. (Smith, D., Germain, C., Gips, C.: Care of the Adult Patient, ed. 2. Philadelphia, J. B. Lippincott, 1971)

CLASSIFICATION OF NEOPLASMS

Neoplasia usually begins in a single focus, although it may arise in several adjoining areas. Occasionally, neoplasia is systemic. In the reticuloendothelial system, for example, neoplastic overproduction of leukocytes (leukemia) may involve bone marrow throughout the body. Neoplasia may be minimal, with tumors just visible macroscopically; on the other hand, the tumor mass may grow wildly, invading and destroying surrounding tissues. In the latter case, complete surgical removal is difficult, and should any neoplastic cells remain following surgery, the tumor will probably recur. In addition, neoplastic cells carried through the blood and lymphatic vessels form new tumors in sites far removed from the primary lesion. Neoplasms in the intermediate area between the two extremes show varying growth rates, varying tendencies to destroy neighboring tissues, and varying rapidity of penetration into the lymphatic and blood vessels.

Because neoplasms vary so greatly in their characteristics, particularly their potential for change, some sort of classification is needed. Classifying tumors is not always a simple matter, but it is important to do so since the tumor type has a bearing on treatment and prognosis.

Tumors are first divided into two main groups, *benign* and *malignant.* Some tumors cannot readily be placed in either category, and occasionally a tumor is transformed from benign to malignant over a period of time.

CLASSIFICATION
NOT ALWAYS
CLEARCUT

Next, they are classified histogenically, that is, according to the tissue where the lesion originated. In some cases it may be impossible to determine the histogenesis. Generally, tumors are named according to their probable histogenesis, their anatomical site, and, of course, whether they are benign or malignant; e.g., a fibrosarcoma is a malignant tumor arising in fibrous tissue, and a leiomyoma is a benign tumor arising in smooth muscle.

BENIGN AND MALIGNANT TUMORS

The essential feature of all malignant and, to a lesser extent, benign tumors is failure of the mechanism that controls the cell mass and lack of functional contribution of this tissue. With a few exceptions, benign and malignant tumors differ in several specific respects, including clinical effects, structure, growth, metastasis, and recurrence.

Clinical Effects

The benign, or simple, tumor is significant clinically chiefly because of the pressure it exerts on other tissues as it increases in size. These growths cause death only infrequently, usually by accident of position. For example, a tumor growing within the cranial cavity, however slowly, sooner or later will cause death. A benign tumor may indirectly cause serious damage or death by producing a secondary disease, as may occur when a functionally active benign tumor of glandular tissue causes secondary disease by overproduction of hormones; this is the case in adrenal adenomas.

No matter where the malignant tumor, or cancer, grows, if neglected, it usually kills by destroying tissues, interfering with physiological functions, causing hemorrhage or ulceration in infected areas, and producing secondary starvation.

BENIGN TUMORS RARELY LETHAL; MALIGNANT TUMORS OFTEN SO

Structure

Benign tumors are well *differentiated* (specialized in form, character, or function) and may perfectly reproduce the structure of their tissue of origin, whereas malignant cells tend to *dedifferentiate* (lose specialization and revert to a more primitive form), sometimes to such a degree that the parent structure cannot be determined. Cells may be *pleomorphic*, varying in size and shape. The faster the cell growth, the more primitive are the cells. Some tumors totally lack structural and cellular differentiation; they are described as *anaplastic*. On the other

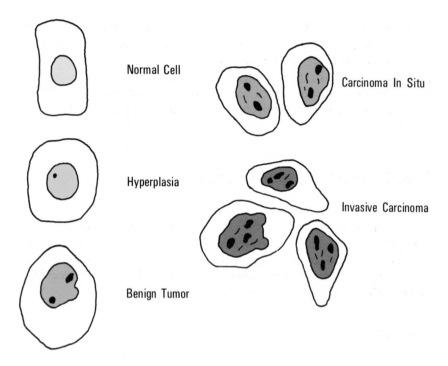

As normal cell progresses to malignant cell, hyperplasia first occurs. Then nuclear and nucleolar material become more prominent. Next, the tumor cells depart further from the form of the tissue whence they sprang. Finally, cells invade adjoining tissues, lymph channels, and bloodstream.

hand, some malignant tumors are so well differentiated as to be almost indistinguishable from normal tissue. The nucleus of a malignant cell is likely to be enlarged, and the nucleolus is large in proportion to the nucleus.

Growth

Benign tumors grow by expansion and frequently are surrounded by a capsule of compressed tissue—a reassuring finding since tumors with capsules are always benign. Although malignant tumors *never* have capsules, the absence of a capsule does not necessarily mean that the tumor is malignant, as many benign tumors, particularly those arising in connective tissue, do not have capsules.

Malignant tumors grow by invasion. They compress and penetrate surrounding tissues, crowding into spaces between tissue cells, and eventually destroying and replacing normal cells. Usually they grow rapidly, whereas benign tumors are relatively slow growing. Sudden rapid growth of a benign tumor may indicate malignant change. Sometimes, however, a benign tumor will greatly increase in size over a period of a few days because of hemorrhage into the tumor, but this is not actual tumor

BODY CELLS

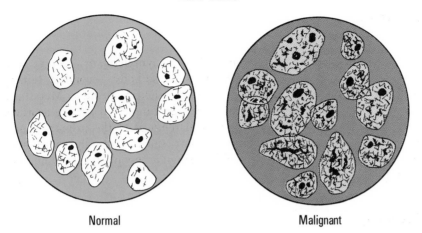

Normal   Malignant

The malignant cells differ from the normal by having considerably more nuclear and nucleolar material; by having greater variation in shape; and by their dissimilarity to the tissue cells that gave rise to them.

growth. The growth rate of a neoplasm may be assessed by the histologic appearance, particularly by the number of mitotic figures present. In benign neoplasms, mitotic figures are absent or scanty, whereas in malignant neoplasms they are usually numerous. The faster the growth, the more numerous the mitotic figures.

HOW A CARCINOMA BECOMES INVASIVE

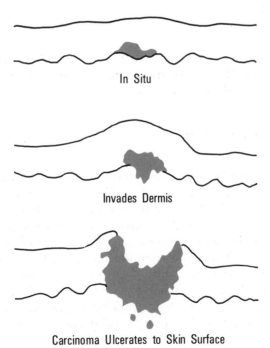

In Situ

Invades Dermis

Carcinoma Ulcerates to Skin Surface

Metastasis

When a malignant neoplasm invades lymphatic or blood vessels, neoplastic cells are carried to other parts of the body. Secondary tumors may grow from these cells in a process called *metastasis*. Metastatic growth *always* indicates malignancy. Benign tumors do not metastasize. Once a tumor has metastasized, surgical removal of the primary tumor is usually useless. Life expectancy is short, since eventually, vital structures will be damaged or destroyed by malignant neoplasms growing in or near them.

Recurrence

Sometimes a malignant tumor reappears following its removal by surgery or treatment by radiotherapy. This means that some of the neoplastic cells escaped destruction and subsequently multiplied, forming another mass. Such cells may lie dormant for a long time, perhaps years, before they cause a recurrence. Similarly, cells in metastatic sites may remain dormant for years before their presence becomes clinically obvious. This occurrence may be associated with hormone dependence, which will be discussed later in this chapter.

HISTOGENESIS

Most tumors originate either from epithelial tissues or from connective tissues. Those that cannot be identified histogenetically are called *anaplastic malignant growths*.

Neoplasms of Epithelial Tissue

Benign epithelial tumors growing on a free surface are called *papillomas*. There are three kinds of papillomas: adenopapilloma, as from the colon; transitional cell papilloma, as from the bladder; and squamous cell papilloma, as from skin. Papillomas are usually rounded, cauliflower-like growths consisting of simple or complex elongated processes with fibrovascular cores. They grow from the surface and are covered by the epithelium from which they arise. The processes form a stalk, which varies in length from one tumor to another, and which attaches the growth to the parent surface. Some papillomas, particularly those of the colon and bladder, tend to undergo malignant change. Infiltration of

PAPILLOMAS
CHARACTERIZED
BY PRESENCE
OF STALK

epithelial cells into the stalk and cores of the processes is important evidence of this change. The stalk and processes may shorten and become more solid with malignant degeneration. Aberration and increasing hyperplasia of cells in the epithelial lining of the processes also suggest malignant change.

Benign epithelial tumors growing in solid glandular epithelium are called *adenomas*. They are well-defined, rounded lesions in the substance of the parent tissue, frequently more solid than the normal tissue, which occur in solid organs, such as the adrenal cortex, pituitary, breast, liver, kidney, and parotid gland. Functional adenomas lead to hypersecretion of the hormone or other substance produced by the parent organ. Although their structure usually resembles that of the parent organ, they may show some irregularity of glandular structure, increased mitotic activity, and solid masses of undifferentiated cells. These features suggest malignant change.

ADENOMA A TUMOR OF SOLID TISSUE

All malignant epithelial tumors are called *carcinomas*. They may be further described by adjectives or prefixes referring to the type of epithelium from which the tumor arose or to the structure of the growth. For example, squamous carcinoma, adenocarcinoma, and transitional cell carcinoma originate from and resemble their respective parent structures. Papillomas that undergo malignant transformation and exhibit some degree of papillary structure and glandular epithelium are known as *papillary adenocarcinomas*.

CARCINOMA A GENERAL TERM QUALIFIED BY TYPE OF EPITHELIUM

Carcinomas, which ordinarily appear pale yellow and rather friable, have a supporting fibrovascular stroma (framework) for their epithelial cells that is said to originate in normal stroma of the parent tissue. Sometimes, particularly in carcinomas of the breast and stomach, the proportion of connective tissue present greatly exceeds that of the tumor cells, such disproportionate growth of fibrous stroma being called *scirrhous*. Scirrhous carcinoma of the breast and of the stomach ("leather bottle" stomach) are examples of such tumors.

Sometimes a diagnosis of carcinoma is based solely on the appearance of the cells. For example, microscopic examination of a skin lesion may show pleomorphic cells with an enlarged nucleus and increased mitotic activity. When these features are so pronounced that a diagnosis of malignancy is justified, the condition is called *carcinoma in situ*. This type of lesion is probably most common in squamous epithelium although it does arise in other tissues as well. Carcinoma in situ is considered to be preinvasive and in all likelihood will become invasive over a period of time.

Some adenocarcinomas secrete the same substance as would be produced by the normal organ and thereby exert functional effects. Cancers of mucous epithelium frequently secrete mucus; they are referred to as *mucoid adenocarcinomas*.

Neoplasms of Connective Tissue

BENIGN
CONNECTIVE
TISSUE
TUMORS
RESEMBLE
PARENT
TISSUE

Benign tumors of connective tissue are named according to their tissue of origin, such as fibroma, lipoma, and chondroma. These tumors are usually pale, solid, and well-defined structures that appear histologically similar to the tissue from which they arise. Aberration of cell type, dedifferentiation of architecture, increased mitotic activity, and early invasion of surrounding tissues indicate malignant change in such tumors.

Malignancies of connective tissue are called *sarcomas*. When the tissue of origin can be identified, the appropriate prefix is used as well, such as fibrosarcoma, chondrosarcoma, and osteosarcoma. Anaplastic malignant tumors of epithelial or connective tissue origin are called *spheroidal cell carcinoma* and *spindle cell* or *round cell sarcoma* to describe the appearance of the tumor cells. Sarcomas are usually grayish-pink in color. Well-differentiated sarcomas resemble to some extent the tissue of origin, but as dedifferentiation increases, they become essentially formless, spindle-shaped or ovoid. High mitotic activity.and pleomorphism of cells are usually apparent. Areas of necrosis are common, and sometimes the tumor may be almost entirely necrotic. Cancers, especially sarcomas, frequently show areas of hemorrhage. A tumor in the wall of a hollow viscus may ulcerate and become infected, resulting in hemorrhage. Ironically, although such tumors possess fantastic powers of growth, they have little regenerative ability; once the surface ulcerates, healing is unlikely.

SARCOMAS
QUALIFIED
ACCORDING
TO TISSUE

Neoplasms of the Reticuloendothelial (RE) System

RE SYSTEM
TUMORS
ALWAYS
MALIGNANT

Tumors of the RE system differ from other sarcomas in their clinical and pathologic characteristics. Neoplasms originating in leukocyte-forming tissue—the leukemias—may be myeloid (granulocytic) or lymphoid (lymphocytic). The blood contains large numbers of white cells, which may be primitive. Plasma cell myeloma (myelomatosis or multiple myeloma) is an important tumor affecting the bone marrow which becomes packed with plasma cells. These deposits may give rise to osteolytic lesions of bone, particularly in the skull, that resemble "punched out" defects. Masses of plasma cells may also be present in soft tissue.

RE system tumors may occur throughout the body. The most important are reticulum cell sarcoma (reticulosarcoma) and lymphosarcoma. Many or all of the lymph nodes, the spleen, and sometimes the liver and bone marrow are affected. Masses of neoplastic cells may also be found in other tissues; lymphosarcoma may, for example, be associated with lymphocytic leukemia.

Hodgkin's disease (multiple lymphadenoma) is generally considered a neoplasm of the RE system. This disease involves the lymph nodes, spleen, liver, bone marrow, and sometimes the skin and other soft tissues.

Neoplasms of the Brain and Nerve Sheaths

Tumors of the neuroglia and of the ependyma are called *gliomas*. Untreated glioma of the brain can cause death from intracranial pressure, and in the spinal cord it is usually fatal because of tissue damage. Hence, gliomas are usually regarded as malignant. The faster growing and more pleomorphic of these tumors are called *glioblastomas*. They vary greatly in growth rate and degree of invasion into surrounding brain tissue, and unlike other malignant tumors, they never metastasize outside the central nervous system. Nerve sheath tumors, such as neurilemmomas, are usually benign.

Neoplasms of Embryonic Origin

In addition to epithelial and connective tissue tumors, there are developmental tumors. These may be subdivided into three main groups: teratomas; tumors associated with aberrant development of one organ; and chorion carcinoma (also called *choriocarcinoma* and *chorionepithelioma*).

Teratomas, which originate from embryonic cells, may be present at birth, and although they usually occur in young persons, they may not become evident until middle age. Teratomas may be either benign or malignant. These lesions often are cystic, in which case they are called *dermoid cysts*. This form is especially likely to be seen in the ovaries. Teratomas of the testes are usually malignant.

Tumors caused by defective embryonal development of a single organ arise in infancy or early life, or may develop prenatally. *All* are malignant. Wilms' tumor of the kidney (nephroblastoma) is of this type, as are neuroblastoma, found mainly in the adrenal medulla, and retinoblastoma, in the eye.

The chorion is the fetal part of the placenta. Chorion carcinoma, which obviously develops after the start of a pregnancy, arises from the epithelial covering of the chorion. This tumor is preceded in many cases by a hydatidiform mole. The mole is essentially innocent, but should it develop into a chorion carcinoma, the carcinoma will be highly malignant.

There are several tumor-like formations that are benign. The hamartoma is a tumor-like nodule consisting of an abnormal arrangement of normal components of an organ. Hemangioma, a benign tumor consisting of newly formed blood vessels, and lymphangioma, composed of newly formed lymph spaces and channels, are similarly classified. These formations do not undergo malignant transformation; they present symptoms chiefly because they displace other tissues.

ROUTES OF SPREAD

INVASIVENESS
MOST
CRITICAL
FACTOR IN
MALIGNANT
TUMORS

The chief obstacles to effective treatment of malignant neoplasms are their ability to grow invasively and their capacity to metastasize. Of the two, invasive growth is the more important, for metastasis could not occur without it. Secondary growths occur frequently in certain sites, whereas other organs and tissues are only rarely involved. The lymph nodes, lungs, liver, and skeleton are common sites of secondary tumor growth, while the spleen and skeletal muscle are relatively immune. Circulatory factors that influence the distribution and localization of all types of particulate matter (for example, embolism) are responsible in large measure for the dissemination of tumors. This is known as *hematogenous spread*. There is also a definite tendency for certain tumors to metastasize to certain tissues. Thus, carcinoma of the lung frequently metastasizes to the adrenal glands and to the brain, while carcinoma of the prostate has a strong tendency to metastasize to bone.

There are some broad differences in the routes of spread of carcinomas and sarcomas. Carcinomas primarily invade the lymphatics, frequently setting up metastatic foci in regional lymph nodes relatively early. In-

HOW CANCER SPREADS

Direct Invasion

Venous

Lymphatics

Implantation

vasion of blood vessels and more distant secondary growth usually occur much later. Sarcomas, on the other hand, spread mainly through the bloodstream and produce distant secondary growths early, quite frequently in the lungs. Tumor cells may be carried through such pathways as the renal tract or the bronchial tree to sites relatively far from the primary tumor.

In making a prognosis following removal of a primary tumor, the extent of spread through the lymphatics to regional lymph nodes is of great significance. Once the tumor cells have reached the first line of regional lymph nodes, they may be carried to the more distant nodes, in some instances reaching most of the groups in the body. Sometimes many groups of nodes, including the superficial ones, are involved before the primary tumor becomes evident clinically. Thus, the patient may show clinical features suggesting a primary lesion of the lymph nodes.

Transcelomic spread takes place when tumor cells that have been shed into a serous cavity implant themselves onto the serosa and form new tumors. Malignant glial tumors spread in this way. The glioma sheds cells into the ventricles and subarachnoid space, and these cells circulate throughout the space via the cerebrospinal fluid, implanting themselves at various sites along the way.

A surgical operation done for the purpose of excising a tumor may instead be the cause of tumor spread. The tumor cells may be "seeded" into surrounding tissues during the course of surgery. Then too, these cells contaminate instruments, gloves, and even the basin of water into which the surgeon dips his gloved hands. Therefore, it is essential that every item that may have become contaminated while biopsy material was being obtained be replaced before subsequent procedures are begun.

CAUSES OF CANCER

Studies in experimental animals have shown that many agents or factors cause or predispose to neoplasia. It is reasonable to assume that in man, some tumors arise as a direct consequence of particular environmental factors. The causative agents are *carcinogens,* and these include chemical agents, physical agents, viruses, and even hormones. Sometimes disease or chronic irritation predisposes to cancer. Genetic factors also play an important role in neoplasia.

SOME CAUSATIVE AGENTS CLEARLY IDENTIFIED

Chemical Carcinogens

In 1775, Sir Percivall Pott observed the high incidence of carcinoma of the scrotum in the chimney sweeps of England, and proposed a *causal relationship* between that carcinoma and the tarry soot left in the chimneys by the low-grade coal then used in domestic fires. One hundred forty years later, in 1915, Pott's theory was substantiated by two Japanese workers, Yamagiwa and Ichikawa, who produced papillomas and carcinomas in the skin of rabbits' ears by the long-continued application of tar. Their work focused attention upon chemical carcinogens.

Further studies showed that carcinomas sometimes developed in patients to whom arsenic—once the mainstay in treatment of syphilis—had been administered over long periods, and in persons whose work involved the use of arsenic. Carcinoma of the urinary bladder was found where aniline dyes were produced. Only a small proportion of the exposed population developed tumors, sometimes after years of exposure, and in some cases the tumors did not appear until years after the final exposure to the carcinogen. These observations fostered the idea that some essential preliminary change occurs prior to the development of malignant disease and that after a long latent period, this type of change might finally result in neoplasia. Indeed, experiments have shown that a tissue exposed to a carcinogen for a short period of time undergoes transient changes. These changes do not in themselves lead to tumor formation. Instead, they regress, leaving no trace. However, there remains a state of predisposition to tumor formation, so that subsequent exposure to a wide range of nonspecific irritant substances, such as phenols, turpentine, chloroform, nonionic detergents, and croton oil, may stimulate tumor growth. Thus, an *initiating agent* renders a tissue susceptible to tumor formation by producing an instantaneous change in the cells—a somatic mutation. Subsequent long-continued exposure to a second carcinogen, called a *promoting agent*, then results in neoplasia. Since neither of these agents can cause neoplasia without the help of the other, they are often called *co-carcinogens*.

Attempts to relate chemical structure to carcinogenic ability have not been fruitful. The various chemicals used in experimental carcinogenesis are not known to share any specific attribute other than their ability to stimulate tumor growth.

The cause-and-effect relationship between tobacco smoking and malignant neoplasms has been proven unequivocally. Pipe smokers and tobacco chewers are vulnerable to carcinoma of the buccal cavity and tongue. Hot food and drink, as well as strong unrefined alcohol, may contribute to the development of carcinoma of the buccal cavity. Carcinomas of the pharynx and esophagus occur predominantly among smokers and heavy drinkers. Carcinoma of the bladder has been demonstrated among cigar smokers, indicating that tobacco contains a carcinogen that is excreted in the urine. Rats have developed malignant tumors after carcinogens isolated from tobacco were painted onto them. Similarly, malignant change has been experimentally induced in the respiratory epithelium in animals by forced inhalation of tobacco smoke. The

United States Department of Health, Education, and Welfare has published statistical evidence associating tobacco consumption with carcinoma of the respiratory, intestinal, and genitourinary tracts.

Physical Carcinogens

Ionizing radiation is acknowledged to be a carcinogen. The pioneers of radiology were frequently the victims of squamous carcinoma of the skin, and more recently, a higher incidence of leukemia has been found among radiologists than in the general public. X-ray examination of the abdomen during pregnancy is a contributing factor in leukemia of early childhood. Prolonged exposure to sunlight has long been known to produce carcinoma of the skin in many instances.

Heat may be carcinogenic. Carcinoma of the lower lip was common in the days when men habitually smoked clay pipes; possibly it was caused by repeated heating of the mucosa. In Kashmir, where the winters are extremely cold, inhabitants who bind small charcoal braziers to their abdomens are likely to develop squamous carcinoma of the abdominal wall.

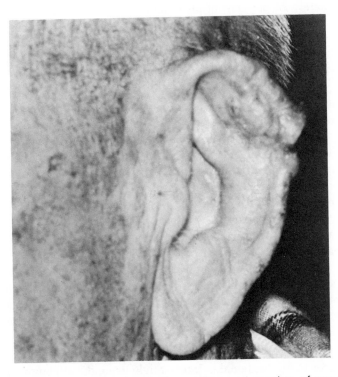

Carcinoma of left ear, showing both swelling and erosion of ear margin. There is danger that a lesion of this severity has already invaded the lymphatics.

Viruses

In 1911, Peyton Rous first induced tumor growth in birds by inoculating them with a tumor extract containing a virus. Subsequently, Rous and others discovered a number of other carcinoma viruses. In 1935, Shope described a papilloma produced in the rabbit by a virus. Since then, other malignant diseases in animals have been found to be of viral etiology. Although we have no definite proof, it is likely that viruses cause at least some types of human leukemia and possibly other types of cancer as well. In fact, many investigators are collecting much evidence for the critical role that viruses may play in causation of cancer, and this exploration is assuming an increasingly important place in our overall understanding of cancer.

Hormones

Hormones may act as carcinogens, i.e., they may both initiate and promote tumor growth. The carcinogenic effect will be manifest only in the organ on which the hormone has physiological effect. For example, approximately 25 per cent of all terminal human cancers develop in the breast, the uterus, the ovaries, and the prostate; yet women whose ovaries were removed early in life do not develop breast cancer, and males similarly do not develop cancer of the prostate when the testes have been removed.

In some way that is not yet entirely understood, an endocrine imbalance initiates the process. After prolonged exposure of the susceptible tissue to the hormones, hypertrophy of the target organ occurs. Nodules develop that are benign at first but later become cancerous. At first, the tumor is hormone-dependent, requiring continual stimulation by the initiating hormone. At some point, the tumor becomes autonomous, no longer requiring hormonal stimulation.

Controversy continues about the possible carcinogenic effect of estrogen therapy for menopausal symptoms. It is strongly suspected that prolonged use of estrogen will induce neoplastic changes in the uterus and the breast, tissues that are extremely sensitive to estrogen.

A few additional points might be cited in regard to the action of hormones in inducing cancer. Estrogen therapy, often employed for the treatment of cancer of the prostate, has occasionally led to carcinoma of the breast in the male subject. Boyd reports that in the African Bantu suffering from liver inadequacy caused by dietary deficits, cancer of the breast and breast enlargement often occur in the male, and fibromas of the uterus in the female. Interestingly enough, although mammary cancer does not appear spontaneously in the rat, it can be stimulated by giving estrogens. Perhaps because of the natural resistance of the rat to cancer of the breast, such a tumor remains dependent on the hormone, whereas in the mouse the carcinoma ultimately becomes independent of hormonal influence.

Premalignant States

Some pathologic conditions tend to eventuate in cancer. Several types of malignant neoplasms in man appear to be causally related to previous disease or chronic irritation of the involved area. The lesions of syphilitic glossitis and the chronic irritation due to gallstones are examples of disease states known to be associated with cancer. Broken or carious teeth that chronically irritate the mucous membranes of the mouth and tongue are associated with carcinoma of the buccal cavity. Patients with ulcerative colitis, in which long-standing colonic ulceration is accompanied by regenerative hyperplasia of the intervening mucosa, develop colonic carcinoma much more frequently than does the normal population. Metaplasia is sometimes associated with malignant neoplasms resulting from chronic irritation. In this process, a specialized epithelium becomes transformed into one more resistant to trauma, such as squamous epithelium. The best known example of this process is the squamous change appearing in the bronchi of heavy smokers. This is the probable cause of carcinoma of the lung in many cases. Senile keratosis and leukoplakia are further examples of malignant metaplasia. Breast carcinoma is preceded in many cases by fibroadenosis, that is, proliferation of cells lining the ducts. Papilloma of the large intestine or of the bladder is considered a premalignant, or precancerous, condition.

CHRONIC IRRITATION A CONTRIBUTING FACTOR

Genetic Factors

It is certain that heredity is a predisposing factor in development of neoplasia. In mice bred for cancer study, a great majority of the females in certain strains (high-cancer strains) develop carcinoma of the breast, while in other strains (low-cancer strains) the incidence is low. The hereditary factor seems to be all-important. It is reasonable to assume that heredity also plays an important role in human cancer; however, good supporting evidence for this view is not available in most cases.

Although there is little evidence to link heredity to any of the common malignant diseases of man, some facts are known. For example, carcinoma of the stomach occurs most frequently in persons of blood group A. In a few human tumors the familial susceptibility is so pronounced that every member of the family will die of a particular type of cancer if he lives long enough. We also know that the genetic material of malignant cells is altered, possibly a result of mutation. All carcinogens, be they

INFLUENCE OF HEREDITY ACKNOWLEDGED ALTHOUGH EXTENT NOT YET CLARIFIED chemical, physical, or viral, probably operate by altering the genetic material of the cells. Variations in chromosome number and form have been found in all malignant neoplasms examined; in fact, none has shown a normal number of chromosomes. Therefore, it seems likely that similar changes occur in most, if not all, malignant tumors.

EFFECTS OF NEOPLASIA

A neoplasm can cause disease or death in several ways. It may distort important anatomical relationships, as by obstructing the lower end of the esophagus or the urethra. It may give rise to an ulcer on a mucous surface, resulting in hemorrhage or sepsis. Or it may produce disease by a more subtle process, known as the *competitive struggle* or *nitrogen trap,* described below.

To build their protoplasm, all growing tissues require raw materials and an energy source. Rapidly growing neoplastic cells, which require large supplies of amino acids and nitrogen for their continuous protein synthesis, compete with normal cells for the available metabolites in the extracellular fluid. Because of their greater ability to metabolize amino acids, the tumor cells win the struggle, and the emaciated normal cells are soon replaced by neoplastic cells. The atrophy and necrosis of normal cells commonly seen at the edge of a rapidly growing tumor are usually attributed to pressure; however, since it is not clear why neoplastic cells are not also affected by the pressure, it appears more reasonable that they are the victors in the competitive struggle for metabolites.

Systemic symptoms, which may result from the primary tumor itself or from metastatic growth, may appear months or even years before the primary growth is found. Several vague symptoms, such as fatigue, weight loss, loss of appetite, and anemia, commonly seen in many clinical conditions are also associated with cancer. We shall not go into them. Apart from these, the most important systemic symptoms may be divided into four main groups: (1) dermatological, (2) vascular, (3) hormonal, and (4) neuromuscular.

NUTRITIONAL COMPETITION BETWEEN NORMAL CELLS AND NEOPLASTIC CELLS

Dermatological Symptoms

Overt signs of carcinoma may be preceded or followed by a wide range of dermatitides and dermatoses. Of these, acanthosis nigricans was the first to be found associated with neoplasia. In this disorder there is increased pigmentation and hypertrophy, causing a dark, velvety thickening of the skin on the neck, groin, and axillae, and frequently around the nipples and umbilicus. In the adult, this dermatosis is associated with a highly malignant, rapidly fatal adenocarcinoma, usually of the stomach. It has been suggested that the dermatologic symptoms may result from an immune response to breakdown products of the tumor, which act as antigens.

Pruritus with hyperpigmentation and dermatitis herpetiformis may be the first clue to neoplasia. Herpes zoster is seen twice as frequently in carcinoma patients as in the normal population. Dermatomyositis may indicate the presence of carcinoma or adenocarcinoma.

Vascular Symptoms

Phlebitis, especially the type known as thrombophlebitis migrans, involving numerous unusual sites may suggest neoplasia long before the tumor is evident. The tumor is most commonly found in the lung or in the pancreas. A migrating phlebitis associated with carcinoma is known as Trousseau's syndrome, for the French physician who discovered this association in himself. The resulting thromboses, which are not affected by anticoagulants, occur in such unusual sites as the neck, upper extremities, and axillae. Thrombosis develops in 30 per cent of the cases before the tumor is obvious; although numerous theories have been offered to explain this phenomenon, none has been proved.

One third of the patients with mucin-producing adenocarcinoma of the stomach, lung, or pancreas also have nonbacterial verrucal endocarditis, an accumulation of fibrin on the heart valves. The carcinoid syndrome, associated with metastatic carcinoma of the liver, is marked by episodic blushing, cardiopulmonary distress, and chronic diarrhea.

Hormonal Symptoms

Certain tumors of nonendocrine origin may secrete agents having a hormone-like action. Sometimes these tumors stimulate the endocrine glands to overproduce the hormones, and thereby bring about a disease state. Cushing's syndrome, gynecomastia, hypercalcemia, and hypoglycemia are examples of such activity.

Cushing's syndrome presents a striking example of hormonal hyperactivity. The lesion is usually an adenoma or a carcinoma of the adrenal cortex, and occasionally is an adenoma of the anterior pituitary; a nonendocrine tumor may produce a similar clinical picture. In Cushing's syndrome due to a nonendocrine tumor, there is frequently severe hypokalemic alkalosis and other features rarely seen in the classic form. An anaplastic oat-cell bronchial carcinoma is the causative lesion in 80 per cent of such cases. The most likely explanation for this phenomenon is that the bronchial tumor secretes sufficient circulating ACTH-like material to promote increased adrenal output of cortisol with suppression of normal pituitary ACTH.

Gynecomastia stems from disturbed estrogen production and may be the only clinical symptom of bronchogenic carcinoma or hepatoma. The tumor apparently secretes gonadotropin, which is elaborated normally only by the pituitary and placenta.

Neoplasms of the breast, lung, and kidney give rise to various metabolic disorders, of which hypercalcemia bears mention. Five to 10 per cent of cases of squamous carcinoma of the lung manifest hypertrophic pulmonary osteoarthropathy. Hypoglycemia is a frequent finding in retroperitoneal fibrosarcoma. Polycythemia sometimes accompanies a benign or malignant tumor of kidney or other organs.

Neuromuscular Symptoms

Carcinomatous neuromyopathies occur in about 5 per cent of all cases of bronchogenic carcinoma. In visceral carcinoma, it is not known how the associated neuromuscular symptoms are produced, as they do not result from metastasis or direct pressure of the tumor. The neurological symptoms may appear long before the tumor is diagnosed and may subside when the tumor is removed.

One of the important neuromuscular syndromes found with carcinoma is corticocerebellar degeneration. This disorder comes on quickly and progresses so rapidly that within a few weeks after onset, the patient cannot walk or stand. Peripheral neuropathies, which may be motor, sensory, or both, and subacute spinocerebellar degeneration are also associated with cancer. In all of these, there are degenerative changes in the corresponding neurones, but the cause cannot be explained.

Carcinomatous myopathies provide another example of the remote and unexplained effects of neoplasia. The effects may be muscular only, as in polymyositis, or neuromuscular, producing a myasthenia-like syndrome.

DISEASE MODEL: CARCINOMA OF THE STOMACH

Carcinoma of the stomach is an important cause of death due to cancer in the United States. It afflicts all age groups but is most commonly seen in patients 50 to 69 years of age. The lesion may develop in any part of the stomach, but it is seen most often in the antrum, lesser curvature, cardia, and fundus. Occasionally there are multiple tumors.

The carcinoma is spread by several routes. There may be direct invasion to the liver, pancreas, and transverse colon and, via the lymphatics, to lymph nodes. Metastasis to lymph nodes occurs early. Because the tumor grows within the wall of the stomach, it frequently invades the lower esophagus. The carcinoma cells are also carried by the transcelomic route throughout the peritoneal cavity, so that a secondary tumor of the ovary often develops. Cells carried by the bloodstream most commonly lead to metastases of liver, lungs, and bone. Pulmonary metastases are often diffuse.

Unfortunately, in most cases there are no early symptoms; by the time the patient seeks medical advice, the tumor has usually spread to tissues outside the stomach. In fact, gastric ulceration, obstruction, necrosis, or immobility may develop before symptoms are noted.

The most commonly observed symptoms are weight loss, pain or indigestion, weakness, loss of appetite, and vomiting, of which weight loss (usually 10 to 15 pounds when the patient is first seen) is the most common. Pain, loss of appetite, vomiting, and difficulty in swallowing contribute to inadequate caloric intake.

Abdominal pain is poorly localized and may be described by the patient as "pressure," "fullness," "ache," or "bloating." The sensation is hard to describe, and many patients refer to it as "indigestion" or "gas." Patients sometimes take it upon themselves to take antacids or other ulcer preparations, which sometimes provide temporary relief. Such symptomatic treatment is dangerous, for the patient, having found relief, may not seek medical attention until it is too late for curative treatment.

Loss of appetite is remarkably common, even when other symptoms that would discourage eating are absent. Or, the patient may feel full after eating one or two mouthfuls of food even if his appetite is normal. The increase in the connective tissue in the stomach lining, rendering the walls rigid and hard—the "leather bottle" stomach—severely limits stomach capacity. The consequent poor nutritional status, plus the anemia that is found in two thirds of the patients, results in marked weakness.

Vomiting may indicate that the neoplasm has invaded the prepyloric area and is causing intermittent obstruction. Vomiting of blood is rare and is not profuse when it does develop. This feature is most commonly associated with tumors of the cardiac region.

As the carcinoma spreads, further symptoms develop. Difficulty in swallowing occurs when the esophagus is involved. Metastases of the liver may produce jaundice. Bone pain may occur as a result of pathologic fracture at a metastatic site.

The only effective treatment modality in carcinoma of the stomach is surgical removal of part or all of the stomach, yet even then, the results are poor. The most favorable data indicate that 70 per cent of patients who undergo "curative" surgery die within 5 years, for a survival rate of only 30 per cent. The 5-year survival rate of all patients with stomach cancer, whether operated upon or not, is 5 to 10 per cent. The growth behavior of the neoplasm is the most important factor influencing prognosis. If the lesion is not confined to the stomach, the 5-year survival rate is only 7 per cent.

Dismal as these figures are, there is a bright side in the picture of gastric carcinoma. For reasons that are not understood, the incidence

GASTRIC CARCINOMA MAY MIMIC OTHER DISORDERS IN EARLY STAGE

of this carcinoma is definitely decreasing in the United States. Dietary habits are thought to be important. To cite one example of this probable relationship: The incidence of gastric carcinoma is high in countries where an important item in the diet is smoked fish. The carcinogen is believed to be not the fish itself, but 3:4 benzpyrene, a chemical agent used in the smoking process. Such findings typify our slow—yet measurable and definite—progress in the battle against cancer.

CLINICAL CONSIDERATIONS

In recent years, great advances in medical science have virtually eliminated a number of fatal diseases and have extended the normal life span. With an increasing number of people reaching old age, the incidence of cancer has risen proportionately. Although many cancers can be treated successfully by surgical removal or radiotherapy (x-ray or radium), cancer is still a leading cause of death. Until that bright day when cancer can be considered a disease of the past, the nurse or other medical attendant undoubtedly will have to care for many of its victims.

CANCER PATIENT NEEDS SUPERIOR CARE BY ALL HEALTH WORKERS

With an understanding in depth of how the disease develops and progresses, one can do much to benefit the patient. From the prophylactic standpoint, the patient who has a suspicious lesion can be advised to have it checked by a physician. Should surgery be deemed advisable, the

INCIDENCE OF CANCER BY SITE AND SEX ✱

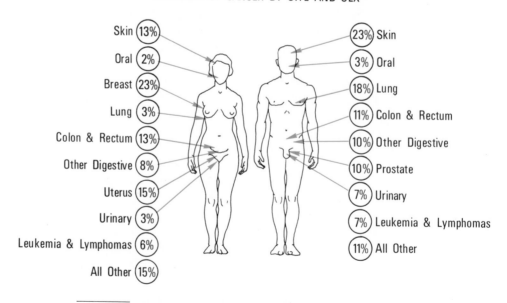

Skin (13%)   (23%) Skin
Oral (2%)   (3%) Oral
Breast (23%)   (18%) Lung
Lung (3%)   (11%) Colon & Rectum
Colon & Rectum (13%) (10%) Other Digestive
Other Digestive (8%) (10%) Prostate
Uterus (15%)   (7%) Urinary
Urinary (3%)   (7%) Leukemia & Lymphomas
Leukemia & Lymphomas (6%) (11%) All Other
All Other (15%)

* Ca—A Cancer Journal for Clinicians. January–February, 1971.

surgeon will take every possible precaution to halt the process, by removing the lesion in its entirety along with a cuff of normal tissue.

Some patients have had a recent history of weight loss. One who understands the competitive struggle between neoplastic and normal cells knows that an advancing malignancy will ultimately result in cachexia and that everything possible must be done to sustain body weight and to conserve energy. Proper nutrition is of prime importance. Everything possible should be done to see that the patient receives an attractive, high-protein, vitamin-rich diet, adequate not only to maintain his nutrition, but to help him gain weight. Since anorexia is so frequent, the patient should be encouraged to eat. If he indicates a desire for certain foods, every effort should be made to provide them if they are not contraindicated by his condition. If oral intake is not possible, one makes sure that feedings by other routes are given at the intervals prescribed by the physician. The patient should be observed for signs of diarrhea or abdominal distress; such findings should be reported to the physician.

Conservation of energy is extremely important, and attendants can do much in this respect. The bedfast patient may become constipated or develop a fecal impaction. When a patient is expending a great deal of energy in bowel movements, administration of a gentle cathartic or enema will make the bowel movement easier, thus conserving the patient's energy. Pain is another source of energy expense in some patients. If the physician has left a p.r.n. order for pain medication, the drug should be administered as indicated by the patient's condition. The patient should be observed to see that he derives the desired effect.

Emotional stress contributes to energy expenditure. Therefore, the patient should be given full psychological support. Then too, his family cannot be ignored but must be given the same considerate interest and assistance as he. With a thorough knowledge of neoplastic disease, one can help family members to understand what they are facing and how to deal with it.

In the later stages, energy conservation is no longer an active therapeutic goal but a matter of personal comfort to the patient. Maintenance of an adequate fluid balance also contributes to the patient's comfort and should be undertaken even if parenteral administration becomes necessary.

Every effort should be made to prevent bedsores from developing in the cachectic patient. Necrotic tissue provides an excellent medium for bacterial growth, so all open lesions should be treated with precise aseptic technique. An infected necrotic ulcer can rarely be controlled satisfactorily since the cachectic patient is unable to heal.

It is most important for the health worker to have wide knowledge of both benign and malignant disease in order to participate in therapy. For example, he should know how important it is to observe the patient meticulously for untoward signs and symptoms following treatment and to report any unusual effects to the physician.

For the patient who has been successfully treated, one can be helpful in referring him to community agencies concerned with rehabilitation. And finally, one should be aware of the possibility of recurrence and should emphasize the importance of regular checkups to the patient and his family.

Much can be done to benefit the patient, even if his disease is terminal. A broad knowledge of neoplasia is an absolute necessity if one is to be truly competent in caring for patients with neoplastic disease.

TOPICS FOR DISCUSSION

1. Is there one criterion that distinguishes absolutely between a benign and a malignant neoplasm?
2. What is it that keeps so many people with early neoplastic lesions from consulting the physician?
3. Is a routine annual physical examination sufficient to detect early neoplasms?
4. Would you favor educational seminars to enable lay people to detect the early signs of cancer?
5. Does cancer have one or many causes?
6. Fifty years ago, many people considered it a disgrace to have a malignant tumor. Do you have any ideas about why this was so?
7. How do you account for the great increase in the incidence of neoplasms in the United States?
8. If a person has once had a malignancy, even a skin carcinoma, that was entirely removed, will he be susceptible to others? Why?
9. Name some growths that have not been established as either neoplastic or non-neoplastic.
10. What does the term "nitrogen trap" mean to you? In this connection, do neoplastic cells have anything in common with bacteria?
11. Why do you think some persons continue to smoke even though they know that the practice positively increases their chances of contracting lung cancer?

BIBLIOGRAPHY

Books

Hopps, H.: Principles of Pathology. New York, Appleton-Century-Crofts, 1964.
The Merck Manual of Diagnosis and Therapy. Rahway, New Jersey, Merck Sharp & Dohme Research Laboratories, 1966.

Sodeman, W., and Sodeman, W.: Pathologic Physiology. Philadelphia, W. B. Saunders Co., 1967.

Douthwaite, A.: French's Index of Differential Diagnosis. Baltimore, The Williams & Wilkins Co., 1967.

Levine, M.: Introduction to Clinical Nursing. Philadelphia, F. A. Davis Co., 1969.

Boyd, W.: A Textbook of Pathology. pp. 213–302. Philadelphia, Lea & Febiger, 1970.

Passmore, R., and Robson, J.: A Companion to Medical Studies. vol. 2, pp. 28.1–28.18. Philadelphia, F. A. Davis Co., 1970.

8

disturbances of fluid and electrolyte balance

Life was born in water and is carrying on in water. Water is life's mater *and* matrix, *mother and medium. There is no life without water. Life could leave the ocean when it learned to grow a skin, a bag in which to take the water with it. We are still living in water, having the water now inside.*
—Albert Szent-Györgyi *

The human body may look—and even feel—like a solid, yet it is approximately two thirds liquid. These liquids, called *body fluids*, are essential to every single one of the billions of body cells. As long as the volume and chemical composition of body fluids remain within certain narrow limits, the body enjoys health. Should these values, however, deviate even slightly from the safe bounds of normal, disease results.

Diseases involving body fluids are called *body fluid disturbances* or *body fluid imbalances*. The disturbances may be primary, such as the sodium deficit that occurs when one sweats profusely and drinks only plain water; or, they may occur secondarily to other conditions, such as the carbonic acid excess (respiratory acidosis) that often accompanies pneumonia. Body fluid disturbances accompany such a host of illnesses that every patient with a serious illness is a potential victim of one or more of them. Even the patient who is only moderately or mildly ill may be stricken. There may be only one imbalance or a combination of two or more.

In this chapter, we shall see that there are several types of body fluids, each having its own unique composition and specialized function. We shall see that body fluids are gained and lost in a number of ways and that abnormal gains or losses greatly affect man's health. In our discussion of body fluid disturbances, we shall employ the *clinical picture approach*

---

* Szent-Györgyi, Albert: Biology and Pathology of Water. Chicago, Ill., Perspectives in Biology and Medicine, Winter 1971. The University of Chicago Press. © 1971 by The University of Chicago. All rights reserved.

introduced by Moyer and later expanded by Snively and Sweeney: 16 basic imbalances will be presented as separate clinical entities. Understanding the basic imbalances is a necessary prelude to understanding the combinations and the interrelationships between imbalances and other disease states. Finally, we shall see that an understanding of body fluid disturbances is quite relevant to daily patient care.

NATURE OF BODY FLUID

Water and certain dissolved substances called *electrolytes* are the chief components of body fluid. Electrolytes are salts or minerals that manifest electrical charges when they are placed in water. Those with positive charges are *cations* and include such substances as sodium (Na), potassium (K), calcium (Ca), and magnesium (Mg). Such substances as chloride (Cl), bicarbonate (HCO_3), sulfate (SO_4), phosphate (PO_4), and proteinate possess negative charges. These are *anions*. The term *ion* includes both cations and anions.

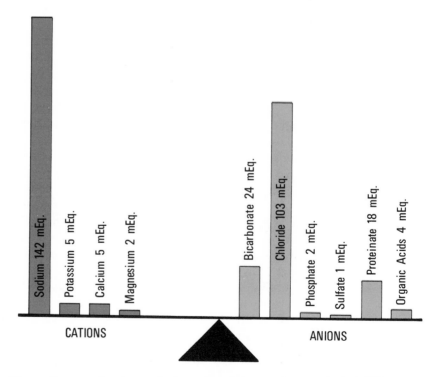

The cations and anions of plasma are shown. Note how the cations expressed in milliequivalents, balance the anions, expressed in milliequivalents.

MICROSCOPIC ANATOMY OF BODY FLUIDS

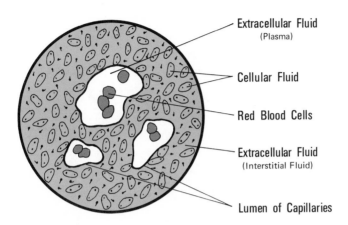

When any electrolyte is dissolved in water, the positive and negative charges balance. The number of positive or negative charges is expressed as an *equivalent*. One equivalent is that quantity of an ionized substance having the same number of charges as 1 gram molecular weight of a univalent substance, such as hydrogen. Essentially, this method allows one to determine the concentration of solutions by measuring the number of molecules of solute rather than the weight of the solute. For convenience, however, the unit of equivalence is usually the milliequivalent (mEq.), 1/1,000 of an equivalent.

The body fluid is divided into two parts. Approximately three fourths of the total body fluid is contained within the body cells. This portion is called *cellular,* or *intracellular, fluid.* The remaining one fourth exists outside the cells and is known as *extracellular fluid.* Plasma accounts for approximately one fourth of the extracellular fluid. The remainder exists as interstitial fluid, being found in the interstitial spaces between cells. Lymph is regarded as a special form of interstitial fluid. Electrolyte composition of plasma, interstitial, and cellular fluid are shown in the table (p. 136).

The extracellular fluid is vital in maintaining the health of body cells. It provides them with a proper environment; it supplies them with substances, such as food, vitamins, oxygen, water, and electrolytes needed for proper function; and it carries away their waste products. Exchanges between cellular and extracellular fluid occur constantly and are of tremendous magnitude. In addition to keeping the cells healthy, extracellular fluid supplies the water and electrolytes needed for secretion and excretion (saliva, gastric juice, intestinal juice, pancreatic juice, bile, nasal secretions, urine, feces, and perspiration). All this activity greatly alters the composition of the extracellular fluid. The chemical regulatory activities carried out by the homeostatic mechanisms maintain the volume and chemical composition of the extracellular fluid within normal limits. Should these mechanisms fail, as they sometimes do, the results can be catastrophic.

EXTRACELLULAR
FLUID
MAINTAINS
CELL
ENVIRONMENT

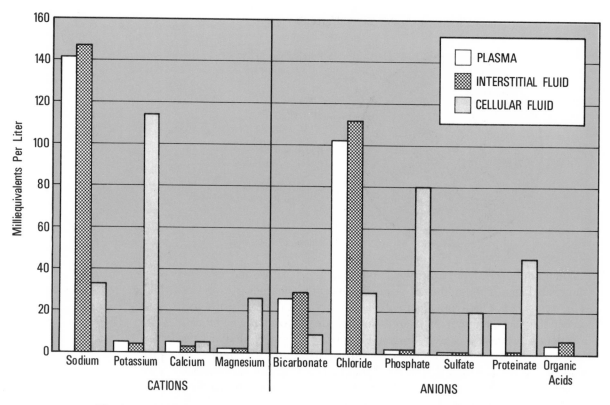

The ions of cellular and extracellular fluid. Plasma contains much proteinate anion, interstitial fluid, almost none; sodium is the chief cation of extracellular fluid, potassium of cellular fluid. The anions chloride and bicarbonate dominate extracellular fluid, phosphate and proteinate, cellular fluid.

GAINS AND LOSSES

The body gains and loses water and electrolytes in various ways. Water alone is gained by drinking distilled water and by oxidation of foodstuffs and body tissues. Softened water, well water, mineral water, most city water supplies, and food provide both water and electrolytes. Hospitalized patients frequently gain water and electrolytes via nasogastric tube, intravenous needle, or rectal tube.

Normal losses of both water and electrolytes occur through the lungs in breath, through the eyes in tears, through the kidneys in urine, through the skin in perspiration, and through the intestines in defecation. In addition, water alone is lost through the skin in insensible perspiration, which goes on constantly. Abnormal losses can occur during illness or injury, as in burn or wound exudate, hemorrhage, vomiting, and diarrhea. Rapid breathing, suction via gastric or intestinal tube, enterostomy, colostomy, and cecostomy also cause great losses of water and electrolytes. Drainage from sites of surgical operations or from abscesses contains both water and electrolytes, as does fluid extracted via paracentesis. Fluids surrounding the brain and spinal cord can be lost if there is an abnormal opening to the outside. Strange as it may seem, fluids may be lost even inside the body. When abnormal closed collections of fluid develop, as in intestinal obstruction, these fluids are just as useless to the body economy as if they were outside the body.

We can see that fluids are gained and lost in many ways. In the healthy adult, the volume of urine excreted is approximately equal to the volume of fluid ingested as fluid; and water derived from solid food and from chemical oxidation in the body approximately equals the normal losses

"STEADY STATE" DISTURBED DURING ILLNESS

IMBALANCES RESULTING FROM LOSS OF SPECIFIC BODY FLUID

Fluid Lost	Imbalances Likely to Occur
Gastric juice	Extracellular fluid volume deficit Metabolic alkalosis Sodium deficit Potassium deficit Tetany (if metabolic alkalosis present) Ketosis of starvation Magnesium deficit
Intestinal juice	Extracellular fluid volume deficit Metabolic acidosis Sodium deficit Potassium deficit
Bile	Sodium deficit Metabolic acidosis
Pancreatic juice	Metabolic acidosis Sodium deficit Calcium deficit Extracellular fluid volume deficit
Sensible perspiration	Extracellular fluid volume deficit Sodium deficit
Insensible water loss	Water deficit (dehydration) Sodium excess
Wound exudate	Protein deficit Sodium deficit Extracellular fluid volume deficit
Ascites	Protein deficit Sodium deficit Plasma-to-interstitial fluid shift Extracellular fluid volume deficit

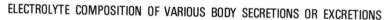

ELECTROLYTE COMPOSITION OF VARIOUS BODY SECRETIONS OR EXCRETIONS

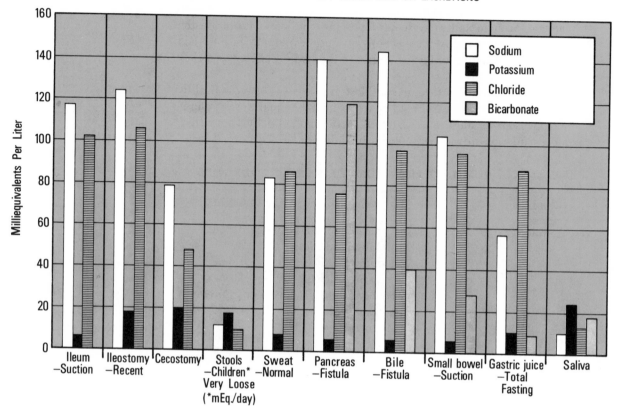

of water through the lungs and skin and in the stool. Thus, the gains approximately equal the losses. During illness, however, gains and losses are not always equal. Intake of food and fluids may cease or diminish, while the normal losses continue. The losses may outweigh the gains by one half liter or more a day. The daily losses are cumulative, so that a serious deficit can develop in a short time. If abnormal losses are occurring as well, as in vomiting or diarrhea, the patient may become gravely ill within a matter of hours. The type of imbalance caused depends upon the kind of fluid lost. Body secretions and excretions vary greatly in their electrolyte compositions and in their total concentrations of electrolytes.

Serious imbalances also occur when the gains are greater than the losses, as when the kidneys are not functioning properly. Excesses are just as dangerous as deficits and can prove fatal in a short period of time.

Thus, *abnormal differences between gains and losses cause body fluid disturbances.*

BASIC IMBALANCES

Because of the constant exchanges between cellular and extracellular fluid, changes in either are reflected in the other. Therefore, imbalances in the extracellular fluid ultimately cause imbalances in the cellular fluid, and vice versa. Since extracellular fluid is readily available and cellular fluid is not, body fluid disturbances are studied, diagnosed, and treated in terms of the extracellular fluid. There are some 16 basic imbalances that can occur; these imbalances involve changes in volume, position, and composition of the extracellular fluid.

Changes in Volume of Extracellular Fluid

Imbalances in the volume of extracellular fluid are either deficits or excesses of both water and electrolytes of the extracellular fluid in approximately the same proportions as they normally exist in that fluid. The Composition of the fluid is not significantly altered in volume disturbances. While we refer to these imbalances as extracellular fluid volume changes, it is important to note that when volume changes occur in the extracellular fluid, there are corresponding changes in the cellular fluid. For example, a volume deficit of extracellular fluid will ultimately cause a volume deficit of cellular fluid as well.

CHANGES IN VOLUME, POSITION, AND COMPOSITION OF EXTRA-CELLULAR FLUID ACCOUNT FOR ALL BASIC IMBALANCES

Extracellular fluid volume deficit   A volume deficit of extracellular fluid represents a pronounced decrease of both water and electrolytes in the extracellular fluid in approximately the same proportions as they normally occur. Other terms frequently used to describe this imbalance are *volume deficit, hypovolemia,* and *dehydration.* The term dehydration is incorrect since dehydration is the loss of water alone.

Volume deficits result from an abrupt decrease in fluid intake, from an acute loss of secretions and excretions, or from a combination of decreased intake and increased loss. The imbalance can strike with savage rapidity and may cause death within a few hours after onset in such diseases as Asiatic cholera.

The deficit usually begins with a loss of secretions and excretions. As the secretions and excretions are depleted, they are replenished by water and electrolytes of the extracellular fluid. Thus, the volume of the extracellular fluid is decreased. With further depletion of extracellular fluid, water and electrolytes are drawn from the cells. This action does not occur immediately, however.

The reduced fluid volume results in an acute weight loss (5 per cent in the child or adult, 10 per cent in the infant), and in oliguria or anuria. The central nervous system is depressed, so that the patient is lethargic or even stuporous. Provided fever is not present, body temperature drops as a result of reduced energy output. The tongue exhibits longitudinal wrinkles or furrows. The skin and mucous membranes become dry. Laboratory studies reveal an increase in the red blood cell count, packed cell volume, and hemoglobin. These values are elevated because extracellular fluid volume deficit does not involve loss of red blood cells; hence, they are more concentrated in the lesser amounts of water and electrolytes.

The goal of therapy in extracellular fluid volume deficit is to restore the volume to normal without altering the electrolyte composition of the fluid. This is done by oral or parenteral administration of a solution formulated to provide electrolytes in quantities balanced between the minimal needs and the maximal tolerances of the patient, plus free water to form urine and to carry out metabolic functions. Such a solution is called a *balanced solution,* or a *Butler-type solution.* When this type of solution is used, the body homeostatic mechanisms retain the water and electrolytes that are needed and excrete the rest.

Extracellular fluid volume excess This imbalance is just the opposite of a volume deficit, that is, an increase of both water and electrolytes in approximately the same proportions as they normally exist in the extracellular fluid. Extracellular fluid volume excess is frequently called *fluid volume excess* or *overhydration.* The latter term is incorrect since it represents an excess of water alone.

Fluid volume excess occurs when the kidneys are unable to rid the body of unneeded water and electrolytes. This inability may result from simple overloading of the body by oral or parenteral administration of excessive quantities of an isotonic solution of sodium chloride. It may result from diseases that affect the function of homeostatic mechanisms, such as congestive heart failure, chronic kidney disease, chronic liver disease with portal hypertension, and malnutrition, in all of which sodium and water are abnormally retained. Whatever the cause, the extracellular fluid becomes excessively salty. The body endeavors to maintain its normal composition of water and electrolytes by drawing water from the cells. The expanding fluid fills tissue spaces beyond their normal capacity, causing pitting edema. Moist rales can be heard in the lungs, and the patient becomes short of breath. The eyelids are puffy and the peripheral veins engorged. The patient may become hoarse, and his pulse bounds. There is also an acute weight gain, which can be in excess of 5 per cent of the normal body weight. The red blood cell count, packed cell volume, and hemoglobin are decreased because the bloodstream is diluted.

The goal of therapy in extracellular fluid volume excess is to return the fluid volume to normal without altering the electrolyte concentration of the fluid. Therapy is directed toward the causative factors. In addition, it may be necessary to withhold all liquids for a time.

Position Changes of Water and Electrolytes of Extracellular Fluid

Although the two types of extracellular fluid—plasma and interstitial fluid—are much alike in composition, there is one important difference: plasma contains a large quantity of proteinate, while interstitial fluid contains only a negligible amount of this anion. Were it not for plasma proteinate, which has a powerful drawing action for water and electrolytes, the great pressure exerted on the blood vessels by the pumping action of the heart would drive the plasma through the capillary walls and into the interstitial spaces. When the proteinate content of plasma decreases or increases, water and electrolytes shift from plasma to interstitial space or from interstitial space to plasma. At other times, unknown forces activated by certain illnesses and injuries produce these shifts. In these cases, the mechanisms responsible for the shifts are obscure.

ROLE OF
PLASMA
PROTEINATE

Plasma-to-interstitial fluid shift   This imbalance involves a movement of water and electrolytes out of the plasma and into the interstitial fluid. It is sometimes called *hypovolemia,* and is closely related to shock and edema. The shift is frequently seen following a severe trauma, massive crushing injury, perforated peptic ulcer, or on the first or second day following a severe burn.

As the water and electrolytes flow from the plasma into the interstitial fluid, the blood thickens. The patient becomes apprehensive, pale, and weak. His blood pressure drops or is undetectable. The heart speeds up, while the pulse is weak or absent. The extremities become cold. Finally, the patient loses consciousness, and may die. The formed elements of the blood remain in the plasma. Because of the decreased plasma volume, the laboratory values for these elements are increased.

Treatment of plasma-to-interstitial fluid shift is directed to the condition causing it. A localized shift may be relieved by application of a binder. Plasma, dextran, or a solution containing electrolytes in approximately the same composition and concentration as plasma may be administered parenterally to maintain or restore plasma volume.

Interstitial fluid-to-plasma shift   This shift involves an abnormal flow of water and electrolytes from the interstitial fluid to the plasma. It is also known as *hypervolemia.* Interstitial fluid-to-plasma shift frequently occurs following excessive intravenous administration of hypertonic electrolyte solutions, serum albumin, plasma, or dextran. Or, it may occur in the recovery phase of conditions that have previously caused a plasma-to-interstitial fluid shift, such as burns or fractures, in which case the shift is referred to as *remobilization of edema fluid.* Sometimes the shift occurs as a compensatory effort of the body to replace water and electrolytes lost during hemorrhage.

As the fluid moves into the blood vessels, the veins become engorged. The blood pressure first rises, then falls. The lungs fill with water, and the patient experiences air hunger. The pulse bounds, and the patient shows pallor and weakness. Cardiac dilatation and finally ventricular failure ensue. Because of the greater plasma volume, the laboratory values of the formed elements of the blood are decreased.

Therapy of interstitial fluid-to-plasma shift is directed toward relieving the excessive plasma volume. If the condition is critical, phlebotomy may be necessary. The application of tourniquets may be helpful. If the shift results from a compensatory effort to restore plasma volume following loss of whole blood, blood transfusions should be given.

Changes in Composition of Extracellular Fluid

Each of the several electrolytes of the body fluid has special functions in the body. Some play larger roles than others, but all are necessary for the maintenance of life. Their normal concentrations in the body fluids are precisely geared to the needs of the body and must be maintained at the proper levels if the body is to remain healthy. Also vitally important are the concentrations of carbonic acid and base bicarbonate. Disease results when the normal composition of the extracellular fluid is altered.

Sodium

Sodium, the chief cation of extracellular fluid and the second most important cation of cellular fluid, has many important functions in the human body. It is largely responsible for the osmotic pressure of extracellular fluid. Inside the cell, it plays a key role in numerous vital chemical reactions. The tubule cells of the kidney could not function without sodium. Probably through some type of chemical-electrical action, sodium stimulates nerve reactions. In addition, sodium is of major importance in maintaining the acid-base balance of the body. The extracellular fluid normally contains 142 mEq. per liter of sodium.

SODIUM THE MOST ABUNDANT CATION

Sodium deficit of extracellular fluid   Sodium deficit of extracellular fluid occurs when the sodium concentration of the extracellular fluid falls below normal. Other names used to describe this imbalance include *electrolyte concentration deficit, low sodium syndrome, hypotonic dehydration,* and *hyponatremia.*

Sodium deficit may be caused by decreased intake or increased output of sodium, or by increased intake or decreased output of water. It frequently follows excessive sweating associated with the drinking of plain water, administration of a potent diuretic, administration of repeated water enemas, parenteral infusion of an electrolyte-free solution, gastrointestinal suction associated with the drinking of plain water, or inhalation of fresh water (as occurs in fresh-water drowning). Sodium deficit is now recognized as the cause of the mysterious "burn poisoning" that formerly caused the death of many patients with serious burns. The imbalance resulted when the burn victim, who usually has an insatiable thirst, was allowed to drink all the liquids he desired. Since large quantities of extracellular fluid had already been lost as edema fluid in the burned tissues, the ingested liquids served only to dilute the remaining extracellular fluid, thus causing sodium deficit.

As sodium deficit develops the patient becomes apprehensive and may experience a bizarre, indefinable feeling of impending doom. Abdominal cramps and convulsions may occur. In efforts to conserve sodium, the adrenal glands secrete increased amounts of aldosterone, which causes the kidneys to conserve water, sodium, and chloride. This action results in oliguria (depressed urinary output) or anuria (complete absence of urinary output). If the deficit is pronounced, there is vasomotor collapse, with such symptoms as hypotension, rapid, thready pulse, cold clammy skin, and cyanosis. Transfer of water and electrolytes from the diluted extracellular fluid into the cells decreases the volume of extracellular fluid, so there is increased plasticity of the tissues, which then tend to retain whatever shape may have been caused by pressure deformation. This can be demonstrated by applying pressure with the finger or thumb on the skin overlying the sternum. Laboratory studies reveal a plasma sodium below 137 mEq. per liter, plasma chloride below 98 mEq. per liter, and the specific gravity of urine below 1.010.

The object of therapy in sodium deficit of extracellular fluid is to restore the sodium level of extracellular fluid to normal as quickly as possible without causing a fluid volume excess. If the volume is normal or excessive, a 3 or 5 per cent solution of sodium chloride is administered to correct the sodium deficit. If the extracellular fluid volume is below normal, an isotonic solution of sodium chloride may be administered.

Sodium excess of extracellular fluid   Sodium excess, sometimes called *hypernatremia, salt excess, oversalting,* or *hypertonic dehydration,* occurs when the sodium concentration of extracellular fluid rises above the normal level. It is caused by decreased intake or increased output of water, or by increased intake or decreased output of sodium. An acute form may follow excessive administration of concentrated oral electrolyte mixtures. It may occur in any condition in which water is lost in excess of electrolytes, as in profuse watery diarrhea or in tracheobronchitis (in which there are excessive losses of water through the lungs due to fever and deep, rapid breathing). Sodium excess may develop in unconscious patients simply because they do not drink water. It is the cause of death in salt-water drowning.

Long-term or chronic ingestion of large amounts of sodium, as when one salts his food excessively or eats extremely salty foods, can cause sodium excess. Hereditary factors largely determine whether this type of sodium excess will cause hypertension.

With increased concentration of sodium in the extracellular fluid, the mucous membranes become dry and sticky, and the tongue becomes rough and dry. Body tissues become firm. Fever develops, and the patient is intensely thirsty. Laboratory findings show a plasma sodium above 147 mEq. per liter, plasma chloride above 106 mEq. per liter, and a specific gravity of urine above 1.030.

Following the law of osmosis, water from the cellular fluid flows into the more concentrated extracellular fluid. This transfer partially repairs the water deficit in the extracellular fluid, but it leaves the cellular fluid in need of water. The object of therapy in sodium excess of extracellular fluid is to reduce the sodium concentration of the extracellular fluid before it reaches a critical level. Treatment involves administration of a Butler-type solution, which is only one third to one half as concentrated as plasma and which provides free water for formation of urine. This type of solution also provides 5 or 10 per cent carbohydrate to reduce tissue destruction and spare protein.

Potassium

POTASSIUM VITAL IN CELL METABOLISM

Potassium, the chief cation of the cellular fluid, plays an indispensable role in the body, being necessary for transformation of carbohydrate into energy and reassembling of amino acids into proteins. The cells must have potassium to maintain their normal electrolyte content, and it is needed as well for transmission of electrical impulses within the heart. Skeletal muscles and the muscles of the heart, intestines, and lungs could not function normally without the presence of potassium.

The human body contains enough potassium to bring death to several dozens of people were it injected quickly into them. The extracellular fluid normally contains 5 mEq. per liter, or about 70 mEq.; the cellular fluid contains a total of 4,000 mEq. Large amounts of potassium are found in secretions and excretions, sweat, saliva, gastric juice, and stool being particularly rich. The potassium content of urine varies with the intake, but it amounts to at least 40 to 50 mEq. daily.

ABSENCE OF POTASSIUM-CONSERVING MECHANISM MAY CAUSE CRITICAL SITUATIONS

Potassium deficit of extracellular fluid   The human body has an efficient mechanism for conserving sodium, but it has no such mechanism for conserving potassium. Even when the body is in great need of potassium, the kidneys may continue to pour out 40 to 50 mEq. daily in the urine. With such continuing losses, potassium deficit, or *hypokalemia,* can develop quickly when the patient's intake of potassium decreases or stops, and it is a frequent occurrence. Two hospital studies revealed that approximately 20 per cent of the patients had symptoms and laboratory findings of potassium deficit, largely undiagnosed. It is frequent when large quantities of potassium-rich secretions or excretions are lost, such as gastrointestinal juice in diarrhea, and is often associated with renal loss of potassium. The use of powerful diuretics, particularly thiazide diu-

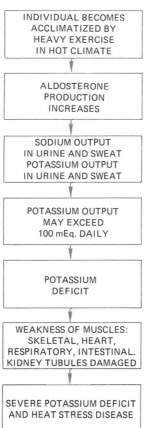

HOW POTASSIUM DEFICIT
DEVELOPS IN
ACCLIMATIZED PERSONS

INDIVIDUAL BECOMES
ACCLIMATIZED BY
HEAVY EXERCISE
IN HOT CLIMATE

↓

ALDOSTERONE
PRODUCTION
INCREASES

↓

SODIUM OUTPUT
IN URINE AND SWEAT
POTASSIUM OUTPUT
IN URINE AND SWEAT

↓

POTASSIUM OUTPUT
MAY EXCEED
100 mEq. DAILY

↓

POTASSIUM
DEFICIT

↓

WEAKNESS OF MUSCLES:
SKELETAL, HEART,
RESPIRATORY, INTESTINAL.
KIDNEY TUBULES DAMAGED

↓

SEVERE POTASSIUM DEFICIT
AND HEAT STRESS DISEASE

retics, without potassium supplementation is probably the leading cause of potassium deficit in the United States. The deficit may be associated with surgical operations, gastrointestinal suction, diseases involving the intestinal tract, periodic familial paralysis, aldosterone-secreting tumor of the adrenal cortex, crushing injuries, broken bones, extensive bruising, and wound healing. Even emotional or physical stress can be the cause. Excessive sweating, fever, and high environmental temperatures are further causes. Potassium loss is a major factor in the development of heat stress disease, which affects people of all ages who are subjected to high environmental temperatures, particularly if they are exercising. Salt tablets are commonly used by factory workers, athletes, and others who are exposed to high environmental temperatures to replace the sodium lost in sweat. Since, however, the body conserves sodium and continues to lose potassium, potassium supplementation is at least as important as sodium supplementation.

Early symptoms of potassium deficit are nonspecific. The patient has malaise, or is "just not feeling well." With progression, the skeletal muscles are weakened, and the reflexes are decreased or absent. Muscle weakness leads to flabbiness; the patient lies flat, like a cadaver. Myocardial symptoms include faint heart sounds, heart block, falling blood pressure, and weak pulse. In the gastrointestinal tract there are symptoms of anorexia, vomiting, gaseous intestinal distention, and paralytic ileus, while weakness of the respiratory muscles produces shallow respiration. The patient may be extremely thirsty. The plasma potassium is below 4 mEq. per liter, the chloride level is often below 98 mEq. per liter, and the plasma bicarbonate is above 29 mEq. per liter. The electrocardiogram also gives evidence of potassium deficit, in a flattened T-wave, depressed S-T segment, and prominent U wave.

Abnormal losses are counteracted by oral administration of a potassium salt and provision of a diet high in potassium. A frank potassium deficit may be treated by oral administration of potassium chloride or other potassium salts or by parenteral infusion of potassium. A balanced, or Butler-type, solution is often administered.

Potassium excess of extracellular fluid Potassium excess, also known as *hyperkalemia,* can result from oral or parenteral administration of excessive quantities of potassium when the kidneys are not functioning adequately. It is often seen with burns, crushing injuries, kidney disease, or adrenal insufficiency. Mercuric bichloride poisoning, which damages the kidneys, can lead to potassium excess.

In a mild case there are symptoms of irritability, nausea, diarrhea, and intestinal colic; if the condition becomes severe there is weakness and flaccid paralysis, perhaps difficulty in phonation and respiration. There is oliguria progressing to anuria. The heartbeat becomes arrhythmic, and finally stops. The plasma potassium is above 5.6 mEq. per liter. A test for renal function will usually show renal impairment. The electrocardiogram reveals a high T-wave and a depressed S-T segment.

When the kidneys are functional, an uncomplicated potassium excess can be corrected by avoidance of additional intake of potassium, either orally or parenterally. If the kidneys are not functioning adequately, a carefully measured replacement solution that supplies fats and carbohydrates but not protein materials, carbonic anhydrase inhibitors, or insulin and dextrose may be given. Ion exchange resins also are useful. In some cases, peritoneal dialysis or hemodialysis may be necessary.

Calcium

Calcium is the most abundant electrolyte in the body. Approximately 99 per cent is concentrated in the bones and teeth, which also contain 75 per cent of the body's phosphorus, while the remainder is distributed throughout the plasma and body cells. The normal concentration of calcium in the extracellular fluid is 5 mEq. per liter.

Calcium is closely associated with phosphorus; they function together to make bones and teeth rigid, strong, and durable. Calcium is also necessary for transmission of nerve impulses. Without it, muscles could not respond and blood could not clot. Enzymes needed to stimulate many essential chemical reactions in the body are activated by calcium, and it is also needed for the absorption and utilization of vitamin B_{12}. In addition, calcium is an ingredient of the cell cement, which holds the cells together.

Calcium deficit of extracellular fluid   Calcium deficit, or *hypocalcemia,* can result from abnormalities in body metabolism, from inadequate dietary intake of calcium, or from excessive losses of calcium in diarrheal stools or in wound exudate. This imbalance is frequently associated with sprue, acute pancreatitis, hypoactive parathyroid glands, surgical removal of parathyroid glands, massive subcutaneous infections, burns, generalized peritonitis, or excessive infusion of citrated blood.

Symptoms include tingling of the ends of the fingers, tetany, abdominal cramps, muscle cramps, carpopedal spasm, and convulsions. Plasma calcium is usually below 4.5 mEq. per liter, and the Sulkowitch test on urine reveals no precipitation. The electrocardiogram and the x-ray film are helpful in diagnosing calcium deficit. If the deficit is severe or is allowed to persist, calcium will be drawn from the bones, so that fractures are apt to occur.

Osteomalacia is an interesting manifestation of calcium deficit. The bones lose their calcium, phosphorus, and other electrolytes, and become soft and pliable. This causes a shrinkage in height. In the first recorded case of osteomalacia, the physician reported that the patient had shrunk some 17 inches in height. The disease is, fortunately, extremely uncommon. Another manifestation of calcium deficit, far more common, is osteoporosis, in which the chemical composition of bone remains normal but bone becomes thinner, lighter, and more porous. The incidence is high among women over 45 years and men over 55.

Acute calcium deficit is treated by intravenous administration of a 10 per cent solution of calcium gluconate. This therapy is of critical importance in tetany or convulsions. A milder deficit may be corrected by a diet high in calcium and oral supplement of calcium lactate.

Calcium excess of extracellular fluid   Calcium excess, or *hypercalcemia,* may result from drinking too much milk or hard water with a high calcium content. It may be caused by tumor or overactivity of the parathyroid glands, multiple myeloma, or excessive administration of vitamin D (over 50,000 units daily) in the treatment of arthritis. Tumors of bone, multiple fractures, and prolonged immobilization also cause symptoms when calcium stores released from bone flood the extracellular fluid. Osteomalacia and osteoporosis, although manifestations of calcium

CALCIUM AND PHOSPHORUS ESSENTIAL IN BONE METABOLISM

deficit, cause symptoms of calcium excess of extracellular fluid in the early stages when calcium is moving out of the bones and into the extracellular fluid.

There is hypotonicity of muscle, flank pain, deep bone pain, bone cavities, and kidney stones. The Sulkowitch test on urine shows heavy precipitation, and the plasma calcium level is usually above 5.8 mEq. per liter. The electrocardiogram and the x-ray study are useful diagnostic tools.

The most extreme manifestation of calcium excess is hypercalcemic crisis, a medical emergency that requires immediate attention if cardiac arrest is to be prevented. The symptoms include intractable nausea and vomiting, dehydration, stupor, coma, and azotemia.

Medical management of hypercalcemic crisis has generally been unsatisfactory, in that because of their slow action or inherent toxicity, none of the many regimens tried has been consistently successful. Inorganic phosphate solutions and sulfate solutions are among the most frequently used. In less critical situations, treatment is directed toward correcting the underlying condition. When other imbalances are being treated as well, only calcium-free solutions should be used.

Magnesium

Most of the body's magnesium is found in the cellular fluid, where its high concentration is maintained in active metabolism. The normal serum level is 1.67 mEq. per liter. Until only recently, magnesium's importance was not understood; we now recognize it as the activator of numerous vital reactions related to enzyme systems. Magnesium activates the systems that enable the B vitamins to function, and is required in enzyme systems associated with the utilization of potassium, calcium, and protein. Magnesium occurs both in bones and in soft tissues and is particularly important in nervous tissue, in skeletal muscle, and in the heart. It has considerable therapeutic value in the correction of arrhythmias and in counteracting the toxic side effects of certain powerful drugs used in treatment of heart disease. In conjunction with hypotensive drugs, it is a useful therapeutic agent in treatment of hypertension. Toxemia of pregnancy, which formerly had a high death rate, responds to magnesium therapy. As further discoveries are made, magnesium may be shown to have other important uses in saving lives and in maintaining health. Since magnesium excess occurs only rarely, we shall not consider it in our study of body fluid disturbances.

Sidenote: MAGNESIUM A COFACTOR IN ENZYMATIC REACTIONS OF CARBOHYDRATE, PROTEIN, AND ENERGY METABOLISM

Magnesium deficit of extracellular fluid   Magnesium deficit occurs when the magnesium concentration of extracellular fluid decreases. It is also referred to as *hypomagnesemia*. This imbalance is not common and is easily mistaken for potassium deficit; it should always be considered when a patient being treated for potassium deficit does not respond to appropriate therapy.

Magnesium deficit may be associated with such conditions as severe renal disease, chronic alcoholism with hepatic cirrhosis, toxemia of pregnancy, diabetes, vigorous drug-induced diuresis, sustained losses of gastrointestinal secretions, diseases of the small intestine that impair gastrointestinal absorption, and prolonged administration of magnesium-free solutions.

The symptoms resemble those of hypocalcemic tetany, i.e., muscle and central nervous system hyperirritability, tremor, choreiform movements, perhaps convulsions. The deep reflexes are hyperactive, and the Chvostek sign is positive. The patient becomes confused and may hallucinate. Tachycardia may occur; the blood pressure rises. The plasma magnesium concentration is below 1.4 mEq. per liter. There is an immediate therapeutic response to magnesium sulfate; this response is helpful in making the diagnosis.

Magnesium deficit is treated by administration of magnesium as magnesium sulfate or other salt. When excessive amounts of magnesium-rich secretions or excretions are being lost, administration of appropriate replacement solutions is useful in preventing a deficit.

TREATMENT MODALITY

Protein

The importance of protein in the plasma has already been described. Protein also plays a vital role in the cellular fluid, for it is essential to all living cells. Without protein, new tissue synthesis and repair of damaged tissue and replacement of destroyed tissue could not occur. It is required for elaboration of enzymes and manufacture of many hormones, as well as for synthesis of some vitamins. In addition, it plays an important role in the immune mechanism since many antibodies are proteins. Because of its unique position in the nutritional arch, it is regarded as the keystone nutrient.

PROTEIN—
"OF FIRST
IMPORTANCE"

Protein deficit of extracellular fluid   Protein deficit results from decreased intake, increased loss, or impaired protein utilization. The condition is also known as *hypoproteinemia* and *protein malnutrition*. It is frequently seen in repeated or chronic loss of whole blood, chronic or repeated infections, fractures, extensive burns, starvation, draining wounds, decubitus ulcers, repeated surgical operations, malignancies, and prolonged gastrointestinal disease.

The symptoms include chronic weight loss, soft flabby muscles, pallor, edema, ready fatigue, and mental depression. Laboratory studies sometimes (but not always) show a plasma albumin below 4.0 Gm. per 100 ml., and a decreased red blood cell count, hemoglobin, and packed cell volume. (These values are significant only if the iron stores are adequate.) Kwashiorkor, or the pluricarencial syndrome as it is called in Latin America, and hypoproteinosis are closely related clinical states.

Protein deficit can be corrected by administration of high-protein foods or by administration of amino acids along with generous quantities of calories in the form of dextrose, alcohol, or both. It may be necessary to use all three agents.

Acid-Base Balance

ACID-BASE BALANCE THE SINE QUA NON OF NORMAL METABOLISM

For the pH, or hydrogen ion concentration, of extracellular fluid to remain neutral, a balance between acids and bases must be maintained. An *acid* is a chemical that can release hydrogen ions, and a *base*, or *alkali*, is a chemical that can accept a hydrogen ion. While hydrogen is present in the extracellular fluid in minute quantities only, it is highly important from the standpoint of health. When the concentration of hydrogen ion lies within a certain narrow range, the extracellular fluid is chemically and physiologically neutral. When its concentration increases (pH decreases), the extracellular fluid becomes acid—this condition is *acidosis*. When the hydrogen ion concentration decreases (pH increases), the extracellular fluid becomes basic, or alkaline—this condition is *alkalosis*.

Union of carbon dioxide with water and electrolytes in the extracellular fluid produces carbonic acid. Base bicarbonate is formed when the cations sodium, potassium, calcium, and magnesium unite with the anion bicarbonate. The concentration of hydrogen ions in the extracellular fluid is determined by the ratio of carbonic acid to base bicarbonate, which normally is 1 to 20. As long as this ratio is maintained, the pH of the extracellular fluid remains normal at about 7.4. It is important to note that absolute quantities of carbonic acid and base bicarbonate are not important in maintaining the balance—*it is the relative quantities that are important*. For example, acid-base balance will be maintained when base bicarbonate is increased, perhaps doubled, as long as the carbonic acid is also increased by the same factor. Or, pH remains normal when both are reduced by the same factor. Imbalances result only when the normal 1 to 20 ratio is upset.

Acidosis results from any condition that increases the carbonic acid or decreases the base bicarbonate. Alkalosis is caused by any condition that increases base bicarbonate or decreases carbonic acid. Two types of disturbances can upset the balance: metabolic, or systemic, disturbances affect the base bicarbonate level, while respiratory disturbances affect the carbonic acid level.

Various laboratory tests have been used to measure the bicarbonate level of the plasma. These include the carbon dioxide content, carbon dioxide capacity, and carbon dioxide combining power. The names of these tests can mislead one unless he recalls that what is being measured is not the carbon dioxide of the plasma but rather the bicarbonate. The reason the words carbon dioxide are part of the name of the test is that in all the tests named, the bicarbonate ($HCO_3{}^-$) is chemically treated so as to release the gas carbon dioxide (CO_2), which is then measured. After allowance has been made for the amount of carbon dioxide (CO_2) dissolved in the plasma, the bicarbonate quantity is calculated on the basis of the carbon dioxide released from the bicarbonate ($HCO_3{}^-$) by the chemical treatment.

Primary base bicarbonate deficit of extracellular fluid   A primary deficit in the concentration of base bicarbonate in the extracellular fluid is called *metabolic acidosis* or *acidemia*. Any clinical event that decreases the amount of base bicarbonate, such as decreased food intake, systemic infection, diabetic acidosis, a ketogenic diet, renal insufficiency, parenteral infusion of an isotonic solution of sodium chloride, or salicylate intoxication after the first stages, can be a factor.

In metabolic acidosis the patient becomes stuporous. In the body's efforts to restore balance by ridding itself of excess carbon dioxide, the breath becomes deep and rapid (Kussmaul's sign). Weakness progresses and, if the imbalance is severe, the patient may lose consciousness. The urine pH is below 6.0, the plasma bicarbonate is below 25 mEq. per liter in adults and below 20 mEq. per liter in children, and the plasma pH is below 7.35.

The lungs may blow off enough carbon dioxide to partially restore balance, while the kidneys excrete carbonic acid and retain bicarbonate. If the compensatory efforts of the lungs and kidneys do not restore balance, the patient may be given bicarbonate or lactate parenterally or an alkaline solution by mouth.

Primary base bicarbonate excess of extracellular fluid   A primary excess of base bicarbonate, referred to as *metabolic alkalosis* or *alkalemia*, can result from any clinical event that increases the amount of base bicarbonate in the extracellular fluid. Loss of a chloride-rich secretion, such as gastric juice, may be the cause. The imbalance can also occur following excessive ingestion of sodium bicarbonate or other alkali or following the infusion of potassium-free solutions. It can appear after the patient has vomited or has had gastrointestinal suction, and may follow administration of adrenocortical hormones. Still another cause may be the use of a potent diuretic that has produced a potassium deficit.

Metabolic alkalosis produces hypertonicity of muscle, tetany, and depressed respiration. The pH of urine is 7.0, and the plasma bicarbonate is above 29 mEq. per liter in adults and above 25 mEq. per liter in children. The plasma pH is above 7.45, and the plasma potassium is below 4 mEq. per liter. If the alkalosis is hypochloremic, the chloride will be below 98 mEq. per liter.

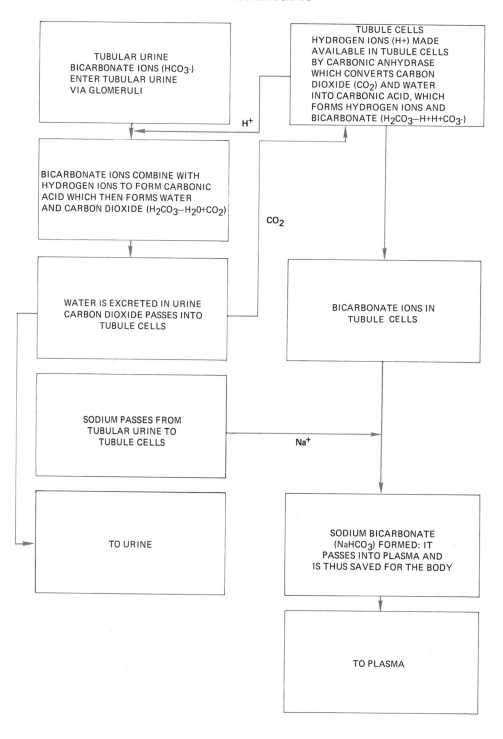

HOW THE KIDNEY
SAVES BICARBONATE

TUBULAR URINE
BICARBONATE IONS (HCO_3^-)
ENTER TUBULAR URINE
VIA GLOMERULI

TUBULE CELLS
HYDROGEN IONS (H+) MADE
AVAILABLE IN TUBULE CELLS
BY CARBONIC ANHYDRASE
WHICH CONVERTS CARBON
DIOXIDE (CO_2) AND WATER
INTO CARBONIC ACID, WHICH
FORMS HYDROGEN IONS AND
BICARBONATE ($H_2CO_3—H+H+CO_3^-$)

H^+

BICARBONATE IONS COMBINE WITH
HYDROGEN IONS TO FORM CARBONIC
ACID WHICH THEN FORMS WATER
AND CARBON DIOXIDE ($H_2CO_3—H_2O+CO_2$)

CO_2

WATER IS EXCRETED IN URINE
CARBON DIOXIDE PASSES INTO
TUBULE CELLS

BICARBONATE IONS IN
TUBULE CELLS

SODIUM PASSES FROM
TUBULAR URINE TO
TUBULE CELLS

Na^+

TO URINE

SODIUM BICARBONATE
($NaHCO_3$) FORMED: IT
PASSES INTO PLASMA AND
IS THUS SAVED FOR THE BODY

TO PLASMA

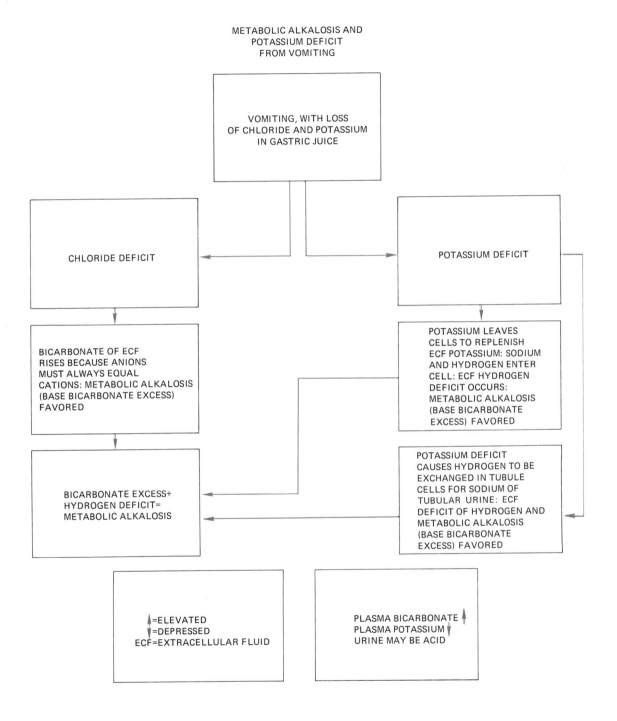

METABOLIC ALKALOSIS AND
POTASSIUM DEFICIT
FROM VOMITING

VOMITING, WITH LOSS
OF CHLORIDE AND POTASSIUM
IN GASTRIC JUICE

CHLORIDE DEFICIT

POTASSIUM DEFICIT

BICARBONATE OF ECF
RISES BECAUSE ANIONS
MUST ALWAYS EQUAL
CATIONS: METABOLIC ALKALOSIS
(BASE BICARBONATE EXCESS)
FAVORED

POTASSIUM LEAVES
CELLS TO REPLENISH
ECF POTASSIUM: SODIUM
AND HYDROGEN ENTER
CELL: ECF HYDROGEN
DEFICIT OCCURS:
METABOLIC ALKALOSIS
(BASE BICARBONATE
EXCESS) FAVORED

BICARBONATE EXCESS+
HYDROGEN DEFICIT=
METABOLIC ALKALOSIS

POTASSIUM DEFICIT
CAUSES HYDROGEN TO BE
EXCHANGED IN TUBULE
CELLS FOR SODIUM OF
TUBULAR URINE: ECF
DEFICIT OF HYDROGEN AND
METABOLIC ALKALOSIS
(BASE BICARBONATE
EXCESS) FAVORED

↑=ELEVATED
↓=DEPRESSED
ECF=EXTRACELLULAR FLUID

PLASMA BICARBONATE ↑
PLASMA POTASSIUM ↓
URINE MAY BE ACID

CLINICAL CONDITIONS AND RESULTANT FLUID IMBALANCES

Condition	Imbalance(s) Likely to Result
Adrenal insufficiency	Potassium excess
Alcoholism, chronic	Magnesium deficit
Asthma	Respiratory acidosis
Burn, early	Potassium excess Plasma-to-interstitial fluid shift
Burn, after third day	Potassium deficit Protein deficit Interstitial fluid-to-plasma shift
Congestive heart failure	Fluid volume excess
Diabetes mellitus, uncontrolled severe	Metabolic acidosis Potassium deficit
Emphysema	Respiratory acidosis
Encephalitis	Respiratory alkalosis
Fever	Fluid volume deficit Respiratory alkalosis
Fractures	Plasma-to-interstitial fluid shift Protein deficit
Gastric disease, repeated vomiting	Potassium deficit Metabolic alkalosis
High external temperature with physiological hyperpnea	Respiratory alkalosis
Hyperaldosteronism	Fluid volume excess
Hyperparathyroidism	Calcium excess
Hypoparathyroidism, primary	Calcium deficit
Fresh water drowning	Sodium deficit
Salt water drowning	Sodium excess
Massive crushing injury	Potassium excess Plasma-to-interstitial fluid shift
Massive infection of subcutaneous tissues	Calcium deficit
Meningitis	Respiratory alkalosis
Multiple myeloma	Calcium excess

CLINICAL CONDITIONS AND RESULTANT FLUID IMBALANCES (Cont.)

Condition	Imbalance(s) Likely to Result
Occlusion of air passages	Respiratory acidosis
Occlusion of major artery, acute	Plasma-to-interstitial fluid shift
Oxygen lack with hyperpnea	Respiratory alkalosis
Pancreatitis, acute	Calcium deficit
Peptic ulcer, perforated	Plasma-to-interstitial fluid shift
Pneumonia	Respiratory acidosis
Pulmonary edema	Respiratory acidosis
Renal disease	Potassium excess Fluid volume excess Metabolic acidosis Calcium deficit
Systemic infection	Metabolic acidosis Fluid volume deficit
Tracheobronchitis	Sodium excess
Trauma, severe	Plasma-to-interstitial fluid shift Protein deficit

IMBALANCES RESULTING FROM MEDICAL THERAPY

Therapy	Imbalance(s) Likely to Occur
Administration of adrenal cortical hormones	Fluid volume excess Potassium deficit Metabolic alkalosis
Administration of potent diuretics	Potassium deficit Sodium deficit Metabolic alkalosis
Barbiturate poisoning	Respiratory acidosis
Early salicylate intoxication	Respiratory alkalosis
Excessive administration of citrated blood	Calcium deficit
Excessive administration of vitamin D	Calcium excess
Excessive infusion of large molecular solution	Interstitial fluid-to-plasma shift

IMBALANCES RESULTING FROM MEDICAL THERAPY (Cont.)

Therapy	Imbalance(s) Likely to Occur
Excessive ingestion of sodium bicarbonate	Metabolic alkalosis
Excessive ingestion of sodium chloride	Sodium excess Fluid volume excess
Excessive parenteral administration of calcium-free solutions	Calcium deficit
Excessive parenteral administration of magnesium-free solutions	Magnesium deficit
Excessive parenteral administration of potassium	Potassium excess
Excessive parenteral infusion of isotonic solution of sodium chloride	Fluid volume excess Metabolic acidosis
Gastrointestinal suction and water drinking	Sodium deficit Metabolic alkalosis Potassium deficit
Mechanical respirator inaccurately regulated (causing too deep or too rapid respiration)	Respiratory alkalosis
Mechanical respirator inaccurately regulated (causing too shallow or too slow respiration)	Respiratory acidosis
Mercuric bichloride poisoning	Potassium excess
Morphine or Demerol in excessive doses	Respiratory acidosis
Oral intake of potassium exceeding renal tolerance	Potassium excess
Prolonged immobilization	Calcium excess
Recent correction of acidosis	Calcium deficit
Salicylate intoxication (later stage)	Metabolic acidosis
Water enemas	Sodium deficit Potassium deficit

The respiratory depression results from compensatory efforts by the lungs to hold back carbon dioxide. The kidneys work to restore balance by excreting bicarbonate and holding back carbonic acid. Chloride should be administered if these efforts fail.

Primary carbonic acid deficit of extracellular fluid   This imbalance, also known as *respiratory alkalosis* or *alkalemia*, can be brought about by any condition that results in an increased rate and depth of breathing, with consequent blowing off of carbon dioxide. Respiratory alkalosis is seen in oxygen lack, fever, extreme emotional states, anxiety, hysteria, intentional overbreathing, and early salicylate intoxication. The excessive blowing off of carbon dioxide reduces the level of carbonic acid, and this gives rise to tetany, convulsions, and finally unconsciousness. The pH of urine rises above 7.0. Plasma bicarbonate is below 25 mEq. per liter in adults and below 20 mEq. per liter in children. Plasma pH is above 7.45.

Since the lungs are the organ source of the imbalance, they cannot participate in corrective efforts. The kidneys, however, excrete bicarbonate and retain carbonic acid. Therapy is directed toward correcting the condition that initially caused the overbreathing. Parenteral infusion of chloride ions to replace bicarbonate ions may be helpful.

Primary carbonic acid excess of extracellular fluid   Primary carbonic acid excess, commonly called *respiratory acidosis* or *acidemia,* is caused by any condition that interferes with normal lung function. Such conditions as pneumonia, emphysema, asthma, occlusion of the respiratory passages, barbiturate poisoning, and morphine poisoning give rise to respiratory depression, with impaired expiration of carbon dioxide. Inspiration of excessive carbon dioxide is also a cause. As the level of carbonic acid in the extracellular fluid rises, the patient becomes disoriented, with symptoms progressing from respiratory embarrassment and weakness to coma. The urine pH falls below 6.0, and the plasma bicarbonate rises above 29 mEq. per liter in adults and above 25 mEq. per liter in children. The plasma pH falls below 7.35.

The lungs obviously are unable to make compensatory efforts, but the kidneys retain bicarbonate and excrete carbonic acid. Administration of bicarbonate or lactate may also be necessary to restore the balance while the primary cause of the imbalance is being treated. Therapy is directed primarily toward the underlying pulmonary disorder.

DISEASE MODEL: INFANTILE DIARRHEA

Infantile diarrhea, a common cause of water and electrolyte disturbances in infants and small children, is well suited to illustrating the development of body fluid disturbances, since it leads to a sequence of imbalances.

The young child's extracellular fluid volume can be rapidly depleted by large losses of liquid stools, especially when these are accompanied by vomiting. Water and electrolytes are usually lost in isotonic proportions, so that fluid volume deficit, or "isotonic dehydration," develops. Sometimes, however, water is lost in excess of electrolytes; this is fluid volume deficit with sodium excess, or "hypertonic dehydration." When electrolytes are lost in excess of water, there is a fluid volume deficit with sodium deficit, or "hypotonic dehydration." Sodium being the chief cation

FLUID
LOSSES
OF
IMMEDIATE
CONSEQUENCE
IN YOUNG
CHILD

of extracellular fluid, a deficit or excess plays a major role in symptom production. Symptoms include the following:

    weight loss

    dry skin with poor tissue turgor

    depression of a patent anterior fontanel

    soft eyeballs having a sunken appearance (due to decreased intra-ocular pressure)

    lethargy

    depressed body temperature (unless there is fever)

    ashen or gray skin and cold extremities (due to inadequate peripheral circulation)

    early hypovolemic shock (weak rapid pulse, decreased blood pressure, oliguria) if treatment is not started promptly

Since intestinal fluids are alkaline, there will be large losses of base bicarbonate, leading to metabolic acidosis, or primary base bicarbonate deficit. If the patient is not eating properly, body fat will be consumed for energy purposes. This leads to accumulation of acidic ketone bodies in the blood, which further contributes to the metabolic acidosis originally caused by the loss of base bicarbonate. A major symptom of metabolic acidosis is an increase in the depth of respiration, as the body endeavors to compensate by blowing off carbon dioxide and thereby reducing the amount of carbonic acid in the blood and increasing the pH. If ketosis of starvation is present, the breath will have an acetone odor.

Since the body is largely unable to conserve potassium, even when abnormal losses are occurring, potassium deficit frequently is an associated problem, giving rise to anorexia, vomiting, weakness, excessive abdominal gas, and flabbiness of muscle.

The first goal of therapy is to increase the extracellular fluid volume enough to prevent or correct hypovolemic shock and to restore adequate renal function. Renal depression is assumed to be present when there has been a recent loss of great quantities of fluid, as indicated by a specific gravity of urine above 1.030 and oliguria or anuria.

THERAPY OF RENAL DEPRESSION

When kidney function is depressed, an initial hydrating solution, or pump-priming solution, having about one third the electrolyte concentration of extracellular fluid, is administered to restore normal function. A typical pump-priming solution provides 51 mEq. per liter sodium, 51 mEq. per liter chloride, and 5 Gm. per liter glucose, prepared by mixing 1 volume of isotonic solution of sodium chloride in 5 per cent dextrose with 2 volumes of 5 per cent dextrose in water. Prepared pump-priming solutions are available.

If the renal depression is due to fluid volume deficit, the initial hydrating solution will restore function. Should this fail, it is assumed that the renal depression was caused by serious renal impairment and not by the volume deficit, in which case attention is then directed toward the renal problem.

Once renal flow is reestablished, the kidneys are again able to excrete organic acids, and the appropriate solutions can then be given to correct the various imbalances. A lactated Ringer's solution with dextrose and added potassium, or a Butler-type, or balanced, solution may be employed. Water and electrolyte requirements in infants and children of different ages and weights vary considerably, so that body surface area is probably the best criterion for determining dosage (except in the case of premature infants) since this method is not based on age or weight. For maintenance purposes, a balanced solution is administered at a dose level of 1,500 ml. per square meter of body surface per day; for correction of a moderate fluid volume deficit, the dose level is 2,400 ml. per square meter of body surface per day; and in severe volume deficit, the dose level is 3,000 ml. per square meter of body surface per day. The solution is administered at a rate of 3 ml. per square meter of body surface per minute.

CLINICAL CONSIDERATIONS

Body fluids play a crucial role in metabolic processes and in nutrition. An understanding of their role therefore gives insight into the body's physiology and the manner in which the function of each body system is coordinated with all other body systems.

When one understands the causes of body fluid disturbances and appreciates the rapidity of their development, he recognizes the need for careful observation of those patients who are likely to manifest such disturbances. In this way, the imbalance can often be corrected in an early stage. An understanding of fluid gains and losses and their roles in disease causation makes clear the importance of maintaining accurate intake-output records. If the health worker has an adequate understanding of the 16 basic imbalances, he can then understand the complex, combined imbalances. Then too, with fluid therapy being employed so frequently in the treatment of hospitalized patients, errors in administration are apt to occur, and a knowledge of which therapy is called for in a given imbalance helps to prevent such errors and may make the difference between life and death.

16 BASIC
IMBALANCES
THE KEY
TO COMPLEX
IMBALANCES

TOPICS FOR DISCUSSION

1. Is the capillary bed the only location in the body where there is normally an interchange between plasma and interstitial fluid?

2. In what way are body fluid disturbances the common denominator of a host of diseases?

3. Do you believe that the study of body fluid disturbances can represent a unifying approach to physiology? Explain your answer.

4. What evidence does the body fluid offer that man's forebears sprang from the sea?

5. What fundamental physiological situation would account for the ready development of potassium deficit?

6. Which electrolyte deficit are alcoholics prone to develop?

7. From the standpoint of diagnosis of body fluid disturbances, why do we focus our attention on the extracellular fluid?

8. What four types of evidence help us in our diagnosis of a specific body fluid disturbance?

9. Why is the milliequivalent so much more useful than the milligram in evaluating the concentration of electrolytes in the body fluids?

10. Why is part of our extracellular fluid, the plasma, contained within the blood vascular system?

BIBLIOGRAPHY

Books

Snively, W., and Sweeney, M.: Fluid Balance Handbook for Practitioners. Springfield, Illinois, Charles C Thomas, 1956.

Weisberg, H.: Water, Electrolyte and Acid-Base Balance. Baltimore, The Williams & Wilkins Co., 1962.

Metheny, N., and Snively, W.: Nurses' Handbook of Fluid Balance. Philadelphia, J. B. Lippincott Co., 1967.

Garrett, T.: Baxter Guide to Fluid Therapy. Morton Grove, Illinois, Baxter Laboratories, 1969.

Snively, W., and Thuerbach, J.: Sea of Life. New York, David McKay Co., Inc., 1969.

Articles

Snively, W., and Westerman, R.: Serum potassium determination. JAMA, *197*:579, 1966.

Snively, W., and Becker, B.: Minerals, macro and micro: dynamic nutrients—part I, the macro-minerals. Annals of Allergy, *26*:167, 1968.

9

diseases of malnutrition

Whatsoever was the father of a disease, an ill diet was the mother.
—George Herbert, *Jacula Prudentum,* 1651

Nutritional deficiency states are among the most widespread of all diseases. These disorders are endemic in poverty-stricken, underdeveloped countries and of surprising frequency in developed countries. They affect rich and poor, young and old. These deficiency states are particularly likely to arise in sick persons, in infants whose diets consist entirely of milk, in children and adolescents during periods of rapid growth, and in women during pregnancy and lactation. Persons who live alone often have poor eating habits and therefore are prime candidates for such illnesses, as are food faddists and weight watchers.

For maintenance of optimal health, the body requires certain amounts of nutrient substances, including protein, carbohydrate, fat, vitamins, minerals, and water. Each nutrient has a specific purpose in the body. Some yield energy for the constant physical, chemical, and electrical activities carried on by the body, others build and repair tissues, while still others regulate various metabolic processes. As we shall see, nutritional deficiencies develop when the body does not receive the essential nutrients in the proper amounts, or is unable to utilize them properly. Diseases of malnutrition are largely deficiency diseases, although excesses of certain nutrients can also cause illness. Often several such disorders occur simultaneously, since a diet unbalanced in relation to one nutrient is apt to be similarly unbalanced in several.

THE CALORIE

The large, or great, calorie, which measures energy or heat, represents the quantity of heat needed to raise the temperature of 1 liter of water 1 degree centigrade, or 1.8 degrees Fahrenheit. The stored fuel in foods is expressed in calories. One gram of pure protein provides

161

4 calories, as does the same amount of carbohydrate. One gram of fat supplies 9 calories, 1 gram of alcohol, about 7. For optimum health, about 15 to 20 per cent of the daily caloric intake should be derived from protein foods, 30 to 35 per cent from fat foods, and 35 to 50 per cent from starch or carbohydrate foods.

Daily caloric requirements vary from one individual to another, with such factors as sex, age, size, activity, environment, and general state of health determining one's caloric needs. Most adults expend approximately 70 calories per hour while resting, 105 calories per hour while standing, and several hundreds of calories per hour while exercising vigorously. When more calories are expended than are taken in, the body begins, literally, to consume its own stores of fat, in order to generate calories for energy. When the fat stores are depleted, solid tissues (chiefly muscles) are chemically broken down and converted into calories. New tissue synthesis and repair of damaged tissues cannot occur since any food consumed is, for the most part, diverted for energy purposes.

CALORIC DEFICIT AND CALORIC EXCESS BOTH CAUSES OF MALNUTRITION

The symptoms of caloric deficit are easily recognized. Obviously, there is hunger and loss of weight. There is mental depression and apprehension, and the slightest effort produces fatigue. Then there are less obvious symptoms, such as shortness of breath. If the caloric deficit continues, protein deficit follows. A diet providing 1,600 calories constitutes a caloric deficit in most adults, while an intake of 1,200 calories or less represents a deficit in all adults.

Caloric excess, as well as caloric deficit, can lead to disease. Unneeded calories are stored in the body as adipose, or fat, tissue for future use. Chronic excesses lead to obesity, which is not only unattractive but also poses a threat to health and longevity. Even minor degrees of overweight—5 or 10 per cent above normal—can be dangerous. Long-standing obesity is known to be a predisposing factor in diabetes, hypertension, myocardial failure, orthopedic disorders, degenerative arthritis of the back and knees, varicose veins, leg ulcers, and postoperative thromboembolism—not to mention its psychic effects. Obesity also increases the likelihood of complications accompanying pregnancy, childbearing, and operative procedures.

In recent years, a plethora of faddist reducing diets proclaiming that "calories don't count" have been widely publicized. Unfortunately, these popular schemes for losing weight painlessly not only are ineffective, but may even be dangerous. The sad truth is that "calories do count," and to lose weight one must achieve a caloric deficit. A sensible, well-balanced diet providing 1,200 to 1,500 calories allows one to lose weight safely. For optimum health this should be supplemented with daily exercise, which helps burn excess calories and tones flabby muscles.

PROTEINS

Proteins are the fundamental structural element of every cell of the body. In their role as enzymes, proteins regulate the breakdown of food for energy and the synthesis of new compounds for repair and maintenance of body tissues. Certain proteins are now known to be the functional element of hormones as well. Many antibodies are proteins (recall Chap. 3) and therefore play an important role in immunity. Obviously, when protein substances are deficient in the diet, the body as a whole suffers in various ways.

Protein malnutrition can result when the diet is protein-deficient, in conditions of increased utilization of protein for energy purposes (as occurs in caloric deficit), or in diseases associated with impaired digestion or absorption, impaired synthesis of plasma proteins, increased catabolism, or excessive loss of body protein. Hypoproteinemia, a deficiency of protein in the body fluids, is described in Chapter 8.

DIETARY IMBALANCES FREQUENTLY ASSOCIATED WITH POVERTY

CARBOHYDRATES AND FATS

Carbohydrates, the most abundant and economical source of bodily energy, constitute approximately 70 per cent, by weight, of the food in the average American diet. They are the chief constituents of baked goods, sugar, syrups, starch, confections, cereals, and fermentation products. The chief function of carbohydrate is to supply calories for energy purposes. Glucose, the principal form of carbohydrate in the blood, is a readily available source of energy. Carbohydrate in excess of bodily needs is converted to fat and stored as fatty tissue.

Fats provide the body with a concentrated source of calories for energy purposes. Adipose tissue protects the body from mechanical injury and serves as a heat insulator.

Carbohydrates and fats are the main sources of calories for energy purposes. A deficiency of them leads to caloric deficit and the burning of protein for energy purposes, whereas an excess results in overweight. Excessive intake of saturated fats (those that remain in a solid state at room temperature) increases the serum cholesterol level, and this is believed to contribute to the development of coronary artery disease, as described in Chapter 12.

VITAMINS

Vitamins—coined from the words *vital amine*—are potent organic compounds occurring in small concentrations in foods. Although they are essential to life, they are needed in only minute quantities for normal body function. With the exception of vitamins A and D, vitamins in excess usually do no harm, as in most instances the excess is simply excreted in the urine. An excess of vitamin A or D (*hypervitaminosis*) can cause damage when given in huge doses for prolonged periods.

Vitamins do not provide calories, but are required for normal growth and reproduction, maintenance of good health, and protection against disease and infection. Thus vitamin deficits may lead to various types of dysfunction. Two types of vitamin deficiency, or *avitaminosis*, can occur. The first type, known as *primary* or *simple* deficiency, results from inadequate dietary intake of vitamins. Primary avitaminosis is rarely seen in developed countries, but it is widespread in developing countries, particularly Africa and the Orient, and may occur during wartime in any involved country. The second type is called *secondary* or *conditional* deficiency. In this case, vitamin supplies are adequate but cannot be utilized properly. Prolonged vomiting, esophageal obstruction, loss of appetite, painful lesions of the mouth, or any condition that causes reduced intake are among the contributing conditions. Chronic pancreatitis and chronic enteritis, for example, hinder absorption of vitamins and thus lead to deficiencies.

Avitaminosis may occur during periods of great demand, as during pregnancy and lactation, infancy, and puberty, and in other conditions that increase metabolic function, such as prolonged fever and hyperthyroidism. Deficiencies also may occur secondary to diseases that reduce storage ability, such as cirrhosis of the liver. Alcoholics with liver disease are prime candidates for vitamin deficiency, not only because they are likely to suffer widespread damage to the liver, but also because they quite frequently substitute alcohol for food. A poorer substitute could scarcely be imagined.

Marginal note: VITAMINS PERFORM SPECIFIC FUNCTIONS IN CELLS AND TISSUES, YET ARE NEEDED ONLY IN MINUTE QUANTITIES

Vitamin A

Vitamin A preserves the visual purple in the rod cells of the retina. This substance is essential for night vision, maintains the integrity of the epithelial surfaces of the body, regulates early bone growth and development, and aids in formation of healthy tooth enamel.

It is unlikely that a deficit of vitamin A would often be primary since the vitamin is widely distributed in foods and since the liver stores vitamin A in large quantities. Rather, avitaminosis A occurs secondary to other conditions, such as pancreatic dysfunction, disease of the biliary tract, sprue, and the malabsorption syndrome. Over a period of several years, liver disease may bring about a deficiency.

In avitaminosis A, columnar epithelium atrophies. This leads to basal cell proliferation, as the atrophied tissue is replaced with stratified keratinizing ("horny") epithelium. This *keratinizing metaplasia* may be seen in the conjunctiva, salivary glands, trachea, bronchi, nasal mucosa, accessory

Marginal note: AVITAMINOSIS A

nasal sinuses, pancreas, renal pelvis, ureters, and uterus. Such serious ocular disorders as xerophthalmia leading to keratomalacia, follicular hyperkeratosis, and nyctalopia (night blindness) may follow. In young animals, vitamin A deficiency retards bone growth.

As with vitamin D, it is possible—though rare—for the body to have too much vitamin A. An excess is harmful, however, only when tremendous doses are taken over long periods of time, as is likely to occur through overenthusiastic administration by parents. Chronic vitamin A toxicity produces symptoms of the nervous system, the skeleton, and the skin, including persistent severe headache with visual disorders; bone pain; pruritus; sparse, coarse hair; fissuring and soreness at the corners of the mouth; and pigmentation. There is rapid clinical improvement when excessive intake is stopped.

HYPERVITAMINOSIS A

Vitamin D

Vitamin D increases the amount of calcium and phosphorus that is absorbed from the lower end of the gastrointestinal tract, so that when vitamin D is deficient, calcium and phosphorus are deficient also. Avitaminosis D may result from an inadequate supply of bile salts, pancreatic insufficiency, the malabsorption syndrome, and liver disease.

In the child, the clinical manifestation of avitaminosis D is rickets; in the adult, it is osteomalacia. There is faulty mineralization of bone, since calcium absorption is dependent on vitamin D. In severe cases, the soft bones are deformed and may fracture easily. Tooth development may be faulty also.

AVITAMINOSIS D

Like vitamin A, vitamin D can cause illness when massive doses are taken for prolonged periods. Hypervitaminosis D produces hypercalcemia and hyperphosphatemia, with calcification of soft tissues. The earliest symptoms include anorexia, nausea, and vomiting, followed by polyuria, polydipsia, weakness, nervousness, and pruritus.

HYPERVITAMINOSIS D

Vitamin E

Of all the vitamins found in the ordinary diet, vitamin E is the most abundant, and as a result, little is known about avitaminosis E in the human. Experimental deficiency has been produced in animals, however, and has been shown to affect reproductive ability. In the male, spermatozoa are destroyed and the entire seminiferous epithelium degenerates. The ovaries of the female animal do not appear to be injured, and the animal is able to conceive. In the rat, however, on about the eighth day following conception, pathological changes occur in the placenta, as a result of which the fetus dies and is absorbed. Vitamin E also aids in preserving the integrity of skeletal muscles.

Vitamin K

Because of its role in blood coagulation, vitamin K is of great clinical significance. The vitamin is necessary for the manufacture of prothrombin, which is essential in the clotting of blood.

Avitaminosis K in man is probably never caused by lack of the vitamin in food. Rather, vitamin K deficiency is a *conditioned* deficiency, which may be brought about by three types of conditions: bowel obstruction; malabsorption of fat, as in pancreatic disease, sprue, celiac disease, and bowel hypermotility; and failure of intestinal bacteria to synthesize vitamin K, as occurs when the normal flora is altered by the action of antibiotics.

For coagulation of blood, which is necessary to stop hemorrhage, the level of the blood prothrombin must be normal. When, however, vitamin K is deficient, plasma prothrombin is low. This is of major clinical significance in obstructive jaundice and hemorrhagic disease of the newborn. The presence of sufficient vitamin K is itself not enough; the vitamin must be absorbed in order to be utilized in the manufacture of prothrombin. Vitamin K cannot be absorbed unless bile is present in the intestine. In obstructive jaundice bile cannot enter the bowel; consequently, vitamin K cannot be absorbed and prothrombin cannot be formed in sufficient amount. Hemorrhage results. The lack of bile accounts for the marked tendency of jaundiced patients to bleed after operations. Not only is there bleeding from severed vessels, there may also be hemorrhages in the skin and mucous membranes, particularly of the bowel. Such bleeding can be prevented by oral or intravenous administration of both bile and vitamin K, or of synthetic vitamin K alone, which is absorbed without the presence of bile. Since, however, prothrombin is produced in the liver, administration of vitamin K is of no avail if the liver is severely damaged, as in cirrhosis or amyloid disease.

Two factors contribute to hemorrhage in the newborn: (1) vitamin K-producing bacteria are not present in the intestine during the first few days of life, and (2) the liver does not produce bile during this period. The infant has received sufficient prothrombin from the mother at birth, but this supply is rapidly depleted. Without prothrombin, severe, even fatal, hemorrhage may take place, particularly within the skull. Hemorrhagic disease of the newborn can be prevented by administering vitamin K to the mother before delivery.

ANTIHEMORRHAGIC
ROLE OF
VITAMIN K

Vitamin C (Ascorbic Acid)

Vitamin C is essential for the health of the ground substance of mesenchymal structures, such as osteoid, collagen, dentine, and the cement of capillary walls.

Avitaminosis C causes scurvy, or scorbutus, with clinical manifestations including delayed healing of wounds, defective bone formation, a pronounced tendency to bleed, and, in experimental animals, defective tooth formation. All are based on the fundamental defect in the metabolism of mesenchymal substance.

Infantile scurvy, or Barlow's disease, is similar to adult scurvy, but the symptoms are primarily caused by bone lesions. Hemorrhages beneath the periosteum produce such tenderness of the legs that the child will scream if his legs are touched, or perhaps even if one enters his room! Bone growth is halted, and the gums may be tender and bleeding. Infantile scurvy usually appears in the second half of the first year and is seldom seen in an acute form after the second year, since by then the diet is more varied.

Vitamin B Complex

The term *vitamin B complex* is used to describe a group of substances now known to be of different chemical compositions and physiological actions but originally thought to be a single factor. In relation to human disease, the most important members of the complex are thiamine (vitamin B_1), riboflavin (vitamin B_2), niacin, folic acid, and vitamin B_{12}. At least three of the B vitamins—thiamine, riboflavin, and niacin—are needed as coenzymes in the Krebs citric acid cycle of energy-transfer reactions in cell respiration.

12 FRACTIONS OF VITAMIN B COMPLEX PRESENTLY RECOGNIZED

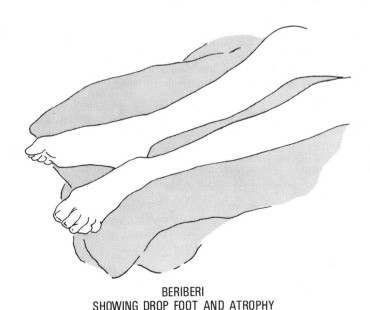

BERIBERI
SHOWING DROP FOOT AND ATROPHY

Thiamine   Thiamine, or vitamin B_1, is the antineuritic or antiberiberi factor. This vitamin B fraction is essential to enzyme systems concerned with carbohydrate metabolism, especially that involving the nervous system. Thiamine deficiency leads to beriberi, manifested by peripheral neuritis, edema, and myocardial weakness—a combination of symptoms found in perhaps no other disease. A cerebral form of beriberi, Wernicke's encephalopathy, usually causes death within a few days after onset. This condition is, fortunately, rare.

Riboflavin   Riboflavin, or vitamin B_2, is sometimes called the *tissue respiratory vitamin* since it is essential for normal cell respiration. It plays a role in the transfer of oxygen from the plasma to the tissue cells. Symptoms of riboflavin deficiency are most conspicuous in the lips, mouth, skin, and eyes. Cheilosis develops early. Its most common form is simple chapping, but in adults an atrophic form is frequently seen in which the exposed mucosa becomes thin and parchment-like. Pallor, erythema, or slight maceration of the mucosa in the angles of the mouth may appear, followed by dermatitis of the adjacent skin. The dermatitis begins in the nasolabial folds and extends to the cheeks in a butterfly distribution. Fissures appear in the affected areas and often leave scars after healing. If the fissures become infected, grayish-white lesions appear—a condition known as perlèche. There is scaling dermatitis about the nose, ears, and scrotum. Lesions of the eye are the most serious. The most common is circumcorneal injection, and in advanced cases, capillaries arising from the limbic plexus invade the cornea, causing opacity and keratitis.

Niacin   Niacin, or nicotinic acid, plays a role in the formation of two coenzymes (known simply as coenzyme I and coenzyme II) that form an essential part of the respiratory enzyme system of cells. Niacin deficiency is believed to contribute to development of pellagra, characterized by dermatitis, diarrhea, and dementia, with corresponding lesions of the skin, alimentary tract, and central nervous system.

Interference with the normal metabolism of the epidermis causes the skin to become reddened, thickened, and hyperkeratotic, followed by peeling on exposed parts of the body, particularly the face and backs of the hands. In the alimentary canal, lesions develop in the mouth and over the tongue and esophagus. These lesions are similar in character, with complete disappearance of the lining epithelium and development of bacteria-filled ulcers. Similar lesions are found throughout the colon. In the nervous system, there is degeneration of the ganglion cells in the cerebral cortex and myelin degeneration of the same tracts in the spinal cord. In the liver there is extensive fatty degeneration at first, followed by a massive accumulation of iron pigment in liver cells, necrosis, and, finally, cirrhosis.

A diet deficient in one vitamin is very likely to be deficient in others,

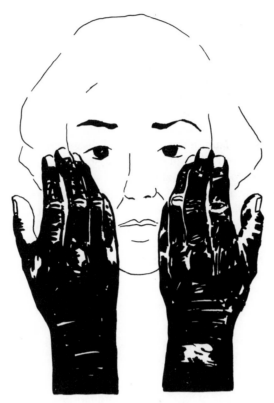

PELLAGRA

so it is not surprising that pellagra, beriberi, and riboflavin deficiency often coexist in man.

Folic acid and vitamin B_{12}　　Folic acid and vitamin B_{12} are growth factors in the maturation of red blood cells in the bone marrow. When these nutrients are deficient, red blood cells are produced much more slowly than normal, and those that are produced are larger than normal, poorly formed, and quite fragile. Pernicious anemia and other megaloblastic anemias can result from such abnormal formation. Body tissues store an abundant supply of B_{12}, however, so deficits develop slowly, perhaps over a period of years.

　　B_{12} is used in treatment of pernicious anemia and also may be helpful in stimulating growth in children who have failed to grow. Folic acid, or pteroylglutamic acid, is useful in some anemias and is specific in treatment of the nutritional anemia produced by tropical sprue. Folic acid is contraindicated in the treatment of pernicious anemia, since it exerts no beneficial effect on lesions of the central nervous system and may, in fact, aggravate them while correcting the anemia and giving rise to a false sense of security.

MINERALS

Minerals can be divided into two groups: (1) those which occur in fairly large amounts (1 gram or more in the average adult) and (2) those which occur only in minute quantities. Those in the first group are termed *macrominerals*. Most of these, including sodium, potassium, calcium, phosphorous, and magnesium, are discussed in Chapter 8, Disturbances of Fluid and Electrolyte Balance, so we shall limit our discussion of macrominerals to iron and zinc.

Minerals present in the body only in trace quantities are called *microminerals, trace minerals,* or *trace elements.* These include copper, manganese, molybdenum, iodine, cobalt, vanadium, and fluorine.

QUANTITIES OF MINERALS IN 70 KILOGRAM MAN

Macrominerals	Grams	Microminerals	Grams
Calcium	1,400	Copper	0.1
Phosphorus	770	Manganese	.02
Potassium	140	Molybdenum	.005
Sodium	105	Iodine	.028
Magnesium	35	Cobalt	.003
Iron	4	Vanadium	.0001
Zinc	2.3	Fluorine	Unknown

Iron

The macromineral iron is required for synthesis of hemoglobin. Nursing infants, premature infants, young children, pregnant women, and women whose menstrual flow is excessive are prime candidates for iron deficit and should be given iron supplements. The adult male rarely needs supplementation unless he is losing blood.

When iron is deficient, hemoglobin cannot be synthesized properly, and the patient develops iron deficiency anemia, with symptoms of pallor, weakness, ready fatigue, dyspnea on exertion, headache, and palpitation. A male with iron deficiency anemia should be examined thoroughly to rule out the existence of infection, cancer, stomach ulcer, or other sources of blood loss or destruction. The anemia is corrected by administration of iron.

Prolonged excessive iron therapy can, however, lead to excess accumulation of iron, as can transfusional hemosiderosis (due to many transfusions) and idiopathic hemochromatosis. The latter, which is apparently linked to an inborn error of metabolism (recall Chap. 2), is a rare disease that predominantly affects males and results in cirrhosis of the liver, bronzing of the skin, diabetes mellitus, and endocrine abnormalities. It is not known, however, whether it is iron per se or other metabolic abnormalities that give rise to the pathologic changes and abnormal distribution of iron.

Zinc

Zinc, a long-ignored macromineral, is now known to be an integral part of red blood molecules, where it assists in carbon dioxide exchange. Zinc is also an essential element of enzymes needed for growth and normal functioning.

In swine, zinc deficiency produces a severe dermatitis known as parakeratosis. In other animals, the deficiency causes loss of hair or feathers, somatic growth failure, atrophy of male gonads, embryonic deformities, and thickening of the skin and esophageal lining.

In man, zinc deficiency is seen in areas of the world in which nutrition is extremely poor. Investigators in Iran and Egypt found decreased zinc levels in the serum and hair of dwarfs who appeared to have iron deficiency anemia. With zinc supplementation body growth and sexual maturation were promoted. Another investigator found subnormal zinc levels in the neck hair of severely burned patients. When healing began, about 100 days postburn, zinc levels returned to normal. In another study, injured patients receiving zinc sulfate healed in 45 days, while in controls healing required 75 days. Patients with arteriosclerosis have been found to have remarkably low zinc levels; however, the significance of this finding is not understood.

According to some reports, dental caries is seen with diets chronically high in zinc. Zinc toxicity is almost invariably associated with the eating of foods that have been stored in zinc-coated containers. Its effects include nausea, vomiting, and diarrhea.

ZINC DEFICIENCY IN HUMANS ONLY RECENTLY RECOGNIZED

Copper

The micromineral copper plays a role in the action of several essential enzymes. It helps activate lipid enzymes systems, particularly those associated with phospholipid synthesis. The element also participates in the absorption of iron from the gastrointestinal tract and in the production and survival of red blood cells.

Patients who have a combination of sprue, iron deficiency, hypoproteinemia, and kwashiorkor develop copper deficit, or hypocupremia. Infants whose diet is restricted to milk may develop hypocupremia since milk contains little copper. The condition responds to copper supplementation, as does nutritional anemia in infants. Experimentally, copper supplementation in mice fed meat diets decreased exchangeability of bone calcium, improved mineralization, and promoted growth.

HUMAN REQUIREMENT FOR COPPER PROBABLY UNDER 2 MG. DAILY

Excesses of copper are toxic, giving rise to gastric disturbances, muscular cramps, tremors, and peripheral neuritis. In one study, elevated copper levels were found in four of nine persons with chronic schizophrenia; the significance of this finding is not known, however.

In hepatolenticular degeneration (Wilson's disease), a rare familial disorder of copper metabolism, the brain, liver, and kidneys show increased amounts of copper. It becomes recognizable when the affected child is 5 to 7 years old. Treatment, consisting of a low-copper diet and agents that prevent intestinal absorption of copper, may not be successful, and the patient may die from the cumulative effects of cirrhosis of the liver and brain degeneration.

Manganese and Molybdenum

The body requires both manganese and molybdenum for bone formation, normal metabolism, and normal growth. Like several other trace elements, manganese activates many essential enzymes. Molybdenum is thought to inhibit tooth decay in animals and children, although other minerals may play a role in this protective action.

Manganese deficiency in man has not been demonstrated. However, fowls lacking the mineral show poor growth, decline in reproductive capacity, faulty bone growth, and nervous disorders. Molybdenum deficiency has not been reported in either man or animal.

Both elements are relatively safe in amounts found in the normal diet, but an excess of either disturbs the chemical balance. Iron metabolism is disturbed by excessive manganese, and that of copper is hampered by excessive molybdenum. Manganese miners absorb manganese dust from the respiratory tract. The symptoms, which include anorexia, headache, apathy, leg cramps, impotence, and speech disturbances, progress insidiously to such a degree that the clinical picture resembles Parkinson's disease. The condition becomes irreversible with severe toxicity.

Cobalt

Cobalt, a component of vitamin B_{12}, is essential for normal production of red blood cells in the bone marrow. Some investigators believe that cobalt speeds regeneration of red cells destroyed by radiation. Cobalt deficiency in man has not been demonstrated. It has been observed, however, that sheep become weakened after grazing on pastures low in cobalt.

In many species of animals, excessive cobalt causes overproduction of red blood cells—true polycythemia—through an unknown mechanism. In man, grave pulmonary symptoms result from inhalation of cobalt dust. Cobalt powder can cause contact dermatitis; and nausea and vomiting result from ingestion of soluble cobalt salts.

Fluorine

Of all the microminerals, fluorine is probably the most controversial. To date, little is known about fluorine metabolism. The element inhibits tooth decay when added to water, when given in a vitamin preparation, when applied directly to the teeth, or when incorporated in toothpaste. It is not known just how this comes about, but it is thought that during the formative years the mineral reduces the solubility of tooth enamel by acids produced by bacteria. According to recent reports, administration of sodium fluorides may result in arrest of osteoporosis and Paget's disease of the bone. Preliminary evidence suggests that extended space flights may lead to rarefaction of bone due to calcium loss. Administration of fluorides may be a means of protecting the skeletal system during such travel.

With excessive fluorine intake, tooth enamel becomes mottled; in fact, dental fluorosis is endemic in a number of communities, particularly in parts of Colorado and Texas where the fluorine content of water is high (above 2 parts per million). In miners who have been exposed to dust containing fluoride for many years, the bones become hard and dense. The effects of acute fluoride poisoning include severe eye irritation, sometimes with blindness; respiratory tract irritation; severe skin burns; and stomatitis. In chronic toxicity there are changes in bone and ligament, anemia, eosinophilia, and skin burns.

CRITICAL LEVEL OF FLUORINE 1 PART PER MILLION

Iodine

Iodine, a component of thyroid hormone, is a many-faceted mineral: applied topically, it is a counterirritant, bactericide, and fungicide; added to water, it is a disinfectant; as found in the thyroxin of the normal thyroid, it prevents cretinism and goiter.

In iodine deficiency, the secretory activity of the thyroid is increased by compensatory effort. The gland becomes enlarged, causing a swelling in the front of the neck. This enlargement is known as *goiter*. Even when iodine is present in sufficient amounts, certain drugs, such as thiourea and thiouracil, prevent the thyroid gland from oxidizing iodide to iodine. There are other factors that also may be contributory toward goiter.

Foods of the genus *Brassica*, such as rutabaga and cabbage, contain a goitrogenic substance. In certain inland areas, such as the Alpine regions of Europe and the Great Lakes area of the United States, the water and soil are lacking in iodine. The use of iodized table salt decreases the incidence of goiter in these areas.

In sensitive persons, ingestion of average therapeutic doses of iodine may cause skin lesions. Large quantities may cause abdominal pain, nausea, vomiting, and diarrhea. As little as 2 to 3 grams of iodine may cause death, but this occurrence is rare.

IODINE ONE OF FIRST MICROMINERALS TO BE RECOGNIZED AS VITAL IN NUTRITION

Vanadium

Vanadium was discovered in 1830, but intensive investigation of its activity began only recently. The element is believed to play a role in tooth enamel protection. Some scientists have suggested that vanadium reduces cholesterol levels in the blood and thereby helps prevent death from arteriosclerosis.

Vanadium deficiency in man has not been confirmed. Excesses have, however, been demonstrated in animals. Toxic symptoms appear when vanadium is administered parenterally, and the rat will die from 0.2 per cent vanadium in the diet. In man, ingested vanadium causes gastrointestinal disturbances. Boiler cleaners exposed to vanadium dust may manifest conjunctivitis, nasopharyngitis, and persistent cough.

Nonessential Trace Elements

RECLASSIFICATION MAY FOLLOW INCREASED UNDERSTANDING OF SOME ELEMENTS PREVIOUSLY REGARDED AS NONESSENTIAL

Several minerals previously thought to be nonessential are now being studied with new interest. One of these elements is chromium. In the rat it contributes to growth, longevity, and resistance to infection, while a deficiency induces a disease resembling human diabetes. With chromium administration the diseased rats live longer than controls.

Another such element is lithium. This mineral has long been known to be highly toxic, but it is now being studied extensively in the prophylaxis of recurrent depression in manic-depressive psychosis. Psychiatrists have so far been unable to explain the apparent effectiveness of lithium in preventing recurrent depression.

Nickel also presents unsolved mysteries. In rats, high intakes of nickel cause dental decay. In man, neither nickel deficiency nor nickel excess has been reported.

Selenium appears to prevent breakdown of polyunsaturated fatty acids; however, it also appears to promote tooth decay. The element is formed by the burning of cigarette paper and is strongly suspected to be a cause of cancer among cigarette smokers.

Several other microminerals used in a host of industrial processes may cause poisoning. These elements include arsenic, lead, antimony, cadmium, strontium, beryllium, mercury, tellurium, and thorium. A second group, though possessing therapeutic properties, may be toxic even when administered carefully. This group includes bismuth, boron, arsenic, barium, antimony, gold, mercury, and lithium. Thus, even the justifiable use of these elements in therapy involves a calculated risk.

Undoubtedly, as research continues, our understanding of both the microminerals and the macrominerals will improve. It is likely that these elements will find wide usage in the prevention and treatment of disease, as well as in the maintenance of optimal nutrition.

WATER

Water is an absolutely essential nutritive substance. One experiencing any other nutritional deficiency can live for a relatively long period, but without water one can live for only a few days. There is no substitute for water in the living cycle—a fact readily appreciated when one considers that the adult body is about 60 per cent fluid. Water can dissolve many substances and is the basis of our body fluids. The body is, in a sense, a bag of more or less solid materials dissolved in a greater quantity of water. Without it, the myriad chemical reactions of the body cannot occur, and in fact no vital function can go'on without water. Therefore, a generous intake of water is essential for optimum body function.

Although water is usually regarded as completely innocuous, about seven times the normal daily intake can be toxic. Excessive water promotes the washing out of electrolytes from the body and is one cause of body fluid disturbances, as described in Chapter 8.

WATER NECESSARY FOR FUNCTIONING OF EVERY ORGAN IN BODY

GENERAL PHYSIOLOGIC AND PSYCHOLOGIC EFFECTS OF MALNUTRITION

Reduction in growth rate is perhaps the best-documented effect of malnutrition. Delayed bone growth contributes to smaller physical size. Although factors other than nutrition can influence physical size, possibly a good indicator of nutritional status is physical size for age. The underdeveloped child has probably been malnourished during some significant period of his development.

In malnourished populations, sexual maturation—particularly menses in females—appears to occur later, whereas in more developed countries, sexual maturation occurs at a younger age with each succeeding generation.

Malnutrition during pregnancy has been implicated in fetal wastage and birth defects, and may be a factor in prematurity. It has also been linked to the high mortality in infants and preschool children, particularly between the ages of 1 and 4, in developing countries.

MENTATION MAY SUFFER MOST SERIOUS CONSEQUENCES OF MALNUTRITION

Recent reports indicate that severe malnutrition during early infancy retards brain development. The brain normally develops by cell division until the infant is about 6 months old, so that malnutrition during this period presumably leads to irreversible impairment, with the brain having fewer cells than a normal brain. Animal studies suggest that once this developmental period has passed, subsequent malnutrition will not necessarily cause irreversible damage. That is, the brain cells may be smaller than normal, but with improved nutrition the brain cells—

hence brain—may grow to normal size. There is also evidence that malnutrition is associated with subnormal intelligence. Testifying in August, 1969, before the U.S. Senate Select Committee on Nutrition and Human Needs, Dr. Charles Lowe stated: "There is no evidence that feeding people makes them smart, but it is indisputable that hunger makes them dull."

Malnourished children and adults alike are apathetic, listless, and unresponsive to external and internal stimuli. This picture may produce various other problems, including impaired learning ability, lowered self-esteem, inadequate social relationships, and unsatisfactory parent-child relationships. According to Dr. David J. Kallen, these effects of malnutrition "tend to produce and perpetuate within the society a disvalued and dysfunctioning group, a section of society for which the social system will have to provide as the economic opportunities for the unskilled, undereducated, and unmotivated become fewer and fewer."

Without any doubt, nutritional deficiency states can produce not only severe physiological effects, but severe psychological and social effects as well.

DISEASE MODEL: CHRONIC PROTEIN DEFICIENCY

Chronic protein deficiency is a consequence of greatly reduced protein intake, greatly increased catabolism, or conditions associated with impaired intestinal absorption, disturbed metabolism of ingested protein, or excessive loss of protein.

The body needs at least 30 grams of good-quality protein per day to maintain *nitrogen balance,* or *nitrogen equilibrium,* that is, the normal state of health in which nitrogen intake (in food) equals nitrogen output (in feces and urine). Loss of 1 kg. of protein represents a negative nitrogen balance of 160 gm. and a body tissue loss of about 4 kg., a loss that is quickly reflected in decreased plasma albumin concentration and a fall in plasma colloid osmotic pressure. Edema gradually develops, first in the dependent portions of the body, then generally. Edema in the wall of the gastrointestinal tract may cause digestive disturbances that result in impaired digestion and absorption of nutrients. Plasma albumin continues to fall gradually and may reach a low concentration.

PROTEIN INTAKE, RATHER THAN HEREDITY, MAY BE MOST IMPORTANT FACTOR IN PHYSICAL STATURE

Weight loss is common, although a patient may actually gain weight as a result of fluid retention. Patients who are protein deficient frequently develop decubitus ulcers. Weakness, anorexia, lethargy, and loss of muscle mass are common. If the deficiency is severe, all vital functions dependent on protein are impaired, including growth, repair of injury, and production of enzymes, antibodies, and certain hormones. Protein deficiency is severe in kwashiorkor, the most prevalent nutritional disease in the world. It affects primarily infants and children. In Central and South

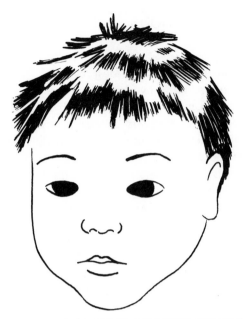

"FLAG SIGN," HAIR OF INDIAN BABY WITH KWASHIORKOR

America it is known as the *pluricarencial syndrome*. Some years ago the senior author photographed a group of children whose protein status was normal and an equal number who were protein deficient. No attempt was made to have the children pose, nor were any instructions given them except to "stand still." All the children well nourished in protein stood erect and smiled; but all the protein impoverished children had woebegone facial expressions and poor posture. This incident illustrates the importance of protein both in emotional equilibrium and in bone and muscle development.

The most satisfactory method of treating chronic protein deficiency is by oral administration of protein in the form of a mixed diet providing high-quality protein, adequate calories, and sufficient amounts of vitamins and minerals. If rapid treatment is necessary, either a high-protein diet alone or a high-protein diet supplemented with an oral high-protein electrolyte mixture may be used. Partial or complete feeding by nasogastric tube may be necessary when food cannot be taken in sufficient quantity. When feeding via oral or nasogastric route is impossible, difficult, or contraindicated, protein may be administered parenterally.

A word of caution: patients with severe protein deficiency who are suddenly and rapidly fed large amounts of food may develop major gastrointestinal disturbances, with nausea, diarrhea, and peripheral vascular collapse. Repletion of body tissues occurs gradually and is exceedingly slow in many chronic diseases, particularly severe liver disease.

CLINICAL CONSIDERATIONS

Nutritional disorders are widespread, yet, because of their insidious nature, they are often overlooked. These deficiency states often are "silent" at first and must be looked for. Obviously, one must have a broad knowledge of these disorders if he is to recognize the significance of vague or poorly described symptoms at an early stage and to correct them before they become full-blown diseases.

Proper nutrition is just as important to the hospitalized patient as any drug or medication he is receiving, and it is up to those caring for him to see that his nutritional needs are met. He should be served attractive, well-balanced meals. If the patient cannot or does not eat what he is served, the physician should be informed. If the patient is receiving nutrients via nasogastric tube or parenterally, care should be taken to see that feedings are given in the proper amounts at prescribed intervals.

Perhaps many nutritional disorders could be prevented by educating patients. Persons involved in providing health care are in an excellent position to offer facts concerning sound nutrition and some practical information as to how to achieve it. A patient who must follow a special diet should be given careful instructions. He will be more apt to stay on the diet if he is told *why* this is important.

Viewing nutrition from the global standpoint, we must face the fact that proper nutrition of the world's hungry millions is essential for man's continued existence. The problem certainly demands a limitation of the world's burgeoning population, as well as the introduction of efficient agricultural methods in backward areas (which include most parts of the world). It also requires education in diet and nutrition. In many parts of Latin America, for example, countless babies are dying every year because their mothers feed them a syrup and water diet despite the fact that cattle sources of milk and meat abound in the hills surrounding the villages. Many steps are being taken to correct these problems, yet the improvement in humankind's overall nutrition is as yet minuscule.

TOPICS FOR DISCUSSION

1. In your opinion, is daily vitamin supplementation always desirable? Why?

2. What are some common fallacies concerning food and nutrition?

3. Why do you suppose fad diets are enthusiastically tried by many people, even though they may be dangerous to health?

4. Who would benefit more from eating the extra portion of meat at the dinner table—a young boy, or a man? Why?

5. Assuming their activities, age, and weight are equal, would an Eskimo and a South Sea Islander have the same caloric requirements? Why?

6. Name some circumstances in which it could be dangerous for an individual to ingest certain nutrients in the amounts considered proper for most persons.

7. Strangely enough, malnutrition has been named as a possible cause of *overpopulation* in some countries. How do you account for this?

8. Suppose you are floating on a raft at sea. From the standpoint of survival, what nutrient substance is the most important?

9. Very few concentration camp victims developed clinical signs of vitamin deficiency. Why is this?

10. What would you expect to happen to a person who ate nothing but carbohydrate foods for 2 months, assuming he drank sufficient quantities of water?

11. What problems would you expect to develop on a diet restricted to fat-free protein foods?

BIBLIOGRAPHY

Books

Snively, W.: Food and Nutrition. pp. 156–171. In Weber, E.: Health and the School Child. Springfield, Illinois, Charles C Thomas, 1964.

Darby, W.: Nutrition. pp. 471–496. In Better Homes and Gardens Family Medical Guide. New York, Meredith Press, 1966.

The Merck Manual of Diagnosis and Therapy. Rahway, New Jersey, Merck Sharp & Dohme Research Laboratories, 1966.

Snively, W., and Thuerbach, J.: Sea of Life. pp. 126–188. New York, David McKay Co., Inc., 1969.

Boyd, W.: A Textbook of Pathology. Philadelphia, Lea & Febiger, 1970.

Articles

Snively, W., and Becker, B.: Minerals, macro and micro: dynamic nutrients—part I, the macro-minerals. Annals of Allergy, 26:167, 1968.

Snively, W., and Becker, B.: Minerals, macro and micro: dynamic nutrients—part II, the micro-minerals. Annals of Allergy, 26:233, 1968.

Sandstead, H., Carter, J., and Darby, W.: How to diagnose nutritional disorders in daily practice. Nutrition Today, 4:20, 1969.

Kallen, D.: Nutrition and society. JAMA, 215:94, 1971.

Luhrs, C., and Behar, M.: Can hungry children learn? Maryknoll, 65:2, 1971.

White, P.: The world stops for the hungry. JAMA, 215:110, 1971.

10

endocrine dysfunction

Scattered widely throughout the body, the endocrine glands differ in several respects from body systems such as the circulatory, respiratory, and nervous systems. First, although the anterior lobe of the pituitary gland is acknowledged to be the "master gland," there is no central "headquarters" controlling all the endocrine glands. Second, the endocrine glands possess no anatomical continuity. Finally, because of their enormous influence on physiological processes, endocrine disorders can have dire effects on sexual development, growth, and carbohydrate metabolism. Endocrine dysfunction is thus one of the basic disease processes. As Edward C. Reifenstein, Jr., a leading authority in the field of endocrinology, has pointed out, "We have come to recognize that there is an endocrine component to all disorders."

Endocrine glands produce hormones, chemical substances that regulate the activities of various body organs. The endocrine glands pour out their hormones directly into the bloodstream, so are called *ductless glands,* in contrast to exocrine glands, such as the sweat glands, which discharge their secretion through ducts. One gland, the pancreas, is both endocrine (production of the hormone insulin) and exocrine (elaboration of pancreatic enzymes that are poured into the small intestine to help digest food).

As blood-borne messengers controlling distant body functions, hormones travel rapidly, although not with the speed of nerve impulses. Still, the endocrine glands and their hormones are in large part dominated by the nervous system, as will be described.

In general, hormones are of two classes: those that exert their effects in the immediate vicinity of the place where they are synthesized and those that act in parts of the body far removed from that place. The first group of hormones is called *local* hormones, the second, *general* hormones. Among the local hormones is acetylcholine, secreted by skeletal nerve endings, which diffuses into nearby muscle fibers and excites them. The gastrointestinal hormones, secreted by the intestinal mucosa, flow to adjacent regions and control secretion of digestive juices and intestinal motility. The hormone histamine, which may be secreted by damaged cells anywhere in the body, causes increased permeability of capillaries in the vicinity; local edema results.

Among the general hormones are the secretions of the pituitary gland; thyroxin, a secretion of the thyroid; adrenal hormones, secreted in the cortex and medulla of the adrenal gland; insulin, secreted by the pancreas; and male and female sex hormones, secreted by the gonads.

REGULATION OF HORMONE PRODUCTION

GENERAL
HORMONES
CONTROLLED
BY NERVOUS
SYSTEM
FEEDBACK
MECHANISM

Normally, production of many general hormones is often regulated by a feedback mechanism. If the feedback causes production of additional hormone, it is said to be *positive* feedback. If it causes production of less hormone, it is called *negative* feedback. For example, an increase in the level of glucose in the blood stimulates the pancreas to produce more insulin. Should the blood glucose level fall, the pancreas would be signaled to produce less insulin. Production of antidiuretic hormone (ADH) is regulated by the sodium level in the plasma, parathormone by the calcium level. Increased activity of the sympathetic nervous system increases production of epinephrine. Plasma volume regulates the production of the hormone aldosterone: a decreased plasma volume increases production of aldosterone, and an increased plasma volume causes a reduction.

Some hormones are regulated by the blood level of other hormones. For example, thyrotropic hormone of the anterior lobe of the pituitary gland regulates production of the hormone thyroxin by the thyroid gland. Glands whose activities are regulated by tropic hormones are called *target organs;* they are more than targets, however, for they can shoot back, thus: the level of hormone from a target organ controls production of the corresponding tropic hormone.

METHODS OF STUDYING ENDOCRINE GLANDS

Many of the basic discoveries concerning the endocrine glands have been made quite recently. Still, many questions remain unanswered, and much investigation is even now underway to provide answers. Various techniques are employed in the field of endocrinology. Physicians make clinical observations of patients with endocrine disorders and correlate these observations with findings at autopsy. Glands are studied after surgical removal. Effects of depressing the secretion of a given hormone by x-ray or radioactive substances are studied. Natural and synthetic hormones are administered to normal persons and to persons whose hormones are believed to be deficient; in this manner, the quantity of hormones being produced by the individual can be ascertained. Body fluids and tissues are analyzed to determine the presence or absence of specific hormones. Electrodes are placed in the hypothalamus to investigate the key interrelationships between the endocrine and nervous systems. In these ways, almost daily progress is being made in our acquisition of knowledge concerning the endocrine glands. Scientific advances in this important field during the last several decades have been astounding, and bright new discoveries can be anticipated during the decades to come.

THE PITUITARY GLAND (HYPOPHYSIS CEREBRI)

The pituitary gland, or hypophysis cerebri, protrudes from the base of the brain, appearing to hang by a narrow stalk. Appropriately, this important gland—it has been called the *master gland*—is securely wrapped in dura mater and nestled safely in the sella turcica (Turk's saddle) of the sphenoid bone. The pituitary gland consists of two primary divisions: the anterior lobe, called the *adenohypophysis* because it is glandular, and the posterior lobe, called the *neurohypophysis* because it is an outgrowth of the hypothalamus, hence derived from the nervous system. The anterior lobe consists of clusters of large cells supported by delicate reticular fibers; capillary-like blood vessels lie between the nests of cells. It has few nerve endings. The posterior pituitary gland, on the other hand, is crammed with thousands of axons that descend into the gland from cell bodies in the hypothalamus. Capillary networks cluster around the ends of the nerve fibers.

HYPOTHALAMIC CONTROL OF PITUITARY ILLUSTRATES NERVOUS DOMINANCE OF ENDOCRINES

Most of the secretory activities of the pituitary gland are controlled by the hypothalamus. In response to messages arriving from both the external and internal environments, the hypothalamus sends messages down the pituitary stalk, ordering the discharge of hormones stored in the posterior pituitary gland and changes in the secretory activity of the anterior pituitary gland.

Hormones of the Anterior Pituitary Gland

At least six hormones of physiological significance are synthesized by cells of the anterior pituitary gland. These include somatotropin, or growth hormone (GH); thyrotropin, or thyroid-stimulating hormone (TSH); adrenocorticotropin, or adrenal cortex-stimulating hormone (ACTH); follicle-stimulating hormone (FSH); luteinizing hormone (LH); interstitial cell-stimulating hormone of the male (ICSH); and lactogenic or luteotropic hormone (LTH). The anterior pituitary secretes

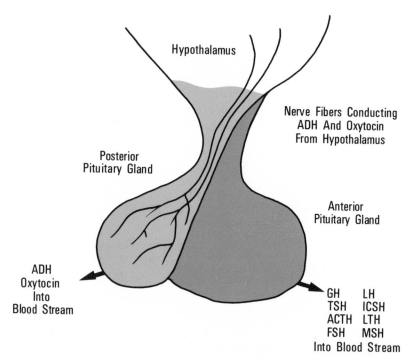

The posterior pituitary gland (neurohypophysis) stores antidiuretic hormone (ADH) and oxytocin. The anterior pituitary gland (adenohypophysis) secretes hormones to stimulate growth (GH), the adrenal cortex (ACTH), ovarian follicles (FSH), corpus luteum (LH), testicular interstitial cells (ICSH), milk production (LTH), and melanocytes (MSH).

still another hormone, melanocyte-stimulating hormone (MSH); its physiological significance is unclear. In common with other hormones, the hormones of the anterior pituitary gland are protein in nature.

Functions of Hormones of the Anterior Pituitary Gland

Somatotropin controls the growth of bones, muscles, and other organs. Thyrotropin stimulates the growth and secretory activity of the thyroid gland. Adrenocorticotropin stimulates the growth and secretory activity of the cortex of the adrenal gland. Follicle-stimulating hormone controls the development of ovarian follicles and the secretion of the female sex hormone estrogen. It also spurs the development of seminiferous tubules and spermatogenesis in the male. Luteinizing hormone controls ovulation, formation of the corpus luteum, and secretion of the female sex hormone progesterone. The corresponding hormone in the male, called *interstitial cell-stimulating hormone*, controls secretion of the male sex hormone testosterone by the testis. Lactogenic, or luteotropic, hormone controls secretion of milk; it also maintains the corpus luteum and stimulates secretion of the female sex hormone progesterone. Melano-cyte-stimulating hormone is concerned with pigmentation of the skin. In Caucasians in whom its production is unduly stimulated, the skin turns dark.

We can thus see that the adenohypophysis exercises control over the hormones of many of the most influential endocrine glands. Since it receives orders via neurohumoral pathways extending to the central nervous system via the hypothalamus, it becomes apparent that the body hormones are to a great extent subject to nervous control.

Functions of Hormones of the Posterior Pituitary Gland

The posterior pituitary gland stores two hormones produced elsewhere. These are manufactured in the hypothalamus, then trickled down the pituitary stalk into the posterior pituitary gland. One is anti-diuretic hormone (ADH), which controls the concentration of the urine and conservation of water by the kidney as it regulates the collecting tubules of the kidneys. The other hormone is oxytocin, which stimulates contraction of the uterus and secretion of milk by the breasts.

Disorders of the Pituitary Gland

Hypofunction of the anterior pituitary gland (hypopituitarism) If the anterior pituitary gland fails to secrete growth hormones, the individual will not grow but becomes a pituitary dwarf. In most cases, however, dwarfism is due to heredity rather than to pituitary failure. The pituitary dwarf stays childlike in all physical respects. Organs, including bones, fail to grow. Sexual development stays that of a young child, even in adulthood. The individual may achieve not more than twice the height of a newborn baby. Sometimes the secretion of growth hormone is diminished rather than absent, causing various degrees of pituitary dwarfism.

In the adult, anterior hypofunction may cause Simmond's disease, with premature senility, a dry wrinkled skin, weakness, mental lethargy, emaciation, loss of pubic and axillary hair, and, perhaps, loss of teeth.

PITUITARY DYSFUNCTON AFFECTS ALL DEVELOPMENTAL PROCESSES

Hyperfunction of the anterior pituitary gland (hyperpituitarism) Excessive secretion of growth hormone occurring before puberty causes gigantism. The condition is brought on by a tumor of the pituitary gland, and results in overgrowth of all parts of the body, including skeletal muscles, internal structures, and the skin.

If hypersecretion occurs after puberty, when the epiphyseal lines are closed, acromegaly results. In this condition there is no increase in height, but there is appositional overgrowth of all tissues. There is thickening of the bones, and the membranous bones grow longer, so that growth is disproportionate. The lower jaw, formed of membranous bone, continues to grow, and the lower teeth separate. The nose and lips enlarge and the

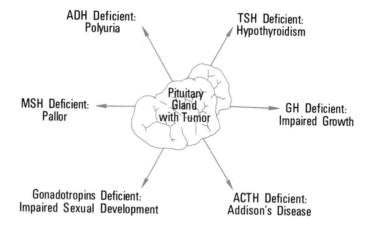

GENERAL PITUITARY FAILURE (PANHYPOPITUITARISM)
(Caused by Tumor)

ADH Deficient:
Polyuria

TSH Deficient:
Hypothyroidism

MSH Deficient:
Pallor

Pituitary
Gland
with Tumor

GH Deficient:
Impaired Growth

Gonadotropins Deficient:
Impaired Sexual Development

ACTH Deficient:
Addison's Disease

face takes on a coarsened look. Overgrowth of the bones of the hands and feet continues, and these organs may become spadelike.

Hypofunction of the posterior pituitary gland (diabetes insipidus)
With inadequate production of hormones of the posterior pituitary gland, the output of urine rises to from 4 to 20 liters a day. It is dilute and sugar free, depending on how much water the patient drinks. Specific gravity of the urine is 1.004 or less. In early times one of the methods used in diagnosis was tasting of the urine, and physicians called this condition *diabetes insipidus* because of the absence of a sweet taste, by contrast with diabetes mellitus, in which the urine tasted as sweet as honey. The patient with diabetes insipidus has an insatiable thirst.

Hyperfunction of the posterior pituitary gland   Posterior pituitary hyperfunction is not a recognized clinical entity.

THE PINEAL GLAND

The pineal gland, or pineal body, is a small conical structure extending backward from the third ventricle just above the roof of the midbrain. Although the precise function of this gland is unknown, it probably is a highly sensitive "biologic clock" that regulates the gonads. Environmental light influences the production of melatonin, a hormone produced only by the pineal gland, and melatonin inhibits activity of the gonads. In one study, girls born blind or who lost their sight during their first year also experienced early onset of puberty, whereas albino girls, who were unduly sensitive to light, showed a great delay in onset of puberty. Children with pineal tumors have a delayed onset of puberty, but in those whose pineal gland is destroyed by a tumor, puberty occurs early.

THE THYROID GLAND

The thyroid gland is located just below the pharynx in the anterior middle region of the neck. The gland consists of two lobes united by a strip, the isthmus, which crosses just in front of the trachea. Septa extend inward to divide the thyroid gland into irregular lobules. The structural unit of the lobule is the follicle.

METABOLIC FUNCTIONS OF THYROID

Production of Thyroxin by the Thyroid Gland

Thyrotropin (TSH) from the anterior pituitary gland stimulates the thyroid gland to produce thyroxin from iodine and the amino acid tyrosine, which are taken up by the thyroid follicles from the circulating blood. Thyroxin is about 65 per cent iodine. Thyroxin then combines with protein to form thyroglobulin. Thyroglobulin is incorporated in a colloid substance that fills the follicles of the thyroid gland. Thyroxin is gradually released from thyroglobulin into the blood as the body needs it. Several months' supply of thyroxin can be stored in the follicles. This explains why one can get along for weeks on an iodine-deficient diet. As thyroxin enters the blood, it promptly combines with a specific plasma protein and is transported as protein-bound iodine to the interstitial fluid and tissue cells.

Thyroxin increases the metabolic rate of all cells. Under its influence, at least 13 different cellular enzymes are produced in increased quantities. Thyroxin therefore stimulates activity of all functions of the body, including those of the cardiovascular system, the nervous system, and the gastrointestinal tract—in short, the total body metabolism.

A second thyroid hormone, triiodothyronine, has functions similar to those of thyroxin. A third hormone, thyrocalcitonin, lowers the level of calcium in the blood.

Disorders of the Thyroid Gland

Hypofunction of the thyroid gland (hypothyroidism) When production of thyroxin is lacking, either because the gland failed to develop during the fetal life or because it atrophied in adult life, the term *hypothyroidism* is applied. An individual can live for many years with complete lack of thyroxin production, but the rate of metabolism is decreased to about one half normal. He becomes lethargic, lacks energy, and may sleep for 12 to 15 hours a day. Constipation, sluggish mental reactions, and obesity follow. In addition to this, a gelatinous mixture of protein and extracellular fluid is deposited in the spaces between the cells. The person appears edematous; for this reason, the state is called *myxedema*. The congenital form is known as *cretinism*.

Hyperfunction of the thyroid gland (hyperthyroidism)   When regulation of the thyroid gland by TSH of the anterior pituitary gland is disturbed, greatly increased amounts of thyroxin are produced—perhaps as much as 25 times normal. Usually this increase is caused by an increase in TSH; but sometimes an adenoma of the thyroid gland will secrete thyroxin independent of control by the anterior pituitary gland. In either case, hyperthyroidism results.

In hyperthyroidism, the basal metabolic rate climbs steeply, to perhaps as much as twice normal. The patient loses weight, develops diarrhea, and becomes extremely nervous and tremulous. The heart rate is greatly increased, with the heart beating so hard that the patient feels it palpitating in his chest. Hyperthyroidism is exceedingly wearing on the individual: it may "burn out" his tissues, leading to degenerative processes in many parts of the body.

Hyperthyroidism is treated by administering a drug that suppresses thyroid function or destroys the thyroid gland, or by surgically removing a large part of the gland. Or, radioactive iodine can be administered. The emission from this isotope either destroys the active tissue or returns it to a normal functional state. In the majority of cases, a single dose is sufficient to provide permanent relief.

In severe cases, exophthalmos, or protrusion of the eyeballs, occurs. Apparently, thyroxin is not involved in this distressing condition. Rather, it is caused by a substance secreted by the anterior pituitary gland, along with the excessive secretion of TSH. The exophthalmos-producing substance secreted by the anterior pituitary gland causes edema, hypertrophy, and finally degeneration of tissue within the orbit. Correction of hyperthyroidism does not entirely eliminate the exophthalmos.

Goiter   In the *hyperthyroid* state, the overactive gland enlarges two to three times and is called *goiter*. Oddly enough, the same thing happens in *hypothyroidism* although the effects are, of course, different. In hypothyroidism the thyroid has more work to do, and therefore it enlarges greatly. Large amounts of colloid substance containing almost no thyroxin are secreted into the follicles. This type of enlarged thyroid gland is called *simple*, or *colloid, goiter;* it may become 15 times as large as a normal thyroid gland, weighing 500 or more grams and occupying a large space in the neck or upper chest. It may obstruct breathing or swallowing.

Persons who live in areas of the world where the soil contains little

BOTH OVERACTIVITY
AND UNDERACTIVITY
OF THYROID
CAUSE
GOITER

iodine, such as the Great Lakes region of the United States, cannot produce sufficient thyroxin, and as a result, the metabolic rate decreases below normal. This increases the output of TSH, which, in turn, goads the thyroid gland to produce more thyroxin. Even this stimulus cannot increase the amount of thyroxin when iodine is missing, but the anterior pituitary gland continues to produce large amounts of TSH. The thyroid continues to enlarge, as more colloid accumulates. The enlarged gland is called an *endemic goiter,* i.e., it is common to the inhabitants of the iodine-deficient region. The addition of a small amount of iodine to table salt will prevent problems. In cretinism, thyroid replacement must be started early in life.

The most accurate test of thyroid function is the protein-bound iodine. Normal PBI range is between 4 and 8 mg. per 100 ml. of plasma. While the basal metabolic rate (BMR) is increased in hyperthyroidism, it is also increased in infections, pregnancy, and other conditions not related to hyperthyroidism.

THE PARATHYROID GLANDS

The parathyroid glands nestle on the posterior surface of the thyroid gland, embedded in the substance of the thyroid. There are usually four parathyroid glands.

Hormones of the Parathyroid Glands

The chief hormone produced by the parathyroid glands is called *parathormone.* They may produce a second hormone, calcitonin. The precise source of calcitonin has been somewhat uncertain. Originally, scientists believed that it was produced by the parathyroids. Then it was discovered that in lower vertebrates calcitonin is manufactured in the ultimobranchial glands located just beneath the parathyroids; these glands are fused with the thyroid and parathyroids in mammals. Thyrocalcitonin and calcitonin are identical, the former being associated with the thyroid and the latter with the parathyroid. Parathormone and calcitonin maintain the correct levels of calcium and phosphorus in the extracellular fluid, thus preserving normal excitability of muscle and nerve tissue. Excitability rises when the serum calcium is depressed, and is depressed when the calcium level rises. Parathyroid hormones are required also for normal bone formation and growth.

Normally, calcium in bone combines with phosphorus in the form of calcium phosphate. But when parathormone is increased, there is an increase in osteoclastic activity. (Recall that the osteoclasts are large cells whose function is to help dissolve unwanted bony tissue during new bone growth.) Thus calcium moves out of bone and floods the blood,

CALCIUM-
PHOSPHORUS
BALANCE
UNDER
PARATHYROID
CONTROL

pours through the kidneys into the urine, and is lost to the body. Just the opposite takes place when parathormone production is decreased: calcium is not mobilized and the tissues are depleted of it. Calcitonin appears to lower blood calcium.

Disorders of the Parathyroid Glands

Hypofunction of the parathyroid glands (hypoparathyroidism) Parathormone secretion may be decreased by inadvertent removal of or damage to parathyroid tissue during thyroidectomy. The serum calcium ion concentration falls so low that tetany (intermittent muscle contractions of the hands and feet, not to be confused with tetanus) develops within 3 days. Prompt treatment is necessary to save the patient. Within a few hours after administration of parathormone or certain vitamin D compounds, sufficient calcium is mobilized from bone to restore normal function. There are also instances of hereditary hypoparathyroidism, which usually is not severe enough to cause tetany, but which may cause chronic depression of bone osteoclastic activity. Bones become brittle, probably because the protein matrix, in the absence of osteoclastic activity, has become old and brittle.

Hyperfunction of the parathyroid glands (hyperparathyroidism) A parathyroid tumor, known as an *adenoma*, may occasionally develop, and, although benign, it can cause serious problems. There is tremendous secretion of parathormone, with overgrowth of osteoclasts. These cells may grow so large and become so numerous that they honeycomb bone, and bones break under little stress; in fact, the patient often is made aware of his disease because of a broken bone. Hypersecretion also increases the calcium level in the body fluids. If this is not too great, the higher calcium level will not cause untoward effects, but if the level rises sufficiently, calcium phosphate will be precipitated in the lungs, muscles, and heart, leading to death within a few days.

THE ADRENAL GLANDS

The adrenal glands are perched just above the kidneys; each has an outer portion, the cortex, and an inner part, the medulla.

Hormones of the Adrenal Cortex

Glucocorticoids The adrenal cortex produces three general types of steroid hormones. First are the glucocorticoids, including cortisol and hydrocortisone. These hormones help preserve the carbohydrate reserves of the body. They also exert a catabolic effect on protein metabolism, promoting mobilization of amino acids from the cells; amino acids then become available for conversion into glucose in the process known as *gluconeogenesis*. Glucocorticoids also promote deposition of glycogen in the liver, mobilization of depot fat, and oxidation of that fat in the liver; the hormones are thus antagonistic to insulin. The glucocorticoids also enable one better to withstand stress. They possess a potent anti-inflammatory effect, tending to limit the destructive effects of inflammation.

Injections of glucocorticoids are utilized in controlling rheumatoid arthritis, although they decrease the individual's ability to combat infection. They have a striking antiallergic effect and see wide clinical use in this area. While the precise mechanism of their anti-inflammatory effect is not known, it may relate to their ability to prevent disruption of lysosome membranes, the cellular organelles that contain powerful digestive enzymes.

Production of glucocorticoids is stimulated by adrenocorticotropin (ACTH) from the pituitary, which in turn is stimulated by impulses from the hypothalamus. A decrease in the blood level of glucocorticoids stimulates the anterior pituitary gland to release ACTH. This, in turn, stimulates the adrenal cortex to increase its secretory activity. As the level of glucocorticoids increases, secretion of ACTH stops in a negative feedback action.

Mineralocorticoids   The mineralocorticoids are involved in maintenance of fluid and electrolyte balance. They are sometimes designated the "salt and water" hormones since they regulate absorption and excretion of sodium, chloride, potassium, and water. By far the most important mineralocorticoid is aldosterone. This hormone acts on the cells of the renal tubules of the kidneys, where it stimulates reabsorption of sodium, chloride, and water and elimination of potassium. Production of aldosterone depends primarily on the intake of sodium; and it is also influenced by the volume of fluid in the body. Thus, an increase in aldosterone secretion occurs when the body is deprived of sodium or when blood or extracellular fluid is lost from the body. ACTH exerts only slight, if any, control over aldosterone secretion.

Sex hormones   The sex hormones are the third general type produced by the adrenal cortex. Several moderately active male sex hormones, the 17-ketosteroids, plus minute quantities of female sex hormones are produced by the adrenal glands in both men and women. Their functions are not known.

Hormones of the Adrenal Medulla

The medulla of the adrenal gland produces a mixture of epinephrine (sometimes called *adrenalin*) and norepinephrine (also called *noradrenalin* and *sympathin*), thus constituting an important link be-

GENERAL HORMONES PRODUCED BY ADRENAL CORTEX UNDER PITUITARY CONTROL

ADRENAL MEDULLARY HORMONES SERVE SPECIALIZED FUNCTIONS

tween the nervous system and the endocrine system. Secretory activities of the adrenal medullary cells fall under control of the sympathetic division of the autonomic nervous system. When stimulated by increased activity of the sympathetic division, the adrenal medulla liberates from two to five times as much epinephrine as norepinephrine. Psychic trauma, hypoglycemia, mild hypoxia, and hypotension are among the stimulating factors. Epinephrine is secreted in increased quantities in emergency states, such as psychic trauma, hypoglycemia, mild hypoxia, and hypotension. In general, its effects are the same as stimulation of the sympathetic division of the autonomic nervous system. It also stimulates production of ACTH, which, in turn, stimulates production of cortisol.

Commercially prepared epinephrine is used widely in the treatment of bronchial asthma, urticaria (hives), cardiac failure, and circulatory collapse.

Norepinephrine differs from epinephrine, since it does not affect carbohydrate metabolism in muscle and liver tissue, nor does it cause hyperglycemia. Norepinephrine is released at the neuroeffector junctions of most sympathetic postganglionic nerve fibers and acts as a chemical transmitter substance, serving to excite or to inhibit effector cells.

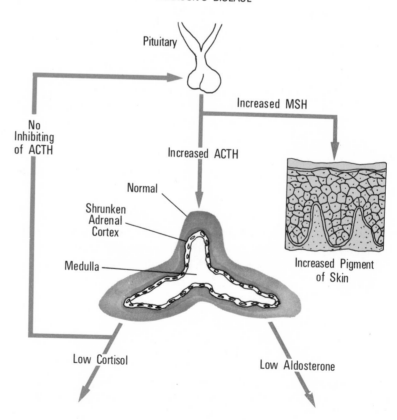

ADDISON'S DISEASE

Pituitary

Increased MSH

No Inhibiting of ACTH

Increased ACTH

Normal

Shrunken Adrenal Cortex

Medulla

Increased Pigment of Skin

Low Cortisol

Low Aldosterone

Disorders of the Adrenal Glands

Hypofunction of the adrenal glands (hypoadrenalism)   The adrenal cortex may be destroyed by disease, usually tuberculosis, or may atrophy. Or it can happen that adrenal overstimulation due to stress causes enlargement, followed by hemorrhage, followed by replacement with scar tissue. Any of these conditions results in adrenal hyposecretion, or hypoadrenalism. When there is chronic insufficient secretion, the condition is known as *Addison's disease.*

In complete adrenal failure (*acute adrenal crisis*), death usually occurs within 3 to 5 days, unless treatment is started promptly, due to lack of aldosterone. This is because kidney reabsorption of sodium depends almost entirely on aldosterone secretion. Administration of the adrenocortical mineralocorticoid, deoxycorticosterone, along with large quantities of salt, can counteract the lack of aldosterone, although the patient remains unable to resist stress. Even a slight respiratory infection, for example, can be fatal. In the chronic form, Addison's disease, the patient becomes progressively weaker, and his skin becomes highly pigmented. His blood pressure falls and he has gastrointestinal symptoms such as vomiting and diarrhea. The adrenocortical hormone, deoxycorticosterone, and salt must be administered.

Hyperfunction of the adrenal glands (hyperadrenalism)   A tumor of the adrenal gland or increased production of ACTH by the anterior pituitary gland can cause hypersecretion of adrenocortical hormones. If the inner zone of the adrenal cortex, the zona reticularis, is stimulated, excessive quantities of male hormones (androgens) are secreted. If the person is a female, masculine characteristics, such as facial hair growth, deepened voice, sometimes baldness, and masculinizing changes of the sex organs develop; the breasts atrophy, and muscularity is greatly increased. If the patient is a boy, his sex organs develop prematurely, as do the changes already mentioned.

If the middle zone of the cortex, the zona fasciculata, is stimulated, symptoms of excess cortisol secretion appear. The condition is called *Cushing's syndrome* or *hypercortisolism.* Proteins and fats are mobilized from storage areas, causing weakness of muscles and tissue fibers; thus the skin becomes thin, and tears of subcutaneous tissue cause the appearance of striae over the abdomen, buttocks, and other parts. Mobilization of protein and fat stimulates gluconeogenesis and the blood glucose concentration climbs; if this causes a high blood sugar level the condition is called *pituitary diabetes.*

When the outer layer of the adrenal cortex, the zona glomerulosa, produces too much aldosterone, primary aldosteronism, or *Conn's syndrome,* occurs. It results from a benign tumor, an adenoma, of the adrenal cortex. There is sodium retention and potassium loss, chiefly via the urine, along with potassium deficit, sodium excess, and metabolic alkalosis. The

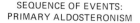

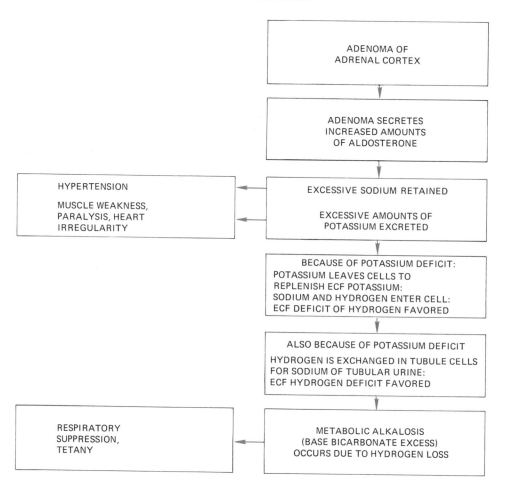

symptoms include general muscle weakness, due to the potassium deficit, and a pounding pulse, due to the hypertension resulting from sodium retention. The plasma sodium is elevated, the plasma potassium is decreased, and the bicarbonate is elevated (base bicarbonate excess, or metabolic alkalosis described in Chap. 8). Daily aldosterone secretion is usually more than 200 mcg. The same clinical picture occurs with diffuse hyperplasia of one or both adrenal glands, or following prolonged ingestion of large amounts of licorice.

So far we have talked about adrenal cortical hypersecretion, but adrenal medullary hypersecretion can occur also. This condition, known as *noradrenalism,* is caused by a pheochromocytoma, a tumor of the adrenal medulla that is usually benign. It produces hypertension, which may be so severe that the systolic pressure may rise to 300 mm.

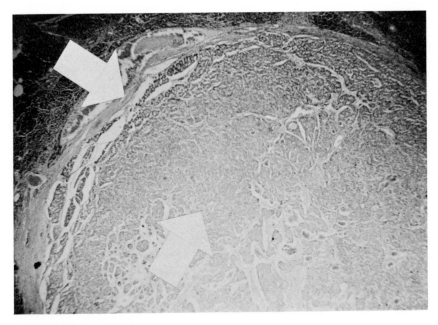

The cells of this encapsulated tumor resemble those of the zona glomerulosa of the adrenal cortex, both in their appearance and their arrangement. Upper arrow points to capsule; lower arrow points to adenoma cells. Such a benign tumor produces primary hyperaldosteronism.

of mercury or more. The patient is extremely nervous and sweats profusely. These symptoms may suggest hyperthyroidism, but the PBI is normal.

ENDOCRINE FUNCTIONS OF THE PANCREAS

The pancreas secretes two important hormones, insulin and glucagon. They are produced by the islets of Langerhans, which are scattered throughout the pancreas in numbers ranging from 20,000 to 2 million. Their cells are of two types: the A or alpha cells secrete glucagon, and the B or beta cells produce insulin.

Insulin is absorbed directly into the blood passing through the pancreas. Production depends primarily on the level of blood glucose. Its function is to regulate carbohydrate metabolism. Insulin lowers the blood sugar by increasing utilization of glucose by the tissues, by stimulating formation and storage of glycogen in the liver, by decreasing gluconeogenesis from amino acids, and by stimulating the formation of fat from glucose. Insulin is antagonized by epinephrine, which stimulates the

ENDOCRINE FUNCTION OF PANCREAS RESIDES IN ISLETS OF LANGERHANS

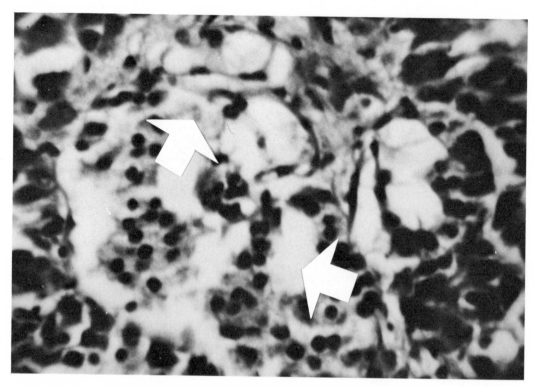

The islets of Langerhans produce insulin. In this slide of a diseased pancreas, the normal structure of the islets is largely replaced by scarring (upper arrow) and vacuolization (lower arrow).

breakdown of glycogen in the liver and produces hyperglycemia; by the glucocorticoids of the adrenal cortex, which stimulate gluconeogenesis; and by thyroxin, which stimulates gluconeogenesis.

Glucagon, the alpha cell hormone, is released into the portal vein when the blood sugar falls too low. This causes a pronounced, though temporary, rise in the blood sugar level by promoting rapid glycogenolysis (splitting up of glycogen) in the liver, so that glucose is released into the blood. Insulin and glucagon operate reciprocally.

Glucose tolerance test   The glucose tolerance test measures the pancreatic response to glucose. In the healthy individual, the blood glucose concentration at the beginning of the test is less than 100 mg. per 100 ml. of blood.

The patient is given 50 grams of glucose. During the following half hour or more, the blood glucose climbs to 130 to 160 mg. per 100 ml. of blood. If the pancreas is functioning normally, large quantities of insulin are produced in less than 1 hour. The blood glucose level falls rapidly, becoming normal in about 2 hours after the initial injection of glucose. The level then drops below normal; this is known as the *hypoglycemic response*. A diabetic, on the other hand, exhibits a *hyperglycemic response,* in which the blood glucose concentration rises to 200 or more mg. per 100 ml. of blood, and may not return to normal for as long as 5 hours or more.

Hypofunction of the pancreas (diabetes mellitus)   As we have described, insulin regulates carbohydrate metabolism. Should the beta cells of the pancreas be damaged so that they are unable to produce insulin, the tissues cannot burn food sugar and convert it into energy, and diabetes mellitus results. The blood glucose level rises to two or three times normal. Large quantities of glucose pass out in the urine because the kidney tubules cannot reabsorb it in the glomerular filtrate. The glucose in the tubular urine reduces reabsorption of water, and the patient loses large quantities of water, as well as glucose, in the urine. Consequently, he is deprived of the energy that would normally be made available from food intake; he loses weight rapidly and becomes weak because his protein and fat stores are being used up. This causes extreme hunger and he may eat voraciously, yet is still not being adequately nourished.

The rapid fat metabolism causes an increase in the quantity of ketone bodies in the extracellular fluid. The pH may fall from the normal value of 7.4 to as low as 6.9. A dangerous acidosis results which may be fatal within a few hours. Immediate treatment of the acidosis and the associated extracellular fluid volume deficit is essential to prevent diabetic coma and death.

Scientists still do not know just what causes the damage to the beta cells, although exposure to certain chemicals and excessive ingestion of carbohydrate are thought to contribute to the development of clinical diabetes. In most instances the diabetic has a parent or other near relative who also has had diabetes.

Through carefully regulated treatment with diet, insulin injections, and other means, the diabetic is no longer threatened by the risk of death from diabetic coma, which used to be the usual outcome, and can look forward to a much longer life span than used to be the case. Yet this prolonged life span gives time for secondary lesions to arise. No matter how carefully the disease is treated, the essential basis of the disease cannot be changed—at least at the present time—and perfect carbohydrate balance cannot be maintained at all times. Thus cholesterol is deposited in the blood vessel walls, and atherosclerosis results. In time the kidneys and the retina are also affected, the kidneys by hypertension and the retina by minute aneurysms of the capillaries which may eventually cause blindness.

Hyperfunction of the pancreas (hyperinsulinism)   When excessive insulin is produced—usually by a tumor of the islet cells—the blood sugar falls to very low levels and hypoglycemia results. Other causes of hyperinsulinism are insulin overdose in diabetes, anorexia nervosa, and extremely vigorous exercise; it may also be associated with certain disorders of pregnancy and lactation. Hypoglycemia occurs because glucose leaves the blood too rapidly or is secreted too slowly. Too much glucose passes into all cells except the neurons. Neuron metabolism breaks down as neurons are first excited and then depressed. During the stage of excitement, convulsions may occur; during the stage of depression, coma, similar to diabetic coma, may occur. It may be difficult to differentiate between these two types of coma.

THE GONADS

The Testes

GONADS
REGULATE
SEXUAL
CHARACTERISTICS
THROUGH
HORMONE
PRODUCTION

The testes are suspended outside the abdominal cavity of the male in a sac, the scrotum, which lies between the upper thighs. Each testis is an oval white body about 1½ inches long and is covered with visceral peritoneum. Beneath this serous membrane is a white fibrous covering. Partitions from this covering pass into the testis and divide it into lobules. In these lobules are tiny coiled seminiferous tubules, which produce spermatozoa, the male sex cells.

Testosterone   Testosterone is produced by the interstitial cells of the testis under the control of interstitial cell-stimulating hormone (ICSH) of the anterior lobe of the pituitary. It controls development of secondary sex characteristics in the male; it also is responsible for development and maintenance of the male organs of reproduction.

The Ovaries

The ovaries are small almond-shaped bodies about 1½ inches long. They are found on either side of the uterus below the fallopian tubes, attached to the posterior surface of the broad ligament of the uterus. The lateral end of each ovary is in intimate contact with the free and open end of the fallopian tube. Each ovary consists of an outer cortex and an inner medulla. The outer layer of the cortex consists of germinal epithelium; immediately below this surface layer is the connective tissue stroma of the cortex. Here ovarian follicles are formed. Each primary follicle consists of a central germ cell, which is surrounded by a layer of epithelial cells. The medulla is composed of loose connective tissue with numerous blood vessels; no follicles exist in this zone of the ovary.

Estrogen   Estrogen, often called the *growth hormone* of the female reproductive system, is synthesized by the cells of the ovarian follicles.

It promotes development of secondary sex characteristics at puberty and maintains them during the reproductive period. Estrogen plays a stellar role during the first half of the menstrual cycle, when it promotes repair of the endometrium following each menstrual period. It causes proliferative development of the endometrium prior to implantation of the ovum and induces cyclic changes in the breast and vaginal mucosa. The production of estrogen is controlled by the follicle-stimulating hormone (FSH) of the pituitary gland.

Progesterone   Progesterone is produced by the cells of the corpus luteum, which develops after the ovum is expelled from the ovary. Production of progesterone is controlled by luteinizing hormone (LH) and luteotropic hormone (LTH) of the anterior pituitary gland. The function of progesterone is to help prepare the uterus for implantation of the fertilized ovum, as well as to nourish and develop the embryo in the early stages of growth. It also supplements the action of estrogen on the mammary glands.

Hypofunction of the testes (male hypogonadism)   If the testes are congenitally absent or nonfunctional, if they are damaged and destroyed by disease or accident, or if the anterior pituitary gonadotropic hormones are lacking, secondary sex characteristics fail to develop. The voice remains high-pitched; there is no growth of hair on the face and trunk. Fat is deposited around the hips, as well as over the breasts and buttocks. The epiphyses close late, and the youth becomes tall, with legs abnormally long in relation to the trunk. His accessory reproductive organs remain small, and he is sterile. Should the testes be destroyed by accident or disease, or surgically removed after puberty, the accessory reproductive organs atrophy.

Hypofunction of the ovaries (female hypogonadism)   When, because of disease or congenital defect, the ovaries are nonfunctional, or when the anterior lobe of the pituitary gland is underactive, the secondary sex characteristics fail to develop, and menstrual cycles are never established. If the ovaries are extensively damaged by disease necessitating their removal after puberty, the uterus, vagina, and external genitalia atrophy.

Menopause   The climacteric and menopause are generally regarded as normal phenomena, although some physicians believe them to closely resemble deficiency diseases due to lack of ovarian hormones. At any rate, between 45 and 50 years of age, women enter the period known as the "change of life." There is a gradual failure of the ovaries to respond to stimulation from gonadal hormones of the anterior pituitary gland. The term *climacteric* covers the entire period of gradual ovarian failure; *menopause* refers to the complete cessation of menstruation. The ovaries no longer produce ova or secrete hormones, and childbearing is no longer possible. The ovaries, fallopian tubes, uterus, vagina, external genitalia, and breasts atrophy. During early menopause, the patient may experience hot flashes or episodes of sweating due to vasomotor instability. Headaches, vague muscular pains, and emotional instability—even depression—may develop.

HORMONES OF THE GASTROINTESTINAL TRACT

STUDY OF
ENDOCRINES
A "FIRST
ORDER OF
BUSINESS"
FOR
MEDICINE

Certain hormones are produced in the walls of the gastrointestinal tract. *Gastrin* has its site of action in the stomach, where it stimulates production of gastric juice. *Enterogastrone* inhibits gastric secretion and gastric motility. *Secretin* stimulates the production of bile and watery pancreatic juice rich in sodium bicarbonate. *Pancreozymin* causes production of pancreatic juice rich in enzymes. *Cholecystokinin* causes the gallbladder to contract and empty. Gastrin is produced in the gastric mucosa of the pyloric region. Enterogastrone, secretin, pancreozymin, and cholecystokinin are produced in the duodenal mucosa.

THE THYMUS

The thymus is a pinkish-gray mass of lymphatic tissue located partly at the base of the neck and partly in the upper thorax behind the sternum. It continues to grow during childhood, reaching maximal size at puberty, and then becomes gradually replaced by adipose tissue. It is not certainly known whether or not the thymus produces any internal secretion, although an active secretion called *thymosin* has been isolated from calf thymus. In mice subjected to whole-body radiation, thymosin stimulates production of lymphocytes and thereby restores immunological competence. It is currently accepted that the thymus is essential for development of immunological competence, i.e., ability to produce antibodies against foreign substances such as pathogenic bacteria. Perhaps it will ultimately be established that the thymus produces an endocrine secretion in the human.

DISEASE MODEL: PHEOCHROMOCYTOMA

Pheochromocytoma, also known as *chromaffin cell tumor,* usually arises in the adrenal medulla, specifically from the chromaffin cells of the sympathoadrenal system. The condition is of medical significance even though it affects well under 1 per cent of patients with hypertension. It is potentially fatal, but it is curable. (In clinical practice most pheochromocytomas are benign.) Most patients are in the fourth to sixth decades. There appears to be a familial tendency to pheochromo-

HORMONES: SOURCES AND CHIEF FUNCTIONS

Hormone	Source	Chief Function
Growth hormone (Somatotropin, GH)	Anterior pituitary	Controls growth
Thyrotropin (TSH)	Anterior pituitary	Controls thyroid
Adrenocorticotropin (ACTH)	Anterior pituitary	Stimulates adrenal cortex
Follicle-stimulating hormone (FSH)	Anterior pituitary	Stimulates ovary and testis
Luteinizing (LH) or interstitial cell-stimulating hormone (ICSH)	Anterior pituitary	Stimulates ovary and testis
Lactogenic or luteotropin (LTH)	Anterior pituitary	Stimulates mammary gland and ovary
Melanocyte-stimulating hormone (MSH)	Anterior pituitary	Causes skin pigmentation
Antidiuretic hormone (ADH)	Posterior pituitary	Conserves water
Oxytocin	Posterior pituitary	Contracts uterus and stimulates mammary gland
Melatonin	Pineal gland	Biologic clock for sexual maturation
Thyroxin	Thyroid gland	Controls metabolism
Triiodothyronine	Thyroid gland	Controls metabolism
Thyrocalcitonin	Thyroid gland	Controls blood calcium
Parathormone	Parathyroid gland	Maintains blood calcium and phosphorus
Calcitonin	Parathyroid gland	Controls blood calcium
Glucocorticoid, anti-inflammatory such as cortisol	Adrenal cortex	Preserves carbohydrate reserves and combats inflammation
Mineralocorticoid, pro-inflammatory such as aldosterone	Adrenal cortex	Conserves sodium and water and eliminates potassium; favors inflammation

HORMONES: SOURCES AND CHIEF FUNCTIONS (Cont.)

Hormone	Source	Chief Function
Epinephrine and norepinephrine	Adrenal medulla	Mimics stimulation of sympathetic division of autonomic nervous system
Insulin	Islets of Langerhans, pancreas	Causes utilization of carbohydrate
Glucagon	Islets of Langerhans, pancreas	Elevates blood sugar
Testosterone	Testis	Develops male sex characteristics and organs
Estrogen	Ovary	Develops female sex characteristics and organs
Progesterone	Ovary	Develops secretory tissue in mammary gland and uterus: maintains pregnancy
Secretin	Duodenal mucosa	Stimulates bile and pancreatic juice
Pancreozymin	Duodenal mucosa	Stimulates rich pancreatic juice
Gastrin	Gastric mucosa	Produces gastric juice
Esterogastrone	Duodenal mucosa	Inhibits gastric secretion and motility
Cholecystokinin	Duodenal mucosa	Contracts and empties gallbladder

cytoma, and there is evidence suggesting dominant inheritance. In about 5 per cent of patients neurofibromatosis is an associated finding. Symptoms arise because the tumor produces epinephrine and norepinephrine in quantities far above those normally produced in the adrenal medulla.

Hypertension, either persistent or paroxysmal, is the most prominent symptom; the blood pressure may rise dangerously. Sweating, blanching or flushing, heart palpitation, and evidence of elevated metabolism such as headaches, apprehension, tremulousness, pain in the chest and abdomen, and paresthesias of the extremities are frequently observed. When the blood pressure becomes extremely high, the patient appears acutely ill;

he is drenched with sweat and his pupils are dilated. Prostration often follows an attack. The manifestations of the disease are diverse; the physician may suspect pheochromocytoma in a patient who manifests sustained or intermittent hypertension combined with excessive sweating, orthostatic hypotension, elevated metabolism, headache, weight loss, elevated fasting blood glucose level, or psychic changes. Various pharmacologic and chemical tests, too technical to describe here, have been developed to aid diagnosis.

Surgical removal of the tumor results in complete relief of symptoms in most cases; exceptions are malignant metastatic tumors and multiple tumors. The blood pressure may remain elevated because of renal damage caused by the prolonged hypertension.

CLINICAL CONSIDERATIONS

Endocrinology is a young science. Insulin, for example, was not discovered until 1922. Aldosterone was not identified until the 1950s. (The senior author remembers this discovery well, for it necessitated virtually complete revision of a manuscript on body fluid disturbances that had already been set in galley proof. It also rendered obsolete virtually every article that had been written on sodium and potassium metabolism prior to 1955.) One might, in fact, compare the rate of growth of the field of endocrinology with the tremendous progress that the human infant makes during his first year of life.

A few hospitals now maintain wards devoted to the study and treatment of endocrine disorders. Here not only the physicians but also the nurses, technicians, and ward attendants are specially trained. The sympathy and understanding of all medical attendants is desperately needed by the patient with endocrine disease. He must undergo rigorous diagnostic studies and must cooperate in programs of therapy that are often quite stringent.

The study of the endocrine glands and their marvelously complex secretions, the hormones, is truly in its infancy. Discoveries in this exciting and important field will greatly enhance our understanding of disease and our treatment of patients. For the investigator who is challenged by the combination of mystery and unlimited opportunity, there is probably no more satisfying field of pursuit than endocrinology.

TOPICS FOR DISCUSSION

1. Might the endocrine glands and the hormones they secrete be regarded as a physiological or functional system rather than a structural or anatomical system? What distinguishes both body fluids and hormonal

secretions from systems such as the cardiovascular, respiratory, and nervous?

2. Does the nervous system completely dominate the endocrine glands? Give reasons for your answer.

3. Why is the pituitary gland called the "master gland"? Is this an appropriate name?

4. Describe some of the communication channels between the nervous system and the endocrine glands.

5. Contrast the physiology of the anterior and posterior pituitary glands. Why is the posterior pituitary called the "neurohypophysis" and the anterior pituitary the "adenohypophysis"?

6. Which hormonal secretions appear most free of nervous dominance? Of dominance by the anterior pituitary?

7. Which hormones are not secreted by discrete endocrine glands?

8. What important organ possesses both endocrine and exocrine secretions? What are the secretions?

9. Could homeostasis be maintained without properly functioning endocrine glands?

10. Imagine a person with no endocrine glands. Assuming he could live for a brief period, how would his physiology be changed from the normal?

11. Name at least two endocrine glands concerning whose function we are still largely in the dark.

BIBLIOGRAPHY

Books

Major, R.: Classic Descriptions of Disease. Springfield, Ill., Charles C Thomas, 1945.

Guyton, A.: Function of the Human Body. Philadelphia, W. B. Saunders Co., 1964.

The Merck Manual of Diagnosis and Therapy. Rahway, New Jersey, Merck Sharp & Dohme Research Laboratories, 1966.

Passmore, R., and Robson, J.: A Companion to Medical Studies. Philadelphia, F. A. Davis Co., 1968.

Selye, H.: Endocrine Aspects of Disease Processes. St. Louis, Warren H. Green, Inc., 1968.

Chaffee, E., and Greisheimer, E.: Basic Physiology and Anatomy. ed. 2. Philadelphia, J. B. Lippincott Co., 1969.

Physician's Desk Reference. Oradell, N.J., Medical Economics, Inc., 1969.

Boyd, W.: A Textbook of Pathology. Philadelphia, Lea & Febiger, 1970.

Brunner, L., et al.: Textbook of Medical-Surgical Nursing. Philadelphia, J. B. Lippincott Co., 1970.

Goth, A.: Medical Pharmacology. St. Louis, The C. V. Mosby Co., 1970.

Tietz, N., et al.: Fundamentals of Clinical Chemistry. Philadelphia, W. B. Saunders Co., 1970.

Articles

Discovered: hormones' helper in the cells. Medical World News, November 13, 1970.

Prostaglandins. Medical World News, August 28, 1970.

Managing vascular disease in the diabetic. Patient Care, December 15, 1970.

Diligence and luck pay off: synthesis of human growth hormone opens many paths in medicine and biochemistry. Science News, January 16, 1971.

11

stress factors in disease

All of us suffer, at one time or another, from stress and are painfully aware of what severe stress can do to us. Even prehistoric man must have associated loss of vigor and exhaustion with stress (although he, of course, did not recognize it as such), as when he had worked strenuously, had been exposed to extreme cold or heat, had been injured, or had been desperately frightened. Perhaps he realized that he had taken all the stress he could when he simply could not go any further. Whenever he did something unusually strenuous, when he swam in ice water, when he fled—perhaps many miles—from an enemy, when he lifted great weights, when he starved or thirsted, he experienced a real hardship. After a while, he found a "second wind," and became used to the travail. But if the trial persisted, he finally could tolerate no more and had to give up. The caveman, being fully occupied with getting enough to eat, not to mention staying alive, probably did not recognize the triple nature of his response to hardship.

Hans Selye, the great physician and investigator who introduced the stress concept in medicine, interprets the caveman's three-step response as a general law that regulates the performance of humans faced with any difficult task. Through Selye's study of this response, a new realm of medicine was opened.

In 1926, as a second-year medical student, Selye was impressed by the realization that patients suffering from diverse diseases had many signs and symptoms in common—the loss of appetite, the generalized weakness, the lack of ambition, the loss of weight, the woebegone facial expression. Whatever the illness, the people were "just sick" and they all looked pretty much the same. Selye inquired into the scientific basis of "just being sick." He wondered if the mechanism underlying the symptoms could be analyzed by modern scientific techniques and decided they could.

Selye was not able to pursue his theories until 1936, when he was working at the Biochemistry Department of McGill University. While searching for a new ovarian hormone in extracts of cattle ovaries, he made a startling discovery: whenever he injected the various extracts with which

DERANGEMENT
OF
NORMAL
HORMONAL
BALANCE
THE
SINE
QUA NON

he was working, they all produced exactly the same symptoms, i.e., enlargement of the adrenal gland, ulcers of the intestinal tract, shrinkage of the thymus gland and of the lymph nodes, and weight loss. At first, Selye thought he had discovered a new ovarian hormone, but then he observed that many poisonous substances produced the same changes. Remembering his early impression of the syndrome of "just being sick," he was struck by the realization that the extracts and drugs he had been injecting were reproducing the syndrome experimentally. He named this the *stress syndrome,* and he used the adrenal enlargement, gastrointestinal ulcers, involution of the thymus and lymphatics, and weight loss as objective gauges of stress.

He then began to develop a nomenclature that has since become famous. To the initial response to stress-producing, or stressor, agents, he gave the name *alarm reaction.* He termed the next stage, in which the individual began to adjust to the stress, the *stage of adaptation,* or *resistance.* This second stage indicated to him that no organism could continuously remain in a state of alarm. Indeed, if the animal could not adapt, it would die. If, however, the animal survived and moved into the stage of resistance, it adjusted to the stress; tolerance built up.

Selye found that in many ways, the second phase, or stage of adaptation, was quite different from the first stage, or alarm reaction. During the alarm reaction, the cells of the shell, or cortex, of the adrenal glands discharged microscopically visible granules of secretion (which contain the hormone) into the bloodstream. The stores of the glands were depleted. But during the stage of resistance, the cortex accumulated a reserve of secretory granules. During the alarm reaction, the blood be-

ALARM
REACTION →
STAGE OF
ADAPTATION →
STAGE OF
EXHAUSTION

TRIAD OF ADAPTATION
(SELYE)

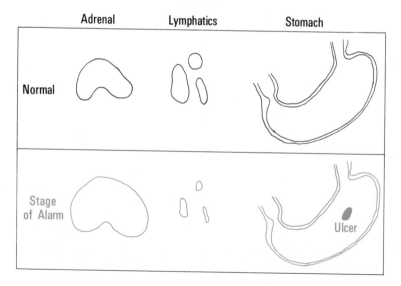

came concentrated and there was a loss of body weight. During the stage of resistance, the blood was diluted and body weight returned toward normal.

After still more prolonged exposure to the noxious agent, the acquired adaptation was lost. The animal entered a third stage, the *stage of exhaustion*. This always followed if the stress was severe enough and was exerted for a long enough period, since there is a limit to the adaptation energy possessed by all living things. Selye adopted a term designed to include the three stages of the response to stresses—*general adaptation syndrome*, sometimes abbreviated GAS. As the name indicates, Selye believed that the chain of events represents an adaptive reaction.

Later, Selye found that stress parallels the intensity with which one pursues various activities. That is, stress increases during episodes of nervous tension, physical injury, infection, muscular work, and emotional crises. This provokes a nonspecific bodily defense mechanism, as will be described.

NATURE OF THE DEFENSES

An essential element in the body's defense against stress is an increase in the secretion by the pituitary gland of adrenocorticotropic hormone (ACTH). This hormone stimulates the adrenal cortex to produce large amounts of adrenocortical hormones, called, by Selye, *corticoids*. These hormones are two in type: (1) cortisone and cortisol, which *inhibit* inflammation, and (2) aldosterone and desoxycorticosterone, which *stimulate* inflammation. These two very different types of hormones have other general effects. The former act mainly on carbohydrate metabolism and are referred to as *anti-inflammatory*, or *glucocorticoid*, hormones. The latter two exert their effect on mineral metabolism and are designated the *proinflammatory*, or *mineralocorticoid* hormones. Apparently, stressed tissues or organs send alarm signals to centers of coordination in the brain, which dispatches further messages to the pituitary and adrenal glands, which produce the hormones mentioned. If the proper amounts of the proper hormones are produced, all goes well; the body is supported in its efforts to combat the effects of the stressor. Sometimes, however, under conditions that will shortly be described, the body responds inappropriately; perhaps too little anti-inflammatory or too much proinflammatory hormone pours into the bloodstream—then these efforts of the body to ward off stress actually cause disease! Selye has termed these disorders the *diseases of maladaptation*, or of *wear and tear*. They result from *faulty adaptation to stress*.

Selye and his coworkers have demonstrated that certain cardiovascular diseases, including malignant hypertension, nephrosclerosis, periarteritis nodosa, and rheumatic diseases, can be produced experimentally in

DEFENSE
AGAINST
STRESS
LARGELY
UNDER
ENDOCRINE
CONTROL

animals by administering overdoses of desoxycorticosterone (DOC) or aldosterone. These substances cause tissue changes identical to those of nonspecific inflammation. Hence, it appears that stress can give rise to conditions that stimulate oversecretion of the hormones.

The diseases of maladaptation include high blood pressure (a special type designated *metacorticoid hypertension*), eclampsia, nephrosis, inflammatory diseases of the skin and eyes, and diseases of the joints. Moreover, the GAS bears a definite relationship to various other disturbances, including allergies, mental derangement, sexual problems, digestive diseases, metabolic diseases (including diabetes), resistance in general, and perhaps even cancer. Intense stress is often followed by the development of acute ulcers of the intestinal tract. (The stress may take the form of burn, prolonged surgery, fracture, cardiac infarct, or brain injury.) In spite of the enormous advances that have been made, knowledge about the general adaptation syndrome is still in its infancy. Selye says, "It is still largely a matter of debate which of the diseases of adaptation are due to an actual overproduction of, or hypersensitivity to, adaptive hormones."

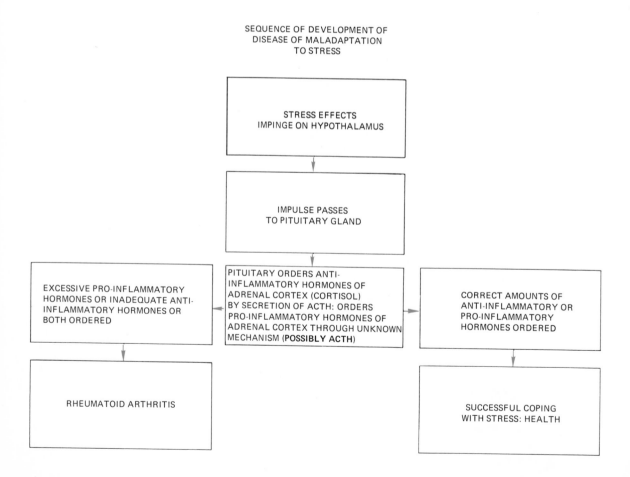

SEQUENCE OF DEVELOPMENT OF
DISEASE OF MALADAPTATION
TO STRESS

STRESS EFFECTS
IMPINGE ON HYPOTHALAMUS

IMPULSE PASSES
TO PITUITARY GLAND

EXCESSIVE PRO-INFLAMMATORY HORMONES OR INADEQUATE ANTI-INFLAMMATORY HORMONES OR BOTH ORDERED

PITUITARY ORDERS ANTI-INFLAMMATORY HORMONES OF ADRENAL CORTEX (CORTISOL) BY SECRETION OF ACTH: ORDERS PRO-INFLAMMATORY HORMONES OF ADRENAL CORTEX THROUGH UNKNOWN MECHANISM (**POSSIBLY ACTH**)

CORRECT AMOUNTS OF ANTI-INFLAMMATORY OR PRO-INFLAMMATORY HORMONES ORDERED

RHEUMATOID ARTHRITIS

SUCCESSFUL COPING WITH STRESS: HEALTH

Different stressors affect different individuals in different ways, such that a given stress may give rise to one lesion in one person but an entirely different lesion in another. Apparently, there exist conditioning factors that can heavily influence the results of stress. This conditioning may stem from genetic elements, age, or sex, or it may arise from some outside influence such as drug therapy. A faulty diet sometimes appears to be a prominent factor. When such conditioning factors are operating, a normally well-tolerated degree of stress can produce disease.

ECOLOGICAL COMPONENT OF STRESS

There exists, in addition to the types of stressors already described, a group that is quite different and that is unique to modern society. These influences might be designated the *ecological stress factors*. In one way or another, all of them have to do with manmade pollution.

In 1969 the United States produced 7 million junked cars, 30 million tons of waste paper, 28 billion bottles, and 48 billion cans. In the large cities, the amount of air pollution caused by car engines is as high as 80 per cent; the automobile is, in fact, said to be the greatest single polluter. Admiral R. J. Galanson, Chief of Naval Materials, has described his experience while aboard a deep submersible craft, 50 miles off the coast of San Diego and 2,450 feet down. As he peered through a porthole to view the wonders of the undersea world—wonders which he might be the first man to see—the first thing he spotted, just 2 feet away on the ocean floor, was an empty beer can.

STRESSORS DUE
TO MAN

Increasingly, the evidence being collected appears to support a causal, or direct, relationship between specific pollutants and specific diseases. Two examples of this association will indicate the scope of the problem. In Japan there have been episodes of numerous human deaths from mercury poisoning; the mercury was discharged from plastics factories into bays, and accumulated in edible shellfish. Outbreaks of upper respiratory infections causing much morbidity and many deaths have occurred—one of the best known being that in Donora, Pennsylvania, in 1948—associated with high levels of air pollution.

There are also long-term effects to be considered. In some situations the cause-and-effect relationship has been proven, as was the case with the uranium miners of Africa. They suffered a high incidence of carcinoma of the lung due to the radioactive uranium. Many scientists fear that there may be an increase in the incidence of leukemia resulting from the increased use of radioactive substances. Noise, congestion, and overcrowding are pollutants, too. All contribute to anxiety and thereby to the overall stress experienced by our urban society.

The effects of noise on hearing have been studied for nearly 100 years, but lately, with our increased appreciation of ecological factors, we have become much more aware of them. Excessive noise traumatizes the hearing apparatus, causing varying degrees of deafness. Much of this damage occurs early in life. In the United States today, at least 10 per cent of the population have hearing deficiencies.

In noisy occupations, such as the heavy machine industry, one out of every two machines produces noise levels above 85 decibels—the level at which hearing loss is provoked. Not to be overlooked are, of course, the steel band, rock and roll, and expressway travel, all of which produce noise levels above 100 decibels. Rock and roll, in fact, exceeds the *maximum permissible* criteria for damage risk.

Then too, pollution, be it in the form of noise, bad air, litter, or any form whatever, helps to create other environmental problems, such as depressed real estate values in residential areas situated near airports, and horrible living conditions in neighborhoods located near oil refineries.

The increase in the number of alcoholics, the alarming rise in drug addiction, and the growing divorce rate certainly suggest that many factors are operating to increase the stress of modern life. Stress may take many forms, and this characteristic makes stress difficult to quantify. The viewpoint is growing, nevertheless, that stress in modern life is of serious proportions and that vast human effort will be needed to deal with it and bring it under control.

DISEASES THAT MAY BE CAUSED BY STRESS FACTORS

Disease	Certain	Likelihood Probable	Possible
Cancer			X
Conjunctivitis			X
Dermatitis			X
Diabetes			X
Intestinal ulcers	X		
Mineralocorticoid hypertension		X	
Nephrosis			X
Rheumatoid arthritis		X	
Toxemia of pregnancy			X

DISEASE MODEL: RHEUMATOID ARTHRITIS

Because stress is so nonspecific, and because it is but one contributor to the overall picture in many diseases, it is difficult to cite a disease model due entirely or even predominantly to stress. Rheumatoid arthritis represents as logical an example as we might cite; nevertheless, stress may not always be its sole cause, and it may not always be an important causative factor.

Rheumatoid arthritis affects women three times as frequently as it does men. It is usually preceded by an illness lasting weeks or months, with symptoms of fatigue, malaise, weight loss, sweating of the palms and soles, rapid heart rate, and stiffness of the limbs. A low fever is noted, and the erythrocyte sedimentation rate is elevated. The white cell count may be increased. The affected joints are tender, swollen, and hot. There is widespread wasting of all connective tissue elements. Anemia and leukopenia may appear. Circulatory disturbances are common. The hands and feet are cold and blue, and, strangely enough, may perspire. There is no infallible laboratory test for rheumatoid arthritis, so that diagnosis must be based upon the clinical picture and on ruling out other arthritic syndromes. However, when the serum of a patient with rheumatoid arthritis is added to a suspension of latex particles mixed with gamma globulin, presence of a *rheumatoid factor* may be revealed by agglutination of the particles. The factor, an antibody-antigen complex, stems from the lymphocytes and plasma cells of lymph nodes and synovial membrane affected by the disease. When the test is positive it indicates rheumatoid arthritis; but when negative it does not rule out such a diagnosis.

The prognosis is extremely uncertain, especially before the rate of progress has been evaluated. The outlook for patients who manifest symptoms early or late in life is poorer than for those in whom the onset occurs in the middle years.

The primary cause of rheumatoid arthritis has not been finally identified, but its manifestations may stem from a faulty production of hormones. Dr. Philip Hench and his associates at the Mayo Clinic suggested this in 1949, when sufficient ACTH and cortisone became available for use in treatment. They found that rheumatic and related inflammations can be largely suppressed by these anti-inflammatory hormones. The relief thereby produced represented a milestone in medical progress.

OLDEST DISEASE KNOWN, YET CAUSATIVE FACTORS NOT FULLY IDENTIFIED

Later, a group of German physicians desired to test the concept of stress therapy in patients suffering from severe rheumatoid arthritis who had not responded to treatment with the usual anti-inflammatory steroids, by testing the combined effect of endogenous anti-inflammatory hormones (produced in the body) and the conditioning action of stress. The stressor was a modified type of insulin shock. These investigators gave a series of insulin shocks to a 44-year-old woman bedridden and crippled by severe chronic rheumatoid arthritis that affected her hands, feet, and knees. After the shock treatment, she was able to walk for the first time in 3 years—a result they ascribed to the production of an alarm reaction, with a discharge of ACTH and anti-inflammatory corticoids by her own endocrine glands. Other physicians, using different types of stresses, arrived at the same findings. These results led Selye to state, "All this makes it quite clear that the rheumatic maladies are really typical diseases of adaptation, because if the body's defenses are adequate the disease is suppressed without any intervention by the physician." Rheumatoid arthritis, then, appears to be due to an inadequate adaptive reaction to stress, the nature of which is not always known.

CLINICAL CONSIDERATIONS

Since the concept of stress as a cause of disease is relatively new, we should not be surprised that such diseases cannot be clearly classified. Yet, the salient features of stress extend to a wide variety of disorders, seen in almost all types of medical practice. Recent work has emphasized the importance of stress in hypertensive disease, for example. Indeed, a mineralocorticoid such as aldosterone can cause hypertensive cardiovascular disease in chicks and rats. In humans, an excess of mineralocorticoids eventuates in both hypertension and hypokalemia, with or without edema. Combined pretreatment with gluco- and mineralocorticoids causes a marked predisposition to necrosis of cardiac muscle, either during stress or after excessive ingestion of fat. Excessive dietary sodium promotes the development of these necroses. Potassium, magnesium, and potassium-sparing agents appear to inhibit the necrosis.

EFFECTS OF STRESS MANIFOLD AND PERVASIVE

The diseases of stress are closely related to psychosomatic disorders. Thus, if the stresses are due to emotional factors, the consequent diseases could just as well be termed "psychosomatic diseases" as "diseases of stress." These disorders are likewise closely related to those produced by specific dysfunction of the endocrine glands not associated with stress factors. Future research in the fascinating area of the stress maladaptation disorders promises to be exciting and productive.

TOPICS FOR DISCUSSION

1. Can you differentiate between psychosomatic disease and disease due to maladaptation to stress?

2. Among the various stresses that are believed to contribute to this group of diseases are infection, exhaustion, structural change, physiological change, and intense emotional experiences. Give a specific example of each. In taking the history of a patient, how would you detect the presence of a stress?

3. Note that the final pathway causing psychosomatic disease appears to be nervous, that is, along the routes of the autonomic nervous system, and that the final pathway of stress disease appears to be largely endocrine, that is, produced by excesses or deficiencies of hormones of the adrenal cortex. What implications do these facts have in relation to therapy?

4. Could you explain hypersensitivity in terms of the stress concept? Some knowledgeable clinicians have attempted to do so, and with considerable logic.

5. In what respects is the therapy of psychosomatic disease similar to that for diseases of stress? In what respects are they different?

6. How would you differentiate between an ulcer caused by psychosomatic factors and a stress ulcer, from the standpoint of cause, treatment, and outlook?

7. Is stress entirely undesirable? Would life without stress be tolerable?

8. Discuss the hazards of excessively prolonged treatment with anti-inflammatory hormones of the adrenal gland.

9. Distinguish between psychic and nonpsychic stresses. Name six of each. Do their effects in producing illness differ?

10. Contrast metacorticoid hypertension with the hypertension of primary hyperaldosteronism (Conn's disease) due to adenoma of the adrenal gland.

11. Is it possible that so-called desensitization in allergic disease is really a form of adaptation?

BIBLIOGRAPHY

Books

Selye, H.: The Stress of Life. New York, McGraw-Hill Book Co., Inc., 1956.
Houston, J., et al.: A Short Textbook of Medicine. Philadelphia, J. B. Lippincott Co., 1968.
Jasmin, G.: Endocrine Aspects of Disease Processes. Proceedings of the conference held in honor of Hans Selye. St. Louis, Mo., Warren H. Green, Inc., 1968.
Earth Day—the Beginning. Compiled and edited by the national staff of Environmental Action. New York, Bantam Books, 1970.

Articles

Editorial: JAMA, 205:112 (September 23), 1968.
Letters to the Editor: JAMA, 206:2523 (December 9), 1968.
Flugarth, J.: Modern-day rock-and-roll music and damage-risk criteria. Journal of the Acoustical Society of America, 45:79 (January), 1969.
Hermann, E.: Environmental noise, hearing acuity, and acceptance criteria. Archives of Environmental Health, 18:784 (May), 1969.

12

the aging process

Physiological processes reach a peak at maturity—about age 30 in man—then gradually fade, or degenerate, to a point beyond which the body cannot survive. This process, commonly called *aging,* occurs in all animals but at different rates of speed according to species. Heredity, diet, and environmental factors are among the forces known to affect the rate of aging in animals, and the rate of aging determines the life span of a species. Man is the longest-living mammal, with a life expectancy of 70 years in the United States.

Over the centuries, many men obsessed with a desire for immortality have wasted their lives in relentless search for the Fountain of Youth, and even today, man endeavors to unravel the mysteries of aging. In recent years, much money, manpower, and time have been expended on gerontology, the scientific study of aging. While understanding of the aging process is still quite limited, it is known that three types of changes contribute to the aging process and that aging of tissues may be either *primary,* i.e., resulting from changes occurring in the individual cell, or *secondary,* i.e., the result of changes occurring in the organism as an integrated unit. In this chapter, we shall see that some body organs have a relatively short life span in relation to others and that still others are capable of living much longer than the normal life span of the individual. We shall see that the visible effects of aging, such as coarse, dry, wrinkled skin with splotchy tan pigmentation; loss of teeth; graying hair, perhaps baldness; stooped posture; signs of worn joints, such as gnarled hands; flabby, atrophied muscles; and so on, are produced by changes in organs and tissues. Some such changes tend to promote characteristic pathologic lesions, such as keratosis and arteriosclerosis. Our disease model, atherosclerosis, will help illustrate how a pathologic process of aging causes disease. Finally, we shall see how the study of aging can be applied clinically.

MECHANISMS OF AGING

While it is not known just what factors initiate changes that occur with age, it is known that three types of changes contribute to the decline in physiologic function: secular changes, senescent changes, and pathologic complications of aging.

Secular Changes: The Natural Result of Wear and Tear

NORMAL
AGING
AN
INEVITABLE
PROCESS

The simple lapse of time produces secular, or natural, changes that increase with advancing age and affect 100 per cent of those in the advanced age groups. It is thought that natural aging occurs as the demands of aging tissues gradually exceed the metabolic support provided by the body. In general, secular changes are associated with changes in the blood supply. If the blood supply diminishes rapidly, the tissue will undergo necrosis or atrophy; if blood supply remains adequate regeneration will occur. Therefore, natural aging involves some correlation between parenchymal and vascular changes, the rate and amount of tissue loss being roughly proportional to the rate and amount of vascular decline in the affected organ.

Secular changes ultimately affect all organs, but they occur first in endocrine-dependent organs, such as the breast, prostate, uterus, ovaries, vaginal tract, and the thyroid, and in tissues in which mitosis is minimal and which become progressively nonvital with the passage of years. Changes in these structures begin at about age 40. The process is inevitable and cannot be prevented. The body makes little effort to compensate for changes that occur with natural aging; regeneration is minimal.

Senescent Changes: Accelerated Aging

STRESS
FACTORS
HASTEN
AGING
PROCESS

Factors that put the total organism under great strain, such as hypertension, excessive physical exertion, and progressive emphysema, accelerate body aging. These factors constitute damaging stresses. According to Selye, we are born with a finite supply of adaptive energy, which is gradually depleted by the wear and tear of life. Superimposed stresses, like those mentioned, serve to deplete the store more rapidly. Stresses are particularly harmful in the presence of other disease conditions, such as starvation, obesity, diabetes, pituitary disease, and loss or deterioration of endocrine organs. The affected organs show changes similar to those of secular aging, but the changes are more pronounced and occur prematurely in relation to the patient's chronologic age.

While all organs are subjected to the depredations of time, accelerated aging most frequently involves slowly mitosing tissues, such as joint cartilage; the elastic membranes of the blood vessels and the lungs; the fibrous structures of the important ligaments, tendons, and joint capsules; the bones; and certain diffusion membranes, such as the synovia and the choroid plexus. Senescent changes also are relatively common in the endocrine-dependent organs, including the breasts, the prostate, the uterus, the vaginal tract, the thyroid gland, and the ovaries. Changes in these organs are related to an imbalance or withdrawal of endocrine stimulation.

In accelerated aging, the scar formation and tissue regeneration provoked by structural damage and loss may be so pronounced as to cause neoplasia, especially in the endocrine-dependent organs.

The most striking example of accelerated aging is progeria, which affects both males and females and becomes apparent during the first year of life. The aging process is so accelerated in this disease that a chronologically young child is physically old. These presenile individuals rarely reach the age of 26 years.

Accelerated aging affects only a minority of people. When its cause is a controllable factor, it can, of course, be prevented. Thus, avoidance of such shortening of the life span can be achieved through medical management of hypertension, maintaining the blood pressure below 150/100 (some physicians prefer 140/90). Also contributing to such prophylaxis are avoidance of extremes of physical exertion, prevention of emphysema (of primary importance is to stop smoking), avoidance of extremes of overweight or underweight, careful medical control of diabetes, and prompt attention to endocrine disturbances. Unfortunately, there are

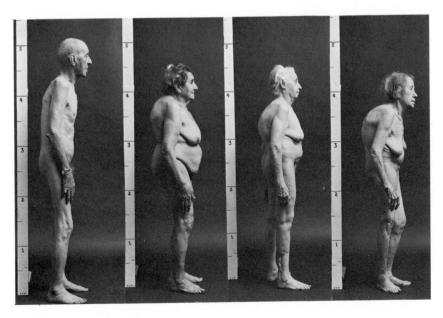

Randomly selected patients from the ambulatory section of a nursing home, illustrating short stature, osteoporotic kyphosis, and relatively long extremities. Ages, from left to right: 82, 78, 79, and 94. From Rossman, I. (ed.): Clinical Geriatrics. Philadelphia, J. B. Lippincott, 1971. (Photo from DeWayne Dalrymple)

some conditions that inevitably lead to premature aging, including familial hypercholesterolemia and progeria.

Pathologic Complications of Aging

Pathologic complications of aging—a term that encompasses the majority of geriatric diseases—also enter into the decline of vital functions. The etiology of many geriatric diseases is uncertain, but there are two general principles that apply to their origin. Some of these disorders, such as osteoarthritis, neoplasia, and malignant hypertension, apparently occur when tissue affected by accelerated aging undergoes fibrous repair or parenchymatous regeneration. Other diseases tend to afflict senile organs. These diseases have a separate etiology and include such entities as reinfection pulmonary tuberculosis in white men over age 50, senile bronchitis, and atherosclerosis.

Whether changes are secular, senescent, or the result of pathologic complications, the functional capacity of tissue decreases either because cell numbers are reduced or because function of individual cells declines. Both factors may participate.

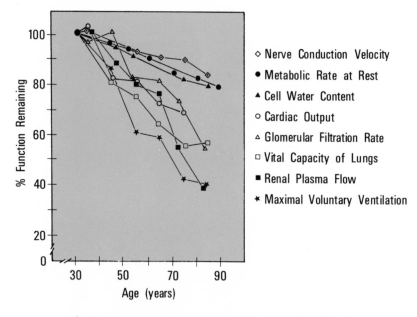

Chart showing the average per cent of various human functional capacity or values remaining at different ages taking 30 years as 100 per cent. (Adapted from Passmore, R. and Robson, J.: A Companion to Medical Studies. vol. 2. Philadelphia, F. A. Davis, 1970)

With loss of cells, there is functional decline of brain, kidney, ovary, skeletal muscle, and heart muscle. Replacement of cells in these tissues is either quite limited or simply does not occur. The rate of cell loss, then, determines the functional life span of the tissue. In tissues in which cell replacement occurs regularly, such as intestinal epithelium, blood cells, and epidermis, cell depletion is not a threat as long as mitotic ability is retained. Aging is much less obvious in these tissues than in tissues in which cells are not replaced, but it does occur. The former type of aging poses no threat to life, however, for these tissues are capable of meeting requirements far beyond the life span of the body.

Aging of a tissue may be either primary or secondary. In primary aging, degeneration is intrinsic to the tissue and occurs independently of other parts of the body. Secondary aging results from changes in other body tissues. Theories advanced suggest that overall aging of the body may occur in one of the following ways:

1. Primary aging in several tissues causes secondary aging in other tissues.
2. A single process in one tissue ages the entire body by causing secondary changes in other tissues.
3. The entire body ages by secondary aging alone, which is brought about by overcrowding of cells within a tissue. The resultant competition for nutrients plus the accumulation of waste products causes an eventual breakdown of cellular integration, with resultant secondary aging of cells and tissues.

Although it is probable that no tissue ages completely independently of the rest of the body, some tissues, such as the ovary, do so to a large degree. Aging of other tissues, such as skin and muscle, is greatly influenced by the body environment.

Aging of Ovaries

The life span of the ovaries is determined by the initial number of ova and their rate of release. Menopause occurs when only a few ova remain. Studies have shown that menstrual cycles do not reappear when old ovaries are transplanted into young mice, but young ovaries transplanted into old mice continue to function normally. Function appears to depend upon normal pituitary action, however, since ovaries from old mice that have undergone hypophysectomy when young are still sensitive to pituitary hormones and produce ova that develop into normal embryos when transplanted into young mice.

The ovaries are not essential to life and can be removed without altering the life span of the individual. However, a cessation of ovarian function is associated with a number of changes commonly regarded as features of aging. In addition, menopause is associated with a rise in serum cholesterol, an important factor in ischemic heart disease.

ABSOLUTE
CELL LOSS
THE YARDSTICK
OF
FUNCTIONAL
DECLINE

Aging of the Endocrine System

Adrenocorticosteroid production drops slightly with age, but plasma corticosterone and cortisol concentrations remain essentially unchanged. There is a decrease in the uptake and turnover rate of radioactive iodine in the elderly, while the concentration of circulating protein-bound iodine and sensitivity to thyroid-stimulating hormone (TSH) remain unchanged.

Although the reproductive hormones were once regarded as a possible source of everlasting life, they cannot prolong life. They may, however, prevent or delay some of the changes that occur with aging. Decreased testosterone production may play a role in muscle atrophy and in the drop in red blood cell count that occurs late in life. Decreased secretion of testosterone without significant changes in plasma corticoid concentration may be responsible for the catabolic processes that occur in the elderly. Castration does not cause premature death, nor does administration of testosterone reverse aging or prolong life. It may, however, restore libido and muscle strength.

EFFECTS OF AGING PROCESS MANIFEST IN ALL BODY SYSTEMS

Aging of the Nervous System

It is estimated that the human brain loses about 30 cells per minute. Although these cells are not replaced, the accumulated loss of itself does not cause death. Between the ages of 30 and 90, central reaction times increase, and the average speed of conduction in peripheral nerves decreases by about 15 per cent. This decrease is due either to loss of fast fibers or to reduced conduction speed of all fibers. The number of fibers in the nerve trunks decreases 30 per cent between the ages of 30 and 90. Changes in the nervous system may play a large role in causing accident proneness and poor response to infection in the elderly, particularly in those with presenile or senile dementia. Since the senile plaques and fibrillary changes present in the neurones in presenile and senile dementia commonly occur in a milder form in most elderly persons, these diseases possibly represent accelerated aging of the nervous system.

Aging of Skeletal Muscle

Irreversible loss of some muscle cells and atrophy of others result in a decrease of approximately 30 per cent in muscle weight and strength between the ages of 30 and 90. While this decline may largely represent inherent aging of the tissue, it is influenced by declining nerve and endocrine function, decreased blood supply, and decreased use of the muscle.

Aging of the Cardiovascular System

After age 30 cardiac output decreases, and as a consequence blood flow to all tissues diminishes. Heart rate falls, and stroke volume decreases by about 0.7 per cent per year. Resting oxygen consumption and carbon dioxide production decrease by about 0.5 per cent per year. Although it is impossible to accurately assess the role of the vascular system in aging, it is felt that decreased cardiac output may play a large role in secular aging. As cardiac function declines, a lack of oxygen and nutrients associated with an accumulation of waste products may cause aging of cells and tissues.

Aging of Skin

The skin, which has a potential life span far beyond that of the individual, is slowly aged by other tissues. Aging skin transplanted into young mice takes on some of the properties of the host, such as the hair regrowth cycle. In young skin transplanted into older mice, the hair regrowth cycle slows to the same rate as the host skin beside the graft. Skin, therefore, apparently ages not because it is old but because it is part of an old animal.

EFFECTS OF AGING IN MAN

It is difficult to distinguish the effects of aging from those of disease, and the older the person, the more likely it is that disease is present. One study revealed that geriatric patients in one hospital had an average of six pathologic conditions each. Another survey showed that the general population aged 65 and over (not sick) had an average of more than three debilitating conditions each.

Diminishing powers of adaptation and increased vulnerability accompany aging, and aged persons show decreased ability to survive trauma. Their resistance to infections is lowered. Any kind of stress exerts a more severe effect upon the aging body than on the young. The aging body also takes longer to correct disturbances in the internal environment.

Effects of Aging in Organs and Tissues

Some pathologic changes regarded as characteristic of the aging process are commonly found in the organs and tissues of aged persons during life or at autopsy. Atrophy of the rete pegs, the epidermal processes that project downward between the dermal papillae, and degeneration of the dermal collagen and elastic fibers cause skin to lose its elasticity and to become atrophic, particularly on exposed parts of the body. Wrinkles, perhaps deep furrows, result. In spite of claims made by the cosmetic industry, this process cannot be prevented, nor is it reversible.

Autopsies performed on elderly persons frequently reveal a significant degree of atherosclerosis. The absence of atherosclerosis in the coronary arteries may be associated with longevity. Atherosclerosis of a minor degree begins in most persons when they are in their twenties, but it usually involves only a few small plaques in the aorta. The condition worsens with age and affects other vessels, such as the coronary and cerebral arteries. Mental confusion in old age is frequently caused by disease in the cerebral arteries, with resultant cerebral ischemia. The process is usually quite slow and may never reach clinical significance. In some persons, however, it progresses so rapidly as to interfere with blood flow through the affected vessel and may result in myocardial or cerebral infarction.

Another vascular change that frequently accompanies old age is arteriosclerosis, a structureless type of thickening of the arterioles. Arteriosclerosis is especially apt to occur in the spleen and kidney. The condition is often present in middle age and is aggravated by hypertension at any age.

ATHEROSCLEROSIS
A FORM OF
ARTERIOSCLEROSIS

Aged persons may shrink as much as 2 inches in height as a result of increased curvature of the spine, atrophy of the intervertebral disks, and flattening of the plantar arches. The dorsal spine is particularly affected; consequently, the shape of the thoracic cage is altered so that it increases in size but decreases in flexibility. The changes in the thoracic cage result in an increased lung volume, while the vital capacity is decreased.

Osteoporosis occurs in most persons over the age of 50, with mild kyphosis a frequent result. Moreover, bones of the elderly break more easily than those of the young, and fractures may not heal as rapidly. Sometimes, however, failure of bones to knit is caused by local ischemia resulting from arterial disease rather than from generalized bony changes. Unfortunately, neither the cause nor the cure of osteoporosis is known.

Sexual vigor decreases in old age. In women the uterus and ovaries atrophy after the menopause. The organs of persons who are quite aged often appear atrophic at autopsy. This finding is usually associated with an increase in the pigment lipofuscin in the cells. When the heart is involved, the condition is known as *brown atrophy.*

The aged person is slow to recognize and respond to stimuli. Although defective perception, caused by deterioration of hearing and vision, and impaired conduction of impulses to effector organs may slow sensory and motor performance, the main delay is in the brain, which takes longer to appreciate a stimulus, identify its nature, and select the appropriate response.

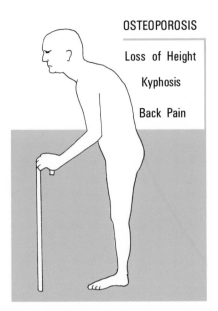

OSTEOPOROSIS

Loss of Height

Kyphosis

Back Pain

Effects of Aging on Mental Function

Until only recently, aging was assumed to be associated with a widespread loss of mental function, with all aspects of intellectual function progressively and irretrievably lost. However, this is not the case. Recent studies have shown that the aging mind is far more resilient than was formerly believed.

Many aged persons display a failure of short-term memory and difficulty in recalling information. This occurs not because the capacity to retain information is diminished, but because the older person is easily distracted by irrelevant stimuli. Inability to concentrate for long periods probably explains why elderly persons have more difficulty with problem-solving tests than do young persons. The impaired short-term retention and comprehension of data often results in learning difficulties. Learning can be achieved successfully, however, if the person is given enough time and is undisturbed.

Aging also may produce changes in personality. For example, an elderly person may become highly suspicious and misinterpret words or gestures as being hostile or antagonistic. This is particularly apt to occur if the individual is deaf or has always had a suspicious nature. In addition, many older persons show a heightened emotional tone and may cry at the slightest provocation.

Older people often tend to feel left out of things and have difficulty in occupying mind and body. Chronic underactivity of the brain leads to apathy and lack of interest. Older people who become more talkative or who complain habitually may only be trying to raise their brain activity to a level nearer the optimum. Similarly, some older people compensate for decreased mental function through increased physical activity or restlessness, which represents a substitution of work for thought.

AGING AND DEATH

> *Have you heard of the wonderful one hoss shay,*
> *That was built in such a logical way*
> *It ran a hundred years to a day?*
> —Oliver Wendell Holmes:
> *The Deacon's Masterpiece*, Stanza 1, 1858

Old age is commonly associated with death. According to Selye, however, no one has ever died of old age per se. Unlike the wonderful one hoss shay, organs and tissues do not all age at the same rate of speed, and aging of one tissue is not necessarily correlated to aging of other tissues. Therefore, some parts wear out faster than others. Somatic death occurs when one vital organ wears out too early in proportion to the rest of the body. Selye states, "Life, the biologic chain that holds our parts together, is only as strong as its weakest vital link. When this breaks—no matter which vital link it be—our parts can no longer be held together as a single living being."

HOMEOSTASIS THE CRITICAL FACTOR

While old age does not in itself cause death, it certainly is a predisposing factor. The functional decline of many processes that results from an overall decline in the functional capacity of tissues causes the body to have a decreased ability to cope with stress and to maintain homeostasis. For example, if an aged person is given a large dose of sodium bicarbonate by mouth, it may take several days for his electrolyte balance to return to normal, whereas a younger person would recover in a matter of hours. In general, functional decline begins at about age 30 and gradually progresses, at a rate of about 0.3 to 1.3 per cent per year. As aging advances, larger and larger deviations from the norm are tolerated before the homeostatic mechanisms come into play. If the homeostatic mechanisms are not activated before the imbalance becomes critical, death may result.

Decreased ability to cope with infection, which suggests a decline in the immunologic system, predisposes to death in elderly persons. The decreased resistance to infection may be related to a reduction of lymphoid tissue, which begins in adolescence. With advancing age, lymph nodes become nodules of fat with only a rim of lymphoid tissue. Studies in animals have shown decreased production and impaired maintenance of adequate antibody levels. In addition, both immediate and delayed hypersensitivity reactions were decreased in severity. A decline in the number of potential antibody-forming cells is believed to cause the decreased immunologic response.

Some terminal diseases of old age are believed to be the direct result of age changes. Malignancy and many age-related autoimmune diseases, such as rheumatoid arthritis, systemic lupus erythematosus, multiple sclerosis, and chronic thyroiditis, may be caused by random mutations that accumulate with age.

DISEASE MODEL: ATHEROSCLEROSIS

Atherosclerosis, a form of arteriosclerosis characterized by intimal thickening, is caused by localized accumulations of lipids. The lesions are known as *atheromas*. Atheromas may develop in any artery, but they are commonly found in the aorta, in the coronary and cerebral arteries, and in the peripheral arteries of the lower extremities. The condition develops insidiously and is probably caused or aggravated by numerous factors.

It is believed that β-lipoproteins, a heterogeneous family of macromolecules containing protein, cholesterol, phospholipids, and triglycerides in varying proportions, are basically responsible for the disease process. Two ideas have been proposed to explain their action: (1) lipoprotein particles of a particular size enter directly into the intimal layer of the artery and thus start the atherosclerotic process; and (2) the chief effect of lipoprotein particles is upon blood coagulability, promoting the development of mural thrombi.

Heredity also plays a role in the development of atherosclerosis, since genetic factors, through control of enzymes and protein concentration, influence both the synthesis and the secretion of lipoproteins by the liver, as well as the structure and elasticity of the arterial wall.

Dietary variations can affect the rate of synthesis and destruction of lipoproteins by changing the metabolism of either the lipid or the protein components.

Sex hormones influence the concentration and ratio of some lipoproteins and may affect the permeability of the vessel wall. Females are much less susceptible to atherosclerosis during the reproductive years than are males of the same chronologic age.

Premature atherosclerosis can occur as a result of diseases in which

HEREDITY
AND
ENVIRONMENT
INFLUENCE
DEVELOPMENT
OF
ATHEROSCLEROSIS

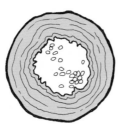

Normal Artery

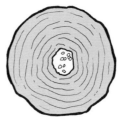

Atheromatous Degeneration
of Artery

fat transport is altered, such as diabetes mellitus, hypothyroidism, and nephrosis. Obesity increases the risk of its development. However, the atherosclerotic condition probably stems from complications or predisposing conditions resulting from obesity rather than from increased adipose tissue per se. Lack of regular exercise and heavy or prolonged use of tobacco may be significant factors in the development of atherosclerosis.

Development of the Disease

Over a period of time, lipids infiltrate the intima and are deposited there, thus forming an atheroma. The earliest lesions of atherosclerosis are the subintimal fatty streaks seen in the thoracic aorta in children. These lesions may regress, or they may grow larger and form plaques. Hemorrhage below the intima or ulceration of the plaque may lead to thrombosis and occlusion of the affected vessel, which results in various signs and symptoms of ischemia. In addition, thrombus formation in the narrowed vessels may cause infarction of adjoining tissue. Canalization may occur, thus allowing the thrombotic process to take place numerous times. Long-standing atheromas may spread into the media, weakening the wall and forming an aneurysm.

In most instances, signs and symptoms of disease do not result from atheromas per se, but from complications of atherosclerosis, including **OCCLUSIVE** stenosis, aneurysm, thrombosis, and, rarely, embolus. Stenosis of coronary **PROCESS** arteries caused by atherosclerosis frequently leads to angina pectoris. **PRECEDES** A thrombosed vessel may cause myocardial infarction. Impaired circula- **CLINICAL** tion to the conduction system may cause cardiac arrhythmias. Con- **DISEASE** gestive heart failure, with or without previous history of infarction, may follow repeated ischemic insults to the myocardium.

Cerebral atherosclerosis is a frequent cause of confusion, forgetfulness, and personality changes in aged persons. Cerebrovascular disease, with or without hypertension, often leads to strokes, which are caused either by thrombosis or by hemorrhage.

Atherosclerosis of the aorta usually does not produce symptoms unless plaques develop in the mouths of one or more major branches, or unless an aneurysm causes pressure or ruptures. Sudden occlusion at the bifurcation results in absent femoral pulses, weakness, pain, and changes in color and temperature of the lower extremities. If occlusion of the terminal aorta is more gradual, intermittent lameness and pain in the buttocks and thighs may occur. Narrowing of the femoral arteries or their branches affects the calves in the same manner, and may even cause gangrene of the toes. Most of the signs and symptoms of atherosclerosis result from occlusions that cause ischemia. Aneurysms that produce abnormal masses or lead to arterial rupture are less common.

Definitive diagnosis of atherosclerosis is generally made following the appearance of an overt complication caused by thrombosis of an artery or infarction of an organ. Patients with signs and symptoms of ischemia, particularly in the arteries of the heart, brain, and lower extremities, can be presumed to have atherosclerosis. Hypercholesterolemia (total blood cholesterol more than 250 mg. per 100 ml.) may suggest atherosclerosis.

While there is no sure method of preventing atherosclerosis, it is possible to modify or control certain factors thought to bear on its development. For example, the substitution of polyunsaturated fats for saturated fats in the diet helps to maintain the serum cholesterol values within the normal range (150 to 250 mg. per 100 ml.). Proper treatment of diseases frequently associated with atherosclerosis is important in controlling its development.

Acute complications of atherosclerosis, such as coronary thrombosis, may be treated with anticoagulants. Angina pectoris may respond to vasodilator drugs.

CLINICAL CONSIDERATIONS

In this century, scientific advances have greatly decreased mortality in infancy and childhood, and as a result, more people are living to an old age. Today, approximately 10 per cent of the total population of the United States is over 65. With an increasing number of people reaching old age, diseases of old age are rising proportionately, and their overall aspects are becoming more serious. In addition, degenerative and involutional changes associated with aging are becoming ever more challenging. The consequence of this relatively recent situation is that geriatrics, the branch of medicine devoted to the problems of old age, looms large as one of the most fruitful fields of study.

Medical science has added years to life; now we must add life to years. Those caring for aged patients can do much in this respect. For example, a patient with incurable arthritis or who has suffered severe stroke may be helped to become self-sufficient to some degree if he is encouraged to do exercises that will restore muscle power and increase functional capacity.

Proper nutrition is of prime importance in aged patients. If the patient has a poor appetite, efforts should be made to encourage him to eat, and to provide instruction on diet, should this be called for. The solution may be as simple as suggesting that he have his dentures checked to make sure that they fit properly.

Many aged patients feel that they are useless and unwanted, and quite often this attitude spells the difference between life and death. Therefore, the patient should be given encouragement and moral support.

By realizing that the patient who is overly talkative or who complains constantly may only be trying to compensate for decreased brain function, one can offer the kinds of understanding therapy he needs. He can be encouraged to participate in civic affairs or other activities (if he is able) that will give him some new interest and perhaps stimulate his brain activity. He also should be encouraged to exercise regularly, though not vigorously.

Patients with terminal diseases should be made as comfortable as possible. They should be made to feel that everything possible is being done and that those caring for them are truly interested in their well-being. If pain is present, careful attention should be directed toward seeing that analgesics are administered at the intervals prescribed.

TOPICS FOR DISCUSSION

1. What is meant by "the wear and tear of life"?
2. What is your opinion of Selye's theory that we are born with a certain supply of adaptive energy and that nothing we can do will replace it?
3. What do you suppose is meant by "retirement disease"?
4. What is meant by premature senility (Alzheimer's disease)?
5. Is the rapidity of aging hereditary?
6. Assuming that the speed with which we age is hereditary, what can we do to retain youth as long as possible?
7. What are some of the desirable forms of exercise for older people? (Read what Dr. Paul Dudley White has to say about this.)
8. Do you feel it is better for an elderly person to live with a group of his age mates or to stay with his family?
9. In what way are some of the unpleasant traits of the elderly defensive?
10. Granted that the most frequent nutritional deficiency in the elderly is that of protein, how can they be persuaded to eat more protein? What specific foods would be best? Should elderly persons take a vitamin supplement?

BIBLIOGRAPHY

Books

Lansing, A.: Cowdry's Problems of Ageing. Baltimore, The Williams & Wilkins Co., 1952.
Selye, H.: The Stress of Life. New York, McGraw-Hill Book Co., 1956.
Geschickter, C.: Some Fundamental Aspects of the Aging Process, pp.

83–105 in VA Prospectus Research in Aging. Washington, D.C., U.S. Government Printing Office, 1959.

Hopps, H.: Principles of Pathology. New York, Appleton-Century-Crofts, 1964.

The Merck Manual of Diagnosis and Therapy. Rahway, New Jersey, Merck Sharp & Dohme Research Laboratories, 1966.

Beeson, P., and McDermott, W.: Textbook of Medicine. vols. I and II. Philadelphia, W. B. Saunders Co., 1967.

Passmore, R., and Robson, J.: A Companion to Medical Studies. vol. 2, pp. 36.1–36.14. Philadelphia, F. A. Davis Co., 1970.

Articles

Over 65. Medical World News, *11*:32J (November 6), 1970.

13

psychosomatic factors in disease

For this is the great error of our day in the treatment of the human body, that physicians separate the soul from the body.
—Plato, *The Phaedrus*

Most of us have at some time experienced an agonizing headache, acute discomfort in the abdomen, a pounding heart, or a drenching sweat because of psychological stress. The discomfort could have stemmed from the prospect of taking a difficult exam, presenting a lecture, or facing criticism from the boss. Although the origin was in the mind, there was nothing imaginary about the physical symptoms—the suffering was all too real. This is an example of psychosomatic illness. The word itself stems from the Greek root *psyche*, meaning mind, soul, self; and the Greek root *soma*, meaning body. We shall see, as we consider psychosomatic illness (sometimes referred to as *psychophysiological* illness), that mind and body are so interrelated that they can hardly be separated. In view of this indivisibility, all illnesses should be considered in relation to the entire person.

INFLUENCE OF PSYCHOSOMATIC FACTORS

Psychosomatic disorders are by no means limited to brief episodes of discomfort such as headache, burning in the pit of the stomach, racing heart, or heavy perspiration, for the mind can exert such influence as to promote organic disease that may be incapacitating or might even be fatal. Fully developed psychosomatic disease is indeed disease, with characteristic symptoms, signs, and physical findings, as well as evidence from x-ray, electrocardiographic, and laboratory studies such as is found in purely organic disorders.

Between 50 and 75 per cent of patients who consult physicians suffer from complaints that are emotional in origin, no matter how frankly

PHYSICAL
DISORDERS
OFTEN
ROOTED IN
PSYCHIC
DYSFUNCTION

physical the symptoms may be. These psychosomatic disorders are not the same as those seen in mentally disturbed persons or persons considered to be merely neurotic. On the contrary, numerous perfectly normal people are afflicted by one or another psychosomatic disturbance at least once during their lifetime. Fortunately, the fear and anxiety that give rise to excessive sweating, clammy palms, parched throat, and pounding heart do not often develop into organic disease; nevertheless, when the emotional stimulus is strong enough and lasts long enough, pathologic changes do occur in body organs.

Psychosomatic illness has widespread effects. In the gastrointestinal system there may be indigestion, loss of appetite, ulcer, diarrhea, constipation, and colitis. Coronary artery disease, high blood pressure, and hardening of the arteries involve the cardiovascular system. Skin diseases, bronchial asthma, and perhaps diabetes and arthritis can originate at least in part in mental, or psychic, distress. Obesity and chronic lower back pain may have psychological causation, as may problems of the menopause, menstrual abnormalities, and frigidity and other sexual problems. Complicating matters is the fact that disorders often labeled psychosomatic can have a physical or a physical-and-psychic origin. For example, the root cause of peptic ulcer may be psychic, originating in some distressing situation, physical, originating in drug usage, or both.

HISTORICAL BACKGROUND

Although great strides have been taken during the last few decades toward an understanding of psychosomatic dysfunction, and research is progressing at a rapid rate, current interest in psychosomatic disease is in some ways a revival of ancient views. At the dawn of medicine, healers regarded mind and body as one and medicine and magic as synonymous. For example, scientists have discovered human skulls 8,000 to 10,000 years old with trephine holes, no doubt drilled by the witch doctor in his efforts to cure the illness by releasing evil spirits from the patient's skull. For more thousands of years, man continued to regard mental and physical diseases as one, as expressed in the magnificent Babylonian-Assyrian culture that flourished in Mesopotamia (circa 2500–500 B.C.), and the great societies established by the Greeks and Romans (400 B.C.–400 A.D.). Even though medicine at this time was dominated by religion and suggestion was a major tool in treatment, medicine was "modern" in the sense that it recognized the indivisibility of mind and body and the influence of mind over body. This concept of the oneness of mind and body persisted through the long Greek period and then through the centuries of Roman medicine. With the downfall of Rome, around 400 A.D., ensued the medieval period when disease was viewed as the direct result of sin, and the ill were regarded

MIND-BODY
CONTINUUM
RECOGNIZED
BY ANCIENTS

as only receiving their just deserts. Brutal and unenlightened though this concept was, it at least recognized the relationship between mental health and physical illness.

Then one of the strangest paradoxes in medical history unfolded. The Renaissance introduced monumental advances in mathematics, chemistry, and physics, dispelling the clouds that had smothered original thought throughout the medieval period. It provided the scientific foundation for the establishment and development of microscopy, biochemistry, bacteriology, and pathology. At the same time, Renaissance medicine took a gigantic step backward. Whereas physicians during the Dark Ages had regarded the psyche as a mystic force that could inflict physical suffering, the Renaissance men, in reaction against this concept, relegated the mind strictly to the province of religion and philosophy. Interest in psychiatry and in the role of mental stress on physical disorders was set aside.

APPRECIATION OF MIND-BODY CONTINUUM LOST IN SCIENTIFIC ADVANCE

As the science of medicine developed further, Louis Pasteur (1822–1895) and Rudolf Virchow (1821–1902) established the scientific basis for the study of disease in the laboratory. The cell became the focus in studying disease. Physical disorders began to be regarded as the result of changes in cell structure. Along with this, the mind-body approach fell into even further disrepute. The disease—not the patient—was treated. The new breed of scientists discredited those who would suggest a correlation between disturbed psyche and physical disease.

Not until Sigmund Freud appeared on the scene in the early 20th century did a more rational view again prevail. His controversial teachings led to a new awareness of the importance of emotions in the causation of not only mental, but physical, disturbances. Although many disagreed with Freud's assertions, it is acknowledged universally that he contributed importantly to efforts to remove the study of the mind from the realm of magic and religion and elevate it to the level of a science. He introduced a vital phase of psychiatry in the form of psychoanalysis, a method of eliciting from the patient an idea of his past emotional experiences and mental life, so as to discover the mechanism by which a pathologic mental state has been produced. Today, psychosomatic medicine, a part of Freud's legacy, emphasizes the interaction between psychological and bodily factors in causing illness, maintaining health, and curing disease.

TWENTIETH CENTURY MEDICINE REDISCOVERS MIND-BODY CONTINUUM

DISTINCTION BETWEEN PSYCHOSOMATIC ILLNESS AND MENTAL ILLNESS

As we examine the background of psychosomatic disease, let us keep clearly in mind several important distinctions. First, psychosomatic illness is *not* mental illness. The overwhelming number of persons suffering from psychosomatic disorders are completely sane and can be either effectively treated or at least helped by conventional medical care, commonsense practices, and, in some instances, psychotherapy. Second, psychosomatic disease is entirely different from hysteria. Let us consider examples of each.

Mary is married to a "tyrant" husband. Her life with him is extremely unhappy, but divorce is out of the question for her since she has no way of making a living. Her suppressed tension and brooding unhappiness cause her to develop muscular spasms in her knees and elbows, although she is not aware of this relationship. The spasms cause circulatory and joint problems and, after a time, arthritis develops. The intense pain and incapacity due to her affliction tend to aggravate her personal problems. Mary's overall situation has been made worse. Her condition has all the characteristics of a *psychosomatic* disorder.

John, an Army private in a battle zone, develops complete paralysis of his legs and is removed to a hospital where a searching physical examination reveals no physical abnormality. He is reacting to a conflict from which he fears death or mutilation and concerning which he feels he has shown cowardice. Thus his paralysis effectively solves his problem by taking him out of the front line action. He feels blameless about his situation. His illness is not psychosomatic, for he has no physical disorder. Rather, he is suffering from *hysteria*, a psychoneurosis characterized by a lack of control over emotions and actions, plus anxiety, and simulation of various physical disorders.

We can see that a major difference between psychosomatic disease and hysteria is that the hysteric "solves" his problem, whereas the victim of psychosomatic disease only adds to his suffering. The symptoms of hysteria, such as paralysis, deafness, and loss of voice, are not accompanied —in the early stages, at least—by actual physical change. Psychosomatic disease, on the other hand, involves organic changes that can progress to a serious or even fatal outcome if the cycle is not interrupted.

Psychosomatic illness is the overt expression of a deep and serious conflict in the mind of the individual. The origin of the conflict is a distressing or anxiety-provoking event or series of events in the patient's life. Emotions in themselves do not cause the illness; rather, they are merely an aspect of the reaction to the damaging events. Indeed, one can develop a psychosomatic illness in which an emotional response is lacking via cerebral reaction to the unhappy experiences. Despite the many gaps in our understanding, we do have some knowledge concerning cerebral initiation of bodily illnesses. Let us consider how these cerebral phenomena are translated into bodily illness.

MECHANISM OF PSYCHOSOMATIC DYSFUNCTION

The nervous system possesses a magnificent functional unity. We can better understand psychosomatic illness by recalling that for study purposes the system has been subdivided into two physiologic divisions. The first is the *cerebrospinal*, or *voluntary*, nervous system, consisting of nerve fibers connecting the central nervous system with structures of the body wall, such as skeletal muscles and skin. It is also designated the *somatic* system. The second is the *autonomic*, or *involuntary*, nervous system, consisting of nerve fibers that connect the central nervous system with smooth muscle, cardiac muscle, and glands. This system innervates the viscera; it is also referred to as the *visceral* system.

AUTONOMIC NERVOUS SYSTEM

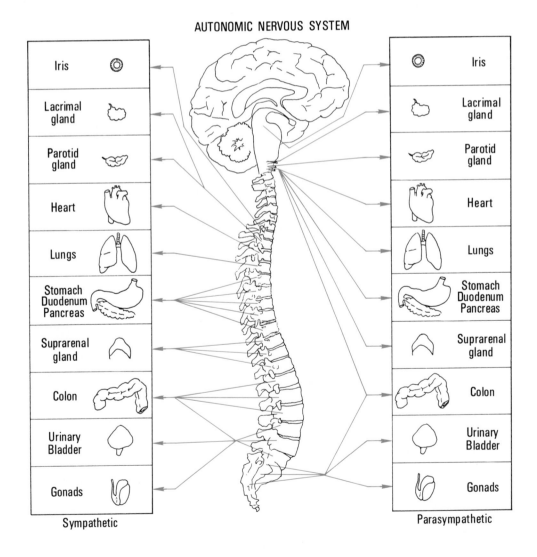

Sympathetic		Parasympathetic
Iris		Iris
Lacrimal gland		Lacrimal gland
Parotid gland		Parotid gland
Heart		Heart
Lungs		Lungs
Stomach Duodenum Pancreas		Stomach Duodenum Pancreas
Suprarenal gland		Suprarenal gland
Colon		Colon
Urinary Bladder		Urinary Bladder
Gonads		Gonads

**AUTONOMIC
NERVOUS
SYSTEM
CHIEF
REGULATOR
OF PSYCHIC
IMPULSES**

Although the cerebrospinal division plays a role in the development of psychosomatic illness, the present discussion focuses attention on the autonomic nervous system. Recall from your basic physiology that the autonomic nervous system consists of nerve pathways primarily concerned with regulating visceral activities, such as the beating of the heart, the movement of food through the digestive system, and the secretory action of glands. This system functions with a certain degree of independence, although it is constantly regulated by cortical and subcortical centers. The cerebral cortex might be likened to a master switchboard in that all nervous impulses are received and analyzed here after they have been sorted and grouped in the thalamus, which is a relay center for incoming impulses and a sensory integrating organ. Most impulses are, however, shunted from the cerebral cortex to the hypothalamus, which then becomes responsible for coordinating the actions of the viscera. The cortex is thus relieved of the necessity of dealing with constant demands for routine visceral adjustments.

Recall that the autonomic nervous system is further divided into sympathetic and parasympathetic divisions. Most of the nerves that control the viscera are supplied by both the sympathetic and the parasympathetic divisions. These divisions have antagonistic effects on individual organs and structures, as occurs, for example, when stimulation of the sympathetic fibers that supply the heart acts to speed up its action, and is followed by stimulation of the parasympathetic fibers which slows the rate of the heartbeat. Both parasympathetic and sympathetic divisions make essential contributions to homeostasis. Stewart Wolf, a pioneer in the field of psychosomatic medicine, has emphasized that traditional concepts concerning the autonomic nervous system need a fresh look. It has been clearly demonstrated that the two systems engage cooperatively in a given response. In this sense, we might say that the two systems are not opposed. Both serve the needs of the body as a whole. In addition to its counterbalancing of parasympathetic effects, the sympathetic division prepares the body for fight or flight when physical danger or emotional crisis intrudes.

**PSYCHIC
DISTRESS
INITIATES
SOMATIC
RESPONSE
IMPULSES**

Consider the series of actions that take place in a cat when confronted by a dog. Impulses from the cat's eyes and nose reach the cerebral cortex, affecting the centers for vision and smell as well as the prefrontal area. Instantaneously, outgoing impulses are dispatched to the hypothalamus, then relayed to lower levels to prepare the cat for the threatened emergency. The entire sympathetic division is thrown into high gear. The pupils dilate. The cat's hair stands on end. Its heart rate accelerates. The blood vessels of viscera and skin constrict, raising the blood pressure and shunting blood into the dilated vessels of skeletal muscle, heart muscle, lung, and brain. The respiratory rate increases and the bronchioles dilate to aid movement of air into and out of the lungs. The level of blood sugar rises. Epinephrine is secreted, thus amplifying and prolonging the activity of the sympathetic division. All these

REVIEW OF AUTONOMIC EFFECTS ON BODY ORGANS

Organ	Parasympathetic	Sympathetic
Pupil of eye	Contracts	Dilates
Ciliary muscle of eye	Excites	No action
Glands of gastro- intestinal tract	Stimulates enzymes	Constricts blood vessels
Sweat glands	No action	Stimulates sweating
Heart muscle	Decreases activity	Increases activity
Coronary arteries	Constricts	Dilates
Abdominal blood vessels	No action	Constricts
Blood vessels of muscle	No action	Dilates
Blood vessels of skin	No action	Constricts or dilates
Lung bronchi	Constricts	Dilates
Lung blood vessels	No action	Constricts mildly
Intestinal lumen	Increases activity	Decreases activity
Intestinal sphincters	Decreases tone	Increases tone
Liver	No action	Releases glucose
Kidney	No action	Decreases output
Body of bladder	Excites	Inhibits
Sphincter of bladder	Inhibits	Excites
Penis	Causes erection	Causes ejaculation
Blood glucose	No action	Elevates
Basal metabolism	No action	Increases
Secretion of adrenal cortex	No action	Increases
Mental action	No action	Increases

changes supply the skeletal muscles and vital organs with increased amounts of blood rich in oxygen and glucose. Peaceful activities, such as digestion, slow down as the cat prepares for offensive or defensive action.

The physiological changes that took place in the cat are closely akin to those which sometimes overwhelm humans. Dr. Walter Alvarez remembers instances of persons apparently dying of fright; in some of these examples the individual died in the operating room before surgery was begun. He recalls an instance in which a rat dropped dead when a dog barked at it, another when a roadrunner fell dead at the sight of a stuffed owl. He recalls cases of Hawaiians being "prayed to death" by a witch doctor. If, under great stress, the functioning of the autonomic nervous system can be so disrupted, it should not surprise us to learn that such stress may give rise to psychosomatic disease.

Individuals vary greatly in their susceptibility to psychosomatic illness. Some overreact to distressing emotional experiences, while others, like the prisoner who thoroughly enjoys his breakfast half an hour before

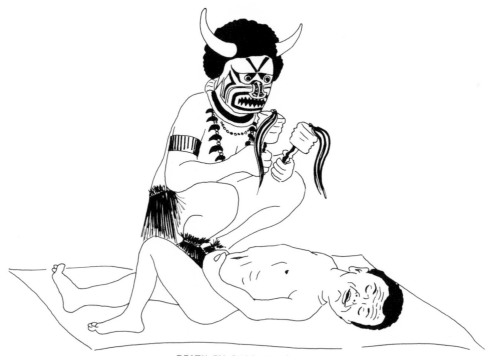

DEATH BY SUGGESTION

he is to be hanged, underreact. Heredity is acknowledged to have a large bearing on the response each individual makes to his life experiences. Temperament stems to a great degree from hereditary factors, and individual temperament certainly has much to do with one's reaction to a specific situation. This heritage might be characterized as the seedbed of psychosomatic illness.

When one considers the number of organs that may be profoundly affected by an emotional upheaval—the lungs, heart, liver, spleen, stomach, pancreas, adrenals, kidneys, intestines, colon, bladder, and sex glands—he can readily understand why a psychosomatic disorder may be the end result of the upheaval.

A partial list of such illnesses would include peptic ulcer, ulcerative colitis, bronchial asthma, essential hypertension, arthritis, migraine, coronary artery disease, the hyperventilation syndrome, and diabetes mellitus. It must be kept in mind, nevertheless, that every one of these can be caused by factors other than emotional turmoil. In such cases, if the underlying cause of the disorder is organic rather than psychic, the psychic component may aggravate the illness or may impede or actually prevent recovery.

In Chapter 11 we considered the diseases of stress, which have their origin in the activities of the pituitary-adrenal axis, a neuroendocrine route. If the stressor is mental or emotional in nature, the disorder may be categorized as psychosomatic. To restate the most important idea of this chapter: the body functions as an integrated whole, in which psychic factors and physical factors are interdependent and interrelated. This unity means that in many instances it is impossible to separate illness components into purely psychic and purely physical ones and in considering illness one should consider the human organism in its totality.

DISEASE MODEL: PEPTIC ULCER

Disagreement exists concerning just which diseases are primarily psychosomatic. Virtually every disease labeled as psychosomatic may also be caused by purely organic factors. For example, peptic ulcer, our disease model, may follow a severe body burn as well as the depredations caused by emotional factors.

As we consider how psychic factors produce peptic ulcer, let us suppose that the person is disturbed because he is trying to work in a position that is considerably beyond his capabilities or for which he is not equipped by training or experience. At first, the developing stress makes him feel merely uncomfortable. Later he has difficulty sleeping. His usually pleasant disposition suffers; he snaps at his wife and children for little or no reason. The vague discomfort appearing after meals he attributes to "acid indigestion" and tries one of the remedies so enthusiastically advertised in the communications media. The discomfort persists, however, and finally becomes noticeable before meals. He finds that eating relieves the discomfort, at least temporarily, but after some time—days, weeks, or months—filling his stomach no longer helps much.

Viewed from the pathophysiologic standpoint, what has happened is that gastric or duodenal irritation has advanced to ulceration. The patient's initial discomfort was but an omen, as it usually is with psychosomatic disease: first the warning, then the fullblown illness. The former represents a temporary alteration in function, the latter a disease, in this case, psychosomatic disease.

In peptic ulcer, when a small area of gastric or duodenal mucous membrane is injured and necrosed, the gastric juice actually digests this tissue exactly as it would digest a piece of meat—the stomach eats itself.

Among the various factors that contribute to peptic ulcer are excessive gastric secretion of hydrochloric acid, excessive secretion of pepsinogen (a substance from the gastric cells which is changed into pepsin by the hydrochloric acid), individual susceptibility to ulcer, and unfavorable environmental factors. Duodenal ulcer is probably more likely to have its origin in psychic factors than is gastric ulcer, according to the available evidence. Vagotomy (cutting the vagus nerve) stops the hypersecretion of hydrochloric acid in patients with duodenal ulcer, but not in those with gastric ulcer.

CIRCULAR NATURE OF SIGNS AND SYMPTOMS ILLUSTRATES INTERRELATION OF PSYCHIC AND SOMATIC FACTORS

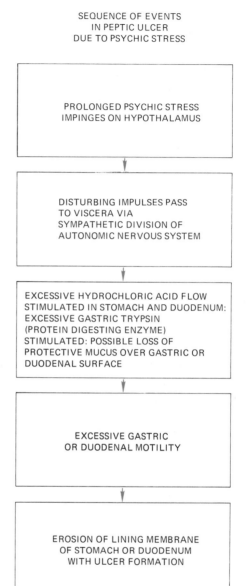

SEQUENCE OF EVENTS
IN PEPTIC ULCER
DUE TO PSYCHIC STRESS

PROLONGED PSYCHIC STRESS
IMPINGES ON HYPOTHALAMUS

DISTURBING IMPULSES PASS
TO VISCERA VIA
SYMPATHETIC DIVISION OF
AUTONOMIC NERVOUS SYSTEM

EXCESSIVE HYDROCHLORIC ACID FLOW
STIMULATED IN STOMACH AND DUODENUM:
EXCESSIVE GASTRIC TRYPSIN
(PROTEIN DIGESTING ENZYME)
STIMULATED: POSSIBLE LOSS OF
PROTECTIVE MUCUS OVER GASTRIC OR
DUODENAL SURFACE

EXCESSIVE GASTRIC
OR DUODENAL MOTILITY

EROSION OF LINING MEMBRANE
OF STOMACH OR DUODENUM
WITH ULCER FORMATION

Peptic ulcer is generally considered a disease of civilization—evidence of its psychosomatic origin. It is rarely seen, for example, in northern India or among the Bantus of South Africa. Before 1900, the incidence of peptic ulcer was far higher in women than in men, but by about 1910, the incidence became equal. At present it is several times higher in men. This again may support the psychosomatic origin of peptic ulcer, for in the 19th century women were severely restricted as regards their personal freedom and had less opportunity for self-expression, while men, on the other hand, enjoyed a highly favored social and economic status. At present women have greater freedom than before, while men are subjected to intensive economic and competitive pressures. The typical ulcer patient is usually described as a tough, hard-driving executive who refuses to acknowledge even to himself his dependence on others. Unconscious conflict ensues and illness results. While this description may fit some patients with ulcer, it certainly fails to adequately describe a great number of them.

As was suggested earlier, one must never lose sight of the fact that organic disorders can also cause peptic ulcer. For example, Cushing's ulcer can occur in brain damage due to trauma, vascular disease, or surgery, especially when the hypothalamic region is involved. A severe burn or other cause of unusually prolonged stress can give rise to a Curling's ulcer. (Both of these are forms of peptic ulcer.) Pancreatic disease may result in ulcer formation. An ulcer may be the first evidence of a parathyroid adenoma. Alcoholics are especially likely to develop ulcers. Various drugs, including corticosteroids, aspirin, phenylbutazone, and indomethacin, can cause ulcers. It is not difficult to see the problems involved in the treatment of peptic ulcer, since this must combine appropriate medical therapy with measures designed to remove or relieve the stressful life situation that brought on the ulcer in the first instance.

CLINICAL CONSIDERATIONS

In managing the patient with a psychosomatic disorder it is of primary importance to appreciate that the illness is real, and its manifestations are organic just as in any illness. While attending this patient, one should try to shield him from unnecessary pain, anger, fear, or worry, since these stimulate the sympathetic division of the autonomic nervous system.

Thorough understanding of the initiating factors is essential. Some physicians prepare a "life chart" on the patient, listing in three vertical columns (1) dates of significant events and his age at their occurrence, (2) his life circumstances and development at significant periods, and (3) the nature of his symptoms, including exacerbations, relapses, and remissions.

There are probably few fields of medicine in which it is more difficult to achieve success than in the management of the patient whose illness is psychosomatic. Merely acquainting the patient with the nature of his problem can be of great help, since "a disease known is half cured," although this alone is not sufficient. Some patients are helped by a strong religious faith. In others, enthusiastic participation in creative activity may provide the key. The great physician, Sir William Osler, advised his patients to live in "daytight compartments," forgetting the problems of tomorrow and the vain regrets of yesterday. Dr. Hans Selye finds his route to satisfaction and happiness in earning the gratitude of others. Helping those less fortunate than themselves has, in turn, helped many patients. Some take joy in new experiences, and in natural things—the sound of a bird, a lovely sunrise or sunset, a walk in a forest. The mountain woman Firelight, in *Christy,* "would interrupt her work to call the children and revel with them in the grandeur of thunderheads piling up over the mountain peaks, heat lightning behind the clouds like fireworks. 'It lifts the heart,' she would say, and that was explanation enough for any interruption!"

Dealing with problems one at a time may aid in reducing tensions. It may thus help to set no time limit on a given task, but rather to work as though an infinite time was available. One should try to help the patient develop enthusiasm for every activity. The patient should be encouraged to think about the happy events of his life rather than the sad ones, as well as to think in constructive ways about his problems. The health worker can help the patient to understand that while there is no universal solution for all problems, none goes on indefinitely and all yield to the passage of time.

It should not be assumed that a psychic disturbance is the crux of

CAN THESE DISEASES SOMETIMES BE CAUSED BY PSYCHOSOMATIC FACTORS?

Disease	Likelihood		
	Certain	Probable	Possible
Anorexia	X		
Arteriosclerosis			X
Arthritis			X
Bronchial asthma		X	
Colitis	X		
Constipation	X		
Coronary artery disease		X	
Dermatitis	X		
Diabetes			X
Diarrhea	X		
Frigidity		X	
Impotence		X	
"Indigestion"	X		
Low back pain			X
Menstrual abnormalities		X	
Obesity	X		
Peptic ulcer	X		

the illness. The patient should be advised to consult a physician who has had broad experience and who is thus able to make a judgment about the probable nature of the illness and its management.

TOPICS FOR DISCUSSION

1. Psychosomatic diseases are sometimes referred to as psychophysiologic diseases. In your opinion which term is more appropriate?

2. Discuss the paradox involved in the magnificent medical discoveries of the Renaissance blocking understanding of psychosomatic ailments.

3. Compare the plight of the patient with psychosomatic disease, who is ill and unhappy, with that of the hysteric, whose disability has enabled him to escape his problem.

4. Discuss the interrelationships between psychosomatic disease caused by messages relayed by the autonomic nervous system and those caused by stress, as Selye uses the term.

5. Name a dozen disorders which could not possibly include a psychosomatic element in their causation.

6. Why are psychosomatic disorders among the most difficult to treat?

7. Is cure *always* possible in psychosomatic disease? Is it *ever* possible?

8. What should be our minimal goal in working with a patient whose disease is psychosomatic?

9. Discuss the reasons why peptic ulcer was chosen as the disease model for psychosomatic disease. Can you suggest another illness that might be suitable?

10. Why are sympathy and understanding of particular importance in dealing with the patient with a psychosomatic ailment?

11. Do the views concerning the functioning of the autonomic nervous system, as set forth by Stewart Wolf, make this activity appear more complex or simpler?

BIBLIOGRAPHY

Books

Dunbar, F.: Mind and Body: Psychosomatic Medicine. New York, Random House, 1947.

Alexander, F.: Psychosomatic Medicine: Its Principles and Application. New York, W. W. Norton & Company, Inc., 1950.

Sadler, S.: Practice of Psychiatry. St. Louis, The C. V. Mosby Co., 1953.

Selye, H.: The Stress of Life. New York, McGraw-Hill Book Co., 1956.

Alvarez, W.: Live at Peace with Your Nerves. Englewood Cliffs, N. J., Prentice-Hall, Inc., 1958.

Freedman, A., and Kaplan, H.: Comprehensive Textbook of Psychiatry. Baltimore, The Williams & Wilkins Co., 1967.

Marshall, C.: Christy. New York, Avon Books, 1967.

Soloman, P., and Patch, V.: Handbook of Psychiatry. Los Altos, Cal., Lange Medical Publications, 1969.

Weekes, C.: Hope and Help for Your Nerves. New York, Hawthorne Books, Inc., 1969.

Articles

Kimball, C.: Conceptual developments in psychosomatic medicine: 1939–1969. Annals of Internal Medicine, 73:307, 1970.

An ache masking depression. Medical World News, 11:54H, (September 25) 1970.

*part
two*

*Representative
Diseases
by Systems*

introduction: causative processes underlying systemic diseases

Having considered 12 fundamental pathophysiological processes that underlie disease, we turn now to the production of disease by these processes.

Not only is one or more of them responsible for the production of disease, a given disease can result from one process in Patient A, and from another in Patient B. Gastric ulcer, for example, can be caused by a burn (a physical agent) or by psychic turmoil (a stress agent).

Furthermore, a disease process can produce effects on more than one body system. Hypertension is an example of the pervasiveness of morbid processes. It is a disease of diverse causes; and it has diverse manifestations. The *cerebral* manifestations include personality changes, stroke, even seizures. Angina pectoris and myocardial infarction are among the potential *cardiac* developments. The occlusive process involves the *peripheral arteries,* and this leads to intermittent claudication. Hypertension appears to be an important predisposing cause of dissecting aneurysm of the aorta. There may be *ocular* disturbances, such as venous thrombosis in the retina. The *kidneys,* always being involved in hypertension, often suffer great damage leading to renal failure. All these events are *end results* of the increased arterial pressure that started the chain of events. Thus hypertensive disease surely is in the front rank among disorders that provoke a "total" response.

The example of syphilis illustrates still another side of a many-faceted disease process. First comes the chancre, appearing at the site of infection, i.e., *genital organs* or *lips.* If treatment is not started, the spirochetes are carried via the bloodstream to distant sites, producing secondary lesions in the *skin, mucous membranes,* and *lymph nodes.* Finally the tertiary lesions develop. These are the most serious, since the entire *nervous system* is now involved.

The key word is *process.* In the Introduction to Part I, disease was described as dysfunction. Going one step further, it becomes evident that *dysfunction* is also *process.* In his study of pathophysiology, the student should keep in mind the question, What process or processes within the body have resulted in the expression of clinical disease? By always posing this question, the student may avoid developing shallow, mechanical notions about the nature of illness. No matter in which field of health practice he chooses to work, this knowledge will enhance his understanding of disease and, of course, his effectiveness as a health worker.

14

common diseases of the musculoskeletal system

The musculoskeletal system represents far more than the structural framework of the human body and its means of locomotion. The bones constitute a dynamic system that participates actively in body metabolism. For example, they store calcium, phosphorus, and sodium, releasing these electrolytes for use elsewhere in the body according to need. The importance of the muscles is shown by the fact that when a body deficiency of potassium (the chief cellular cation) exists, the deficiency is reflected mainly in dysfunction of the muscles—the muscles of respiration, of the skeleton, of the digestive tract, and of the heart.

ARTHRITIS

Arthritis, basically an inflammation involving joints, has many causes. Consequently, it can be divided into various types. We shall focus on adult rheumatoid arthritis as a representative illness.

Rheumatoid arthritis is a chronic systemic disease that affects the entire musculoskeletal system. Joint membranes, cartilage, and skeletal muscle reveal characteristic, though nonspecific, pathologic changes. Women suffer from this disorder two to nine times as frequently as men do. In spite of many theories as to the cause of rheumatoid arthritis, no answer is final. No specific infectious agent has been isolated, nor have hypersensitivity, vascular abnormality, specific metabolic factors, endocrine disorders, or personality patterns been established as causes beyond possible doubt.

PATHOPHYSIOLOGIC PROCESSES WHICH CAN BE INVOLVED IN DISEASES OF THE MUSCULOSKELETAL SYSTEM

	Genetics: Diseases Due to Hereditary Factors	Disease Due to Hypersensitivity and Autoimmunity	Infectious Diseases	Diseases Due to Physical Agents	Diseases Due to Chemical Agents	Neoplasia	Disturbances of Fluid and Electrolyte Balance	Diseases of Malnutrition	Endocrine Dysfunction	Stress Factors in Disease	The Aging Process	Psychosomatic Factors in Disease
Arthritis		■	■						■			■
Bursitis	■		■		■			■				
Cervical Root Syndrome				■								■
Low Back Pain	■	■		■		■		■			■	■
Osteomyelitis				■				■				
Neoplasms of Bone	■			■	■	■						
Muscular Dystrophy	■							■				
Myasthenia Gravis		■										

Pathophysiology

The lesions of rheumatoid arthritis are due to invasion of affected areas by mononuclear cells plus overgrowth of connective tissue. A fibrin-staining material called *fibrinoid* is seen in these lesions. Nodules are found under the skin, over pressure points such as the elbows, over long tendons, or on the periosteal surfaces of long bones. These nodules resemble those seen in rheumatic fever. In a few patients, such nodules are found in the heart. Nearly a third of patients with severe rheumatoid arthritis show inflammation of the pleura and the pericardium.

The onset may be gradual, or explosive, with multiple joint involvement, fever, and prostration. Swelling, pain, and tenderness of the joints of the fingers, wrists, knees, and feet appear, usually symmetrically. The joints may be warm, red, and filled with fluid. Fatigue and weakness are common. The joint and muscle symptoms are most bothersome with physical inactivity, and decrease after activity is resumed. Splinting of adjacent muscles with spasm accompanies pain in affected joints. Usually flexion deformities occur since the flexors are the stronger muscle groups. Because of muscle atrophy both proximal and distal to the swollen joint, these joints often have a spindle-like appearance. Muscle weakness and atrophy stem from the acute rheumatic process in the muscle and from pain. General swelling of the lymph glands occurs in 30 per cent of patients. Anemia develops and the white blood count may be elevated. The erythrocyte sedimentation rate rises. X-ray studies may reveal osteoporosis of the bones adjacent to the affected joints, soft tissue swelling, or actual joint destruction. Cartilage is eroded and destroyed.

Management

The course of rheumatoid arthritis cannot be predicted. There may be periods of great improvement, followed by regression. Occasionally, a severe case ends in invalidism or death. Judicious rest and a well-balanced diet are called for. Salicylates are usually prescribed for pain relief. Adrenocortical steroids are used in severe, rapidly progressing disease, but less hazardous medications should be tried first. Intra-articular injections of hydrocortisone preparations may be useful. Physical therapy to prevent flexion contractures and to restore muscular strength is perhaps the most important part of treatment.

BURSITIS

Bursae (singular, bursa), you will recall, are small clefts lined with synovial membrane, which thus converts them into sacs containing a small amount of synovial fluid. They are located in areas where friction

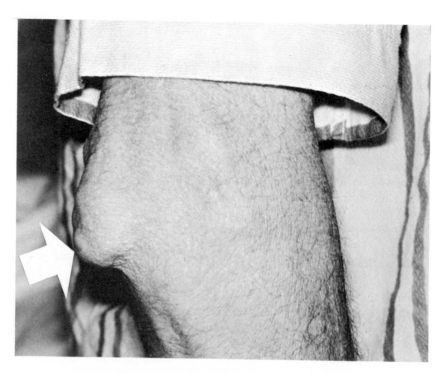

Subcutaneous nodule in rheumatoid arthritis (*arrow*). Such nodules range in size from that of a seed to that of an olive. They may disappear after months or years.

would otherwise develop, usually near a joint. Bursitis, then, is an inflammation of one of these bursae. It may be acute or chronic.

Pathophysiology

OCCUPATIONAL OR PSYCHIC STRESS AN IMPORTANT FACTOR IN MUSCULO-SKELETAL PROBLEMS

An injury, an episode of gout, or an infection can cause bursitis. It is often associated with occupation. For example, miner's elbow affects the olecranon bursa, housemaid's knee the prepatellar bursa, and tailor's or weaver's bottom the ischial bursa. Bursitis also may develop in the deltoid muscle, the Achilles tendon, the patella, the trochanter, and the large toe (in this case it is a bunion).

Acute bursitis usually occurs after injury, prolonged heavy exercise, or infection. The bursa fills with fluid and swells, and this causes tenderness and limitation of motion of the affected area. The chronic form may follow a previous episode of bursitis, repeated injury, or chronic infection. The bursal wall is thickened, and the endothelium degenerates. Later, there may be adhesive inflammation, and calcium may accumulate in the bursa. The muscles overlying the affected area may atrophy. There is pain, swelling, tenderness, muscle weakness, and motion limitation. Mineral deposits can be demonstrated by x-ray study.

Management

In acute bursitis, complete rest and suitable analgesics are indicated. Physical therapy and injections of corticosteroids may be helpful in chronic cases. Deep x-ray therapy may be useful. In some instances, surgical removal of the bursa is indicated. Bursae near the surface can be removed without impairment of function, but deep bursae, especially those that communicate with a joint, are functionally important.

CERVICAL ROOT SYNDROME

This symptom complex results from irritation or compression of the cervical spinal nerve roots in the foramina (canals) between the vertebrae. It is usually caused by poor posture, and occupational and psychic stress may aggravate the postural problem. Injury may cause compression of the intervertebral disks, which may be followed by arthritic spur formation.

Pathophysiology

Pain, numbness, tingling, and weakness are the symptoms, and any or all of them can develop along the distribution of compressed nerve fibers. Depending on the cervical roots affected, symptoms may appear in the shoulders, head, neck, ears, scapula, chest wall, heart, or hand. The patient may experience shoulder pain, stiff neck and shoulders, and numbness of the arm. Movement of the head may be extremely painful. There may be atrophy or contracture of the hand. X-ray findings can well be minimal.

Management

Most patients can successfully counteract mechanical pressure on cervical nerves through postural measures. They should pull in the abdomen and the chin, sitting with the buttocks touching the chair back. They should avoid sitting for long periods with the head tilted back. They will benefit by sleeping flat on the back, using instead of a conventional pillow a hand towel rolled to about 2 inches in diameter or a small cervical pillow. Should they not respond to such simple measures, then physical therapy can be employed. This consists primarily of cervical traction, which can conveniently be carried out at home by use of a device that stretches the neck and thus separates the cervical vertebrae. Prolonged therapy is usually necessary. If disability or pain is severe, surgical operation, consisting of anterior fusion of the vertebrae, may be necessary.

LOW BACK PAIN

Pain in the lower region of the back may be associated with pain radiating to the legs along the course of the sciatic nerve. Among the causes of low back pain are abnormalities elsewhere in the body, such as flat feet, diseased vertebrae, back injury, and a genetically weak back. Disease of the intervertebral disks may also play a role.

Pathophysiology

Pathologic mechanisms producing low back pain are numerous, and in many instances the exact mechanism is far from clear. Menstruation, pregnancy, infection, rectal disorders, prostatic disease, pelvic tumors, and disease of the pancreas may cause back pain. Psychic stress may be a causative factor. Vertebral disease, including tuberculosis of the spine, vertebral infection, vertebral tumors (usually metastatic), arthritis, and osteitis deformans may contribute. In the elderly, osteoporosis is more frequent with debilitating illness, prolonged bed rest, and following the use of certain drugs. Obviously, a fracture of a lumbar or sacral vertebra will cause such pain, as will a vertebral sprain. Herniation of an intervertebral disk gives rise to low back pain radiating down the back of the thigh.

Management

Specific treatment of low back pain is directed toward the cause. Symptomatic therapy includes adequate rest on a firm bed, local heat and massage, local analgesics, salicylates, wearing of a support corset, and weight reduction (if necessary).

OSTEOMYELITIS

Osteomyelitis is a serious bone infection. In most instances it is caused by *Staphylococcus aureus*, and it generally affects the long bones. The infection usually is carried by the blood from another site, although it may follow trauma. Osteomyelitis strikes children mainly, but it may develop in adults by direct infection of bone following a compound fracture. At one time the mortality was high, but today, thanks to antibiotics, death due to osteomyelitis is rare.

Pathophysiology

The organisms invade the blood through a wound, a boil, or another external infection. An abscess forms at that site and produces pus, which spreads along the bone cavity, emerges to the bone surface, and raises the periosteum—the connective tissue covering the bone which, you will recall, provides much of the blood needed by bone. If the infection is not arrested, the bone dies. This dead bone is called a *sequestrum*. The inflamed periosteum now forms new bone (called *involucrum*), which contains many openings (called *sinuses* or *cloacae*) that permit the pus to escape to the surface. If the infection continues to spread, the joint will be destroyed and thrombosis of the marrow vessels may develop.

The first symptoms are sudden pain and high fever. The bone is tender, movement is painful, and action is restricted. The leukocyte count and the erythrocyte sedimentation rate are elevated. Blood cultures may be positive.

PERVASIVENESS OF BACTERIAL PATHOGENS

Management

Prompt and intensive treatment with appropriate antibiotics is most important. In chronic infections, which today fortunately are rare, surgery to remove all dead, infected bone and cartilage may be necessary. Immobilization of the affected part may be desirable.

NEOPLASMS OF BONE

Like tumors arising in other body systems, tumors of bone may be *primary* or *secondary*. Primary tumors may be benign or malignant, whereas secondary ones are, obviously, always malignant. In many instances differentiation between benign and malignant tumors is extremely difficult, and biopsy becomes necessary.

Pathophysiology

The most frequent benign tumors are osteoma, chondroma, and giant-cell tumor. In many respects they resemble the tissue of origin, and most often they develop at the end of one of the long bones. Be-

DISTINCTION BETWEEN BENIGN AND MALIGNANT TUMORS OFTEN A DIFFICULT MEDICAL PROBLEM

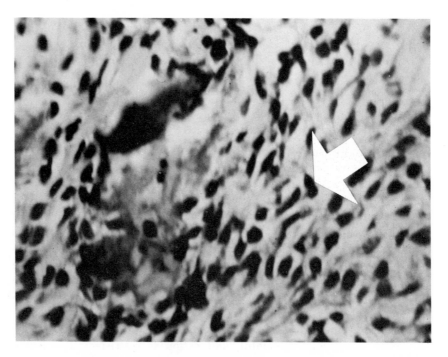

Highly malignant osteosarcoma. Anaplastic cells
(*arrow*) look like horses fleeing from a corral.

cause of the size to which it usually grows, the giant-cell tumor is the
most destructive of the benign neoplasms.

Osteogenic sarcoma, Ewing's tumor, and multiple myeloma are the
major malignant neoplasms of bone. Osteogenic sarcoma most often
develops in the ends of the long bones, and most victims are teenagers.
It is not radiosensitive. Ewing's tumor affects children most often, and
it may begin in any bone. Unlike osteogenic sarcoma, Ewing's tumor is
responsive to radiation therapy, but it invariably recurs. Multiple myeloma, also called plasma cell myeloma, is a tumor of bone marrow rather
than bone. It is a cancer of the middle years. Being multiple, it spreads
very rapidly, producing punched-out areas in the flat bones. Other
malignant bone neoplasms include reticulum cell sarcoma and chondrosarcoma.

Malignant tumors of the breast, lung, prostate, kidney, and thyroid
frequently metastasize to bone. These metastases destroy the bone, so
that a fracture following some minor injury may be the first clue to their
presence.

Management

Every tumor involving bone demands a complete diagnostic assessment of clinical history, symptoms, physical findings, x-ray examination, blood studies, and biopsy (when safe and indicated). All deserve full consideration. If operation is carried out, studies of the removed specimen, both macroscopic and microscopic, may further contribute to diagnosis. Nowhere in the field of oncology does more uncertainty exist than in the case of bone tumors. In general, neoplasms of bone represent a dismal chapter in medicine. Some are so malignant that even the most mutilating operations are futile. Chemotherapy is sometimes beneficial, but much research is needed in this area.

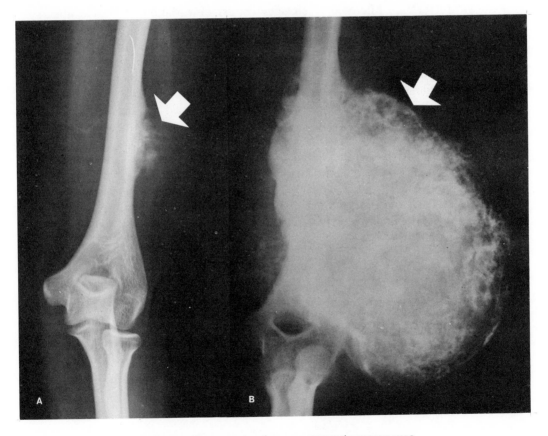

A, On routine examination, a pregnant woman was found to have an early osteogenic sarcoma of the right humerus (*arrow*). Surgical operation was advised, but she refused. *B*, When she returned a year later during a second pregnancy, the bone tumor was found to be greatly enlarged (*arrow*) and her arm enormously swollen. She recovered following amputation of her arm and shoulder.

MUSCULAR DYSTROPHY

The term *muscular dystrophy* really refers to a group of diseases generally classified as the *primary muscular dystrophies*. All are hereditary, due to a genetic disorder of muscle metabolism, and all are characterized by progressive weakness due to degeneration of muscle fibers. The skeletal muscles are primarily involved, although others, including cardiac muscle, may be also.

Pathophysiology

FUNDAMENTAL
ABNORMALITY
STILL
ELUDES
INVESTIGATION

Microscopic changes consist of variation in muscle fiber size, degeneration of fibers, increase in connective tissue, and deposition of fat. Two distinct major varieties of muscular dystrophy are recognized. The *pseudohypertrophic*, or *Duchenne*, form affects only very young boys. Inheritance is sex-linked and recessive. Symptoms such as waddling gait, frequent falls, and difficulty in rising usually appear when the child starts to walk, and he is usually confined to a wheelchair by early adolescence. The calves and other muscles appear to hypertrophy, but this enlargement is due to replacement of muscle fibers by fat.

The *facioscapulohumeral*, or *Landouzy-Dejerine*, form affects both sexes, and is inherited as a dominant trait. The disease usually starts in adolescence. Shoulder girdle weakness is more prominent than leg weakness, and its progression is slower than the Duchenne form.

Myotonic dystrophy and *ophthalmoplegic dystrophy* are less common forms of muscular dystrophy.

Management

Unfortunately, no specific drug therapy exists. Ambulation should be prolonged by muscle-strengthening exercises, by corrective surgical measures, and by proper braces. Those involved in the care of such patients should help them, through providing psychological support, to be as independent as their condition permits.

MYASTHENIA GRAVIS

The cause of this serious chronic disease is unknown. There is extreme muscle fatigue with repeated movements, which is quickly relieved by rest. Even such minor exertion as combing the hair may be so tiring that the patient must stop and rest. The disease mainly affects young adults, and is more common in women than in men.

Pathophysiology

The basic problem is a defect in the transmission of impulses from nerve to muscle cell. The weakness of the ocular muscles produces drooping eyelids and double vision. In some cases a sudden attack of dyspnea followed by collapse occurs and may be fatal, but more often the disease goes on for some years. Difficulty in swallowing and in walking are common. The deep reflexes and normal sensation are preserved, and muscular atrophy is rare. About 25 per cent of patients experience remission of several years' duration.

Management

Bed rest, and exclusion of unnecessary effort, are important in treatment. Neostigmine bromide, administered on a fixed schedule, usually controls the symptoms to a considerable degree. An eye patch to eliminate double vision and "lid crutches" for ptosis are helpful measures. It is necessary to mince the patient's food because of the difficulty in swallowing.

TOPICS FOR DISCUSSION

1. What psychologic factors might influence the onset of rheumatoid arthritis? What psychologic disturbances might rheumatoid arthritis cause? Do you see the possibility of a vicious circle here?

2. What hormones are involved in regulating the content of the electrolytes of bone?

3. Gout appears frequently in the pages of medical history. Obviously, it was once a prevalent disorder, especially among a certain group. How do you account for the fact that it is relatively rare (though not so rare as some suppose) today?

4. Osteomyelitis accounted for much death and disability until about 1940. How do you account for this fact?

5. What organs can serve as the primary origin of a bone tumor?

6. List the diagnostic techniques by which you would distinguish between a benign and malignant bone tumor.

7. Using a general textbook of medicine or a diagnostic nomenclature, make a list of all forms of muscular dystrophy and atrophy.

8. What bone disorders can result from body fluid disturbances?

9. What muscular disorders can result from body fluid disturbances?

10. Review the three types of muscles. Which are controlled by the voluntary nervous system and which by the involuntary (autonomic) nervous system?

11. What major body muscle continues to function at a reasonably efficient level even though all its nerve connections have been severed?

12. Women suffer from rheumatoid arthritis several times as frequently as do men; what possible explanations can you offer?

15

common diseases of the nervous system and the sensory system

The nervous system is the "command post" of the human body, exerting general control over all its activities. The entire nervous system is divided into two great systems: the cerebrospinal or voluntary nervous system (also known as the *somatic system*) and the autonomic, or involuntary nervous system (also referred to as the *visceral system* since it supplies internal organs).

Within the brain and spinal cord, where nerve fibers are not surrounded by neurilemma sheaths, regeneration of injured fibers is impossible. This deficiency seriously hampers therapy and makes complete recovery impossible in such diseases as poliomyelitis and such injuries as transection of the spinal cord. This is one reason why nervous system disorders are difficult to treat and why the final results of treatment are often unsatisfactory. Highly important in the nervous system are the sense organs which enable us to maintain contact with the external environment. Representative disorders of these organs therefore deserve a place in this chapter.

CONVULSIVE SEIZURES

A convulsion, or seizure, may be a *symptom* of some underlying cause (such as infection) or a manifestation of epilepsy. In either case, the seizure is due to an irritation of nerve cells which causes them to discharge abnormal electrical patterns. A single seizure is fairly common in childhood in association with many infections, whereas in epilepsy seizures recur periodically. No explanation for the seizure can be found in 75 per cent of affected adults, although it is agreed that some sort of brain lesion, possibly a scar resulting from birth trauma, is responsible.

PATHOPHYSIOLOGIC PROCESSES WHICH CAN BE INVOLVED IN DISEASES OF THE NERVOUS SYSTEM

	Genetics: Diseases Due to Hereditary Factors	Disease Due to Hypersensitivity and Autoimmunity	Infectious Diseases	Diseases Due to Physical Agents	Diseases Due to Chemical Agents	Neoplasia	Disturbances of Fluid and Electrolyte Balance	Diseases of Malnutrition	Endocrine Dysfunction	Stress Factors in Disease	The Aging Process	Psychosomatic Factors in Disease
Convulsive Seizures	■		■	■	■	■						
Neuritis			■	■	■	■		■	■		■	
Neuralgia						■						
Narcolepsy												
Encephalitis		■	■									
Herpes Zoster			■									
Cerebrovascular Disease			■			■		■			■	
Parkinsonism			■	■	■						■	
Neoplasms of the Brain						■						
Neoplasms of the Spinal Cord						■						
Huntington's Chorea	■											
Glaucoma	■											■
Sympathetic Ophthalmia		■		■								
Iritis			■	■	■							
Retinal Detachment	■			■	■							
Deafness	■		■	■					■	■	■	
Meniere's Disease			■								■	
Meningitis			■									
Syphilis	■		■									
Rabies			■	■								
Cerebral Palsy	■		■	■			■					

Pathophysiology

A convulsion may occur during any of the following states: high fever; central nervous system infection; chemical disturbances, such as hypoglycemia; poisoning due to drugs such as strychnine, or to gases such as carbon monoxide; episodes of breath-holding; brain tumor; congenital brain abnormalities; brain edema, perhaps from eclampsia; skull fracture; hypersensitivity; degenerative brain disease; and withdrawal from hypnotics, tranquilizers, and alcohol. In many of these conditions, the convulsions are transient and cease once the morbid process is arrested; if, however, the disorder is associated with a lesion of the central nervous system, the convulsions may recur periodically for many years, perhaps throughout life.

The seizure is caused by an acute disturbance, either focal or generalized, in cerebral function. Hughlings Jackson, one of the pioneers in the study of convulsive disorders, came to the conclusion that in most cases the seizure develops from a focus or group of abnormally excitable neu-

HIPPOCRATES
DESCRIBED
EPILEPSY
IN FIFTH CENTURY
B.C.

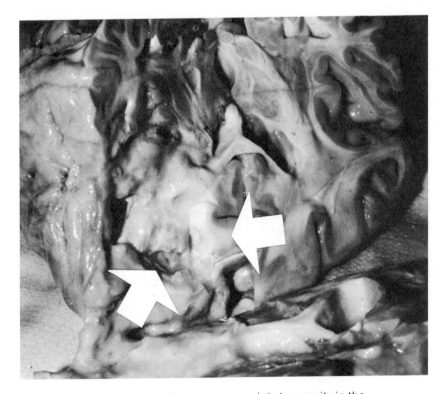

Brain abscess. Lower arrow points to a cavity in the abscess; upper arrow, to outer border of the abscess. Such an abscess can give rise to epileptic convulsions.

rons, and many modern studies support Jackson's view. The focal lesion may be an area of diseased tissue in the cerebrum, such as a brain abscess which discharges abnormally in response to certain stimuli. As the discharge spreads along the brain pathways to other areas of the brain, there is a convulsion, which often is accompanied by loss of consciousness.

Seizure states are classified as grand mal (French for great sickness), petit mal (little sickness), psychomotor (focal), infantile spasm, and epileptic equivalent. The grand mal seizure may be either local or general. There is usually a *prodromal* phase lasting minutes to hours and characterized by anxiety or depression, followed by an *aura* such as an unpleasant odor or a strange body sensation. Then the patient cries out, loses consciousness, and has convulsions ranging from a mild muscle rigidity to generalized violent movements. The attack usually lasts from 2 to 5 minutes, during which the patient may bite his tongue and be incontinent. When he regains consciousness he is groggy and does not remember what has happened. In the petit mal attack, there is merely clouding of consciousness lasting from 1 to 30 seconds. This type occurs most often in children. In psychomotor attacks, both the muscles and the mental processes are affected. Many of these patients suffer from mental disorders. This type of attack is characterized by hallucinations, mental confusion, and automatic movements. Infantile spasms, limited to the first 3 years of life, are manifested by sudden flexion of the arms, forward bending of the trunk, and extension of the legs, lasting only a few seconds. This type is associated with cerebral deterioration. Various behavioral abnormalities, which are recurrent and usually bizarre, are referred to as *epileptic equivalents*.

Management

The first step in management of convulsive seizures is careful diagnosis. The cause or precipitating factors should be removed if possible. Physical and mental hygiene should be stressed. Management of individual convulsions is limited to preventing self-injury or injury to others. If possible, the tongue should be protected; clothing about the neck should be loosened, and a pillow should be placed under the head. A number of anticonvulsant drugs are useful in the management of convulsive disorders. All must be individually prescribed and the side effects must be understood.

NEURITIS

Neuritis is actually a syndrome of sensory, motor, reflex, and vasomotor symptoms caused by lesions of nerve roots or peripheral nerves. Since "neuritis" means "inflammation of a nerve," it follows that any disorder that disturbs normal nerve function can cause neuritis. Mechanical agents include direct blows, penetrating injuries, and compression or damage to nerves by fracture or dislocation of bones. Pressure on a part, as may occur during deep sleep or anesthesia, may cause paralysis, as may pressure due to tumors, bone overgrowth, casts, and crutches. Vascular disorders, such as inflammation of a blood vessel, arteriosclerosis, hemorrhage into a nerve, or reaction to physical agents such as cold or radiation, are other factors. Direct invasion of organisms into one or more nerves is still another cause; localized infectious neuritis is seen in leprosy, tetanus, and tuberculosis. Polyneuritis (affecting many nerves) is often associated with herpes zoster, typhoid fever, diphtheria, malaria, and mumps. Toxins can cause inflammation of one or several nerves. Metal poisoning, e.g., lead, arsenic, gold, thallium, and mercury, is often the cause; in some instances nonmetallic poisoning, e.g., alcohol, carbon monoxide, carbon disulfide, benzene, emetine, carbon tetrachloride, tetrachloroethane, may be responsible. Metabolic disorders, such as thiamine deficiency, diabetes, pernicious anemia, and toxemia of pregnancy usually affect several nerves.

Pathophysiology

Mild damage to a peripheral nerve causes swelling of the axon and myelin sheath; severe damage causes their fragmentation. The connective tissue sheath may proliferate. If infection is present, inflammatory cells will infiltrate the affected area. With vascular lesions there is endothelial proliferation, vascular occlusion, and hemorrhage. Regeneration of peripheral nerves varies with the nature of the lesion, usually going on at the rate of 2 to 4 cm. a month.

The sensory symptoms include tingling, pins and needles, burning, and stabbing pain. The first motor symptom may be weakness, but this may progress to paralysis, with atrophy of affected muscles. Vasomotor symptoms may include hyperemia, sweating, and formation of bullae. The skin may be pale and dry. Osteoporosis may develop. Trophic changes are common in severe, prolonged cases. Laboratory findings may shed light on the cause, e.g., the finding of stippled red blood cells may suggest lead poisoning. X-ray films of the bones will show changes due to trauma, malignancy, or hypertrophic arthritis.

Management

It should be recalled that neuritis is a symptom rather than a specific disease entity. Treatment must, therefore, be directed toward the cause, whether physical damage, neoplasia, vascular disorders, infection, or metabolic disturbances.

NEURALGIA

INNOCUOUS
ACTIONS
MAY TRIGGER
MALIGNANT
EVENTS

In neuralgia there are severe spasms of pain along the distribution of a peripheral sensory nerve. There is no structural change in the nerve—unlike the situation in neuritis.

Pathophysiology

Trigeminal neuralgia, or tic douloureux, refers to brief attacks of excruciating pain along the course of one or more branches of the trigeminal nerve. The cause is not known. The intense pain is usually described as stabbing or shooting pain. At first the attacks last for 1 or 2 minutes and are followed by relief lasting weeks or months, but thereafter these symptom-free intervals become shorter. "Trigger zones" about the nose or mouth bring on an attack when touched. Almost any irritation, such as exposure to cold, washing the face, talking, eating, or drinking can set off an episode. However, sensation over the distribution of the nerve appears to be normal.

Glossopharyngeal neuralgia is a rare syndrome characterized by recurring attacks of severe pain in the back of the throat, tonsils, back of the tongue, and the middle ear. No organic pathology can be found. Pain, beginning in the throat and base of the tongue and radiating to the ears, is spasmodic and excruciating. An attack may last from seconds to minutes and can be precipitated by such innocuous acts as swallowing, chewing, sneezing, coughing, yawning, and talking.

Management

Nerve root section is the surgical treatment in both trigeminal neuralgia and glossopharyngeal neuralgia. In recent years antiepileptic drugs have been employed with some success in trigeminal neuralgia, as has injection of alcohol. Pontocaine spray may provide relief in glossopharyngeal neuralgia. In either case, medical treatment is generally given a trial before surgery is undertaken.

NARCOLEPSY

Narcolepsy is a chronic syndrome involving recurrent episodes of sleep that can take place at any time, or momentary muscle paralysis that usually affects the patient during periods of emotional excitement. Such transient muscular paralysis may precede sleep episodes. The patient is readily awakened. Although the cause is unknown, it has been preceded in some cases by acute epidemic encephalitis, head trauma, or acute systemic infections.

Pathophysiology

No precise pathophysiologic findings have been observed. Narcoleptic sleep differs from normal sleep only in its frequency and untimely onset. Narcoleptics appear unable to resist the impulse to fall asleep; they fall asleep from a few to many times a day. Some will sleep 6 to 8 hours during the day plus 8 to 10 hours at night. Various transient paralyses occur during periods of emotional excitement. The patient may drop the pole when a fish strikes his line, or he may fall when he laughs or becomes angry. No abnormalities appear in the blood or cerebrospinal fluid. The electroencephalogram is normal. The syndrome is of lifelong duration but does not shorten life.

NARCOLEPSY USUALLY A BENIGN THOUGH LIFELONG DISORDER

Management

Various stimulants, ranging from tea or coffee to such drugs as methyl phenidate and dextroamphetamine, are recommended.

INFLAMMATORY DISEASES OF THE BRAIN AND SPINAL CORD

This group of diseases includes encephalitis (inflammation of the brain), myelitis (inflammation of the spinal cord), and encephalomyelitis (inflammation of both the brain and the spinal cord). As several types of each of these subgroups have been identified, a modifying word is usually added to indicate the specific mechanism or causative agent, such as herpes zoster myelitis or postmeasles encephalomyelitis.

Pathophysiology

Encephalitis may be due to several agents, including bacteria, viruses, fungi, and others. Although many of the 150 known viruses carried by arthropods can cause human encephalitis, in most instances the infection is inapparent or produces only generalized symptoms rather than clinical encephalitis. Of the several *arthropod-bor*ne virus (arborvirus) encephalitides, only St. Louis encephalitis and Western equine encephalomyelitis have been identified in the United States. Their onset and symp-

MENINGES ALWAYS INVOLVED

toms are similar. In infants the onset is abrupt, with a high fever, convulsions, and generalized rigidity. In older children and adults the onset is more gradual, with headache, chilliness, muscle pain, and gastrointestinal or respiratory symptoms. Within a day or two, coma, disorientation, and delirium may develop. The temperature, averaging 102° to 103° F., returns to normal by the tenth day. Several viruses other than those carried by arthropods may also produce human encephalitis. An example of a fungal encephalitis is that caused by *Histoplasma capsulatum*. We described this fungus in Chapter 4. Histoplasmosis may give no symptoms, may be benign, or may be progressive and possibly fatal. If the disease process spreads to involve the brain, it is referred to as *histoplasmosis encephalitis*.

Myelitis—spinal cord inflammation—may be due to one of several viruses (as in poliomyelitis), to disease involving the meninges (as in syphilitic myelitis), or to an unknown cause (as in acute multiple sclerosis).

Such common viral illnesses as measles and chickenpox, which usually do not affect nervous tissue, may in some cases be followed by lesions appearing in the meninges and white matter of the brain. This occurrence is referred to as *postinfectious encephalomyelitis*. Similar lesions found following vaccination for smallpox or rabies are called *postvaccinal encephalomyelitis*. In both, the characteristic symptoms of encephalitis are present, but because of the complicating factors the mortality is higher than in uncomplicated encephalitis.

Management

Since the classification of inflammatory diseases of the brain and spinal cord includes numerous entities, it is obvious that specific treatment modalities must be tailored to the individual case. Essential supportive measures that apply to all cases include bed rest, a quiet environment, and attention to diet.

MENINGITIS

MENINGITIS
A DISEASE
OF CROWDED
LIVING
CONDITIONS

Meningitis—inflammation of the meninges, the membranes covering the brain and spinal cord—is caused by a number of microorganisms, most commonly the meningococcus, streptococcus, pneumococcus, and tubercle bacillus. Epidemics of meningococcal meningitis occasionally occur in crowded institutions, army camps, and prisons. One form, influenzal meningitis, affects young children almost exclusively.

Pathophysiology

Meningitis is spread by carriers, who disseminate the organisms in air droplets following sneezing or coughing (recall Chap. 4). The organisms enter the body through the nose and throat in most instances. The illness usually begins as a cold or a sinus inflammation; this is followed by intense headache, stiffness of the neck, high fever, and vomiting. A rash is often present. In fatal cases the patient may become delirious, stuporous, and finally comatose. There is a *fulminant* form, in which the course is so violent and so rapid that the patient dies within 24 hours of the onset of severe symptoms.

Management

The mortality is quite high—above 50 per cent—in untreated cases. Today, however, the sulfonamides and penicillin are generally successful in treatment. General care measures are extremely important, and include careful attention to fluid intake and output, oral hygiene, and frequent turning.

SYPHILIS

Syphilis is included among diseases of the nervous system because its most serious—often tragic—consequences are manifested in the central nervous system. The general characteristics of syphilis were described in Chapter 4. If modern antibiotic treatment is given early, the patient will be cured; but in the absence of such treatment, about 10 to 15 per cent of patients will experience severe central nervous system effects many years later—in fact, nervous system involvement may not be manifest until long after they have forgotten that they ever had the disease. The term *neurosyphilis* is used to describe this form of syphilis; the heart, bones, skin, and viscera may also be attacked.

EARLY
TREATMENT
IS OF
THE
ESSENCE

Pathophysiology

The spirochetes of *Treponema pallidum* always produce their effects locally, rather than at a distance (as through toxins). The spirochetes invade the nervous system and its coverings early in the course of infection whether or not nervous system involvement is manifest later. Yet symptoms of neurologic disease are not necessarily present for some time. The most serious consequences of nervous system involvement are general paresis (dementia paralytica), tabes dorsalis (locomotor ataxia), and optic atrophy. Impaired memory, lack of insight, delusions, and hallucinations may be observed in *general paresis*. Disintegration proceeds rapidly until finally the patient reaches the stage of complete dementia. In *tabes dorsalis* the spirochete destroys the dorsal columns of the spinal cord, so that the victim loses his muscle sense and his joint sense. He walks unsteadily, needing to look at the ground with every step, and cannot keep his balance. He experiences other sensory disturbances as well, including severe leg pains and abdominal pain. The outer portions of the optic nerve are involved in *optic atrophy;* the process continues until finally the central part of the nerve is destroyed and the patient becomes blind.

Management

Penicillin in massive doses often arrests the progress of the disease and relieves the symptoms. Another antibiotic is employed if the patient is sensitive to penicillin.

HERPES ZOSTER

Herpes zoster is an acute infection of the central nervous system involving primarily the dorsal root ganglia. It is also known as *shingles* and *acute posterior ganglionitis.* It is characterized by a vesicular eruption and neuralgic pain in the cutaneous areas supplied by the peripheral sensory nerves arising in the affected root ganglia.

Pathophysiology

Herpes zoster results from infection with a filtrable virus closely related to or the same as that of chickenpox. It may be associated with poisoning due to carbon monoxide, arsenic, or bismuth, and it may appear in the course of tuberculosis, pneumonia, Hodgkin's disease, or uremia. The virus is always the causative organism, and the presence of a local lesion or systemic disease is required to activate it. Chills and fever, malaise, and gastrointestinal disturbances are noted for the first 3 or 4 days. On the fourth or fifth day, characteristic lesions appear in the form of groups of vesicles on the cutaneous distribution of one or more posterior root ganglia, often in the thoracic region. One attack confers immunity. Postherpetic neuralgia may follow and may persist.

Management

No specific treatment is available. In some cases antibiotics and vitamin B_{12} have been beneficial. Local comfort measures and control of secondary infection are carried out.

RABIES

Although the reader will probably never see a victim of rabies, the disease is mentioned in this book in part because it is almost invariably fatal (the first recorded instance of recovery occurred in 1971) and in part because practically every case is preventable. Educational campaigns, vaccination of dogs, registration and control of dogs to the fullest possible extent, and bat control programs are among the measures required to eliminate rabies.

Pathophysiology

Rabies is mainly a disease of dogs, cats, wolves, bats, and certain other mammals but it is occasionally transmitted from a rabid animal to man. The virus is found in the saliva of rabid animals. A bite or scratch gives the virus entrance. The virus moves from the wound site along the nerves to the spinal cord. The symptoms include tremendous excitement, rage, and spasm of the pharyngeal muscles, especially at the sight of water—giving the popular name, hydrophobia (fear of water), to the disease. General paralysis and death follow.

Management

Prevention is of prime importance. If a suspected animal has bitten a person, the animal should, if at all possible, be confined for 14 days to see if signs of rabies develop. If the animal has inadvertently been killed, its brain should be examined microscopically for the presence of Negri bodies, which constitute proof of rabies. Negative findings on a killed animal do not rule out rabies since sufficient time may not have elapsed for Negri bodies to develop. If rabies is proved, rabies vaccination (the Pasteur treatment) is started immediately. If rabies is merely suspected, those concerned are faced with a difficult decision: rabies vaccination can, in a small number of cases, cause a fatal reaction; but rabies is almost invariably fatal (only one well-documented case of recovery has been reported). Usually, if the disease does develop, only general supportive care can be given.

CEREBROVASCULAR DISEASE

This disorder, also known as *apoplexy, stroke,* and *cerebrovascular accident (CVA),* describes any functional abnormality of the central nervous system that is due to pathology of the individual cerebral vessels

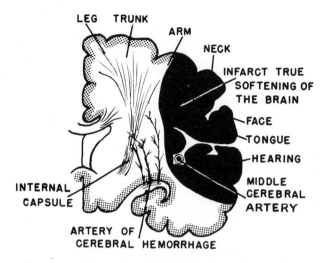

LEG TRUNK
ARM
NECK
INFARCT TRUE
SOFTENING OF
THE BRAIN
FACE
TONGUE
HEARING
MIDDLE
CEREBRAL
ARTERY
INTERNAL
CAPSULE
ARTERY OF
CEREBRAL HEMORRHAGE

A cross section of the left hemisphere of the cerebrum through the motor area. The middle cerebral
artery is represented as plugged by a thrombus.
That part of the brain (black area) supplied with
food by this artery has died. This patient would
have paralysis of the right side of the face, the
tongue, and the neck and part of the arm; he would
be unable to talk or understand what was said to
him.

or the cerebrovascular system. The basic lesion may be cerebral hemorrhage, thrombosis, embolism, or vascular insufficiency.

Pathophysiology

Rupture of an arteriosclerotic vessel usually is the cause of
hemorrhage into the brain; less often aneurysm, injury, acute infection,
a blood disease, brain damage from poisons, or syphilis will be the cause.
In the case of arteriosclerosis or aneurysm, a large, single hemorrhage is
the usual outcome, while diseases of blood and poisoning produce small,
diffuse hemorrhages.

In *cerebral thrombosis*, atherosclerosis is the chief lesion, caused by
occlusion (blockage) of a blood vessel. Fever, syphilis, meningitis, and
encephalitis are other possible factors.

In *cerebral embolism*, a blood clot or bacterial vegetations from a heart
wall or valve are released. The embolus passes into the left carotid artery,
to lodge in the middle cerebral artery. This is the situation in most cases,
although in others a fat embolus, due to fracture of a long bone, may
be the cause.

Cerebrovascular insufficiency may follow a sudden decrease in blood pressure, and the victim may faint or manifest neurologic signs. Intracerebral hemorrhage causes destruction of brain tissue from extravasated blood. Cerebral thrombosis or embolism causes necrosis of brain tissue.

Early symptoms of cerebrovascular disease may include dizziness, vertigo, nausea, and vomiting, to be followed by convulsions and coma. Specific symptoms develop suddenly, reaching maximum intensity in hours or even minutes. Depending on the site of the lesion, these symptoms may include hemiplegia (paralysis on the side opposite the damaged area), hemianesthesia (absence of sensation), or aphasia (speech disturbance). The outcome depends on the size and site of the lesions. Although sudden death is rare, intensive care followed by a long period of rehabilitation is necessary in most cases.

Management

Skillful nursing care is of prime importance. Nutrition and fluid balance must be maintained. Although specific therapy is not available, much can be done in the way of physical therapy and vocational therapy to help the patient achieve the maximum self-sufficiency which his condition permits.

PARKINSONISM

Parkinsonism, also known as *Parkinson's syndrome, paralysis agitans,* and *shaking palsy,* is a chronic disorder of the central nervous system which causes brain degeneration. Characteristically the patient manifests slow, unskillful, unpurposeful movement, weakness, muscular rigidity, and tremor ("pill-rolling").

Pathophysiology

The cause in most cases is unknown, but it is probably a degenerative disease. Many cases were seen following the pandemic of encephalitis that occurred in 1917. Poisoning due to carbon monoxide or manganese can produce a Parkinson-like syndrome, as can head injury or overdosage with tranquilizers. The disease is characterized by a loss of cells from the basal ganglia.

50,000
NEW CASES OF
PARKINSON'S
DISEASE
EVERY YEAR

The patient's countenance is wide-eyed, unblinking, and staring. His facial muscles do not move, his mouth is held slightly open, and he drools. He walks with slow, short, shuffling steps, his arms flexed, adducted, and held stiffly at the sides, and his trunk bent slightly forward. Movement of all voluntary muscles is extremely slow, and tremor is characteristic. Speech may be severely impaired. Despite all these difficulties, the patient's mind remains clear. Although the disease is slowly progressive, the patient may not become incapacitated for many years.

Management

A number of drugs have proved useful in the management of Parkinsonism. In recent years a new drug, L-dopa, has shown great promise. A few years ago a surgical operation involving production of a lesion in certain nuclei of the thalamus was introduced; it provides considerable relief in some cases.

CEREBRAL PALSY

This term refers to any impairment of nervous function due to brain injury before birth, during birth, or in early infancy. Many problems of pregnancy, such as maternal infection and bleeding, seem to have an important bearing on the occurrence of cerebral palsy, as do difficult labor and neonatal hypoxia. The incidence of cerebral palsy is fairly high—six cases per 1,000 live births. This statistic suggests that much remains to be learned about pregnancy and childbirth.

Pathophysiology

There is spastic (hypertonic) weakness of muscle, so that the child's muscles are stiff and his movements awkward. The child has little control of fine movements (those needed for reading and writing, for example). In some cases mental retardation is associated with the palsy. The disorder is categorized according to the extent of involvement, i.e., quadriplegia if all four limbs are affected, hemiplegia if the arm and leg on the same side are affected, spastic diplegia if both legs are affected.

Management

The goal in treatment is to help the child develop his maximal capabilities. Many specialized techniques of physical therapy and educational training are required. In some cases orthopedic surgery may be beneficial.

HUNTINGTON'S CHOREA

Huntington's chorea, also known as *hereditary chorea* and *chronic chorea*, is a hereditary disease that is incurable and fatal. This fortunately rare disease progresses from symptoms of abnormal movements to final total dementia and death.

Pathophysiology

The disorder affects both sexes and is transmitted as an' autosomal dominant. The early symptoms usually are noted in the fourth to sixth decades of life but may develop in youth or old age. The onset is gradual, being marked by such personality changes as obstinacy, moodiness, and lack of initiative. These may precede or accompany the onset of choreiform movements, which appear first in the face, neck, and arms. All these motions are completely purposeless and lacking in direction. The facial muscles contract to produce grotesque grimaces. Speech becomes hesitating and explosive, and gait is so disorganized that walking becomes impossible. Tendon reflexes are increased. Some patients are euphoric, while others are spiteful and destructive. Thought becomes impossible, and the powers of attention, memory, and judgment are impaired. Finally complete dementia sets in.

Management

Persons with a family history of Huntington's chorea should certainly not have children. No treatment has been of real benefit. As the disease reaches an advanced stage, the patient must be confined to a psychiatric facility.

NEOPLASMS OF THE BRAIN

By far the largest number of brain tumors are *primary*, originating within the brain, while a much smaller number are either *secondary* to primary tumors elsewhere in the body or are skull tumors that have ulcerated into the cranial cavity. The most common brain tumors have been classified as follows:

Benign
  Meningioma
  Pituitary adenoma
  Dermoid

TUMORS OF
BRAIN AND
SPINAL CORD
USUALLY
OMINOUS

Craniopharyngioma
Cystic astrocytoma
Hemangioblastoma
Acoustic neuroma, acoustic neurofibroma
Malignant, primary
Glioma
Malignant, secondary
Breast
Lung
Thyroid
Kidney
Skin (melanoma)

Pathophysiology

The general central nervous system symptoms stem from actual invasion and destruction by the tumor, and from the secondary effects of increased intracranial pressure and cerebral edema; these symptoms include headache, nausea, vomiting, choked disk, convulsive seizures, and mental symptoms ranging from drowsiness to bizarre behavior. The specific symptoms vary according to the location of the tumor. For example, a tumor of the motor cortex causes convulsive movements of one side of the body, and a tumor of the occipital lobe causes blindness of half of each eye.

The distinction between benign and malignant tumors does not hold for those involving the brain. A brain tumor may be benign from a histologic standpoint yet, because of the effects of pressure, may be malignant to the patient if it cannot be removed.

Management

Treatment of brain tumors is through surgical therapy, radiotherapy, or both. Total surgical removal is possible in some cases, while in many others only partial removal is possible, and provides temporary relief of the severe symptoms. Some tumors are radiosensitive and radiotherapy may afford considerable relief for a time.

NEOPLASMS OF THE SPINAL CORD

Spinal cord tumors arise from the cord substance and are called *intramedullary* tumors, or from the surrounding tissue, in which case they are *extramedullary*. These extramedullary tumors are classified as *intra-*

dural, that is, arising from the meninges and spinal roots, and *extradural,* arising from the vertebrae or tissues of the extradural space. Like tumors elsewhere in the body, spinal cord tumors may be benign or malignant, and primary or secondary.

Pathophysiology

Histologically, spinal cord tumors resemble brain tumors. The symptoms include sharp pain along the distribution of the spinal roots arising from the cord in the tumor area, along with increasing paralysis below the level of the lesion.

Management

Some spinal cord tumors, most often the benign intradural extra-medullary ones, can be surgically removed. In many other instances, however, surgery cannot be carried out and such temporary relief meas-ures as radiotherapy and chemotherapy will be employed.

GLAUCOMA

In this disorder there is increased intraocular tension with results ranging from slightly impaired vision to complete blindness. Glaucoma may be primary, or secondary to other ocular disturbances. We shall discuss only primary glaucoma.

BOTH PHYSICAL AND EMOTIONAL FACTORS MAY CONTRIBUTE TO INCREASED INTRAOCULAR PRESSURE

Pathophysiology

While the exact cause of primary glaucoma is not known, certain predisposing factors are recognized, including vasomotor and emotional instability, farsightedness, and heredity. The increased intraocular tension stems from a disruption in the formation and reabsorption of aqueous humor in the form of an obstruction that prevents normal control of volume and pressure of intraocular fluid. In acute (narrow-angle) glau-coma, the anterior chamber of the eye is shallow and the aqueous humor cannot reach the canal of Schlemm. In chronic (wide-angle) glaucoma, which is the more common type, the anterior chamber is of normal depth but a physical obstruction preventing access to the canal of Schlemm causes inadequate drainage.

Management

Oral glycerine may abort an acute attack of narrow-angle glaucoma. Miotics are instilled to contract the pupil and draw the iris away from the cornea, and thereby allow the aqueous humor to drain. Surgical procedures may also be employed.

In wide-angle glaucoma, miotics and pilocarpine are effective, but more powerful miotics must be used with great care, as they may precipitate retinal detachment. The patient should try not to become fatigued or emotionally upset, and should not smoke tobacco or ingest large quantities of fluids.

SYMPATHETIC OPHTHALMIA

In this disease there is a severe bilateral inflammation of the uveal tract, which includes the iris, the ciliary body, and the choroid, following trauma to the ciliary body of one eye.

Pathophysiology

AUTOIMMUNITY
OPERANT IN
SYMPATHETIC
OPHTHALMIA

Sympathetic ophthalmia is an autoimmune disease, i.e., based on the response of the antibody-producing mechanism in contact with the antigen, or foreign protein. It follows accidental or surgical trauma to the eye, usually in the form of perforation of the globe with injury to the ciliary body. Uveitis of the injured eye—the *exciting* eye—develops days to weeks before the other eye—the *sympathizing* eye—becomes involved; symptoms of pain on exposure to light, lacrimation, blurring of vision, neuralgic pain, and eyeball tenderness develop in the sympathizing eye from several weeks to perhaps several years after the original injury. Removal of the exciting eye before the onset of uveal irritation in the other eye usually prevents the development of sympathetic ophthalmia; but should the latter occur, there would be active inflammation in the sympathizing eye, finally ending in blindness of both eyes.

Management

Effective treatment of the injured eye is of primary importance. If sight in that eye is destroyed the eye is removed; this must be carried out before the other eye becomes affected or it is of no value. In some cases administration of corticosteroids and atropine is effective.

RETINAL DETACHMENT

A retinal detachment is a partial or complete separation of the retina from the choroid.

Pathophysiology

Retinal detachment occurs most commonly in near-sighted persons. Trauma often precedes the development of retinal detachment, and, as we mentioned earlier, the use of powerful miotics may be a factor. The patient notices flashes of light, then has the sensation that a curtain is moving across the eye. The extent of visual loss depends on the exact location of the detachment. Ophthalmoscopic examination reveals irregularities in the level of the retina, retinal folds and tears, and occluded blood vessels.

Management

Surgical treatment is undertaken as soon as possible, the objective being to create a scar that seals the retina in place as it heals. Since the patient's eyes will be bandaged for a few days following the operation, strong psychological support will be necessary.

DEAFNESS

Deafness, which may be total or partial, is classified as *conductive* or *perceptive*.

Pathophysiology

Among the causes of *conductive deafness* are anomalies of the external auditory canal, eardrum, middle ear, and eustachian tube, any of which interferes with conduction of sound waves to the inner ear. Other causes are mechanical obstruction of the external auditory canal, perforation, scarring, or inflammation of the eardrum; ankylosis of the middle ear bones; middle ear inflammation; otosclerosis of the oval window margin leading to the inner ear; and obstruction of the eustachian tube due to inflammation. In children the most common cause is excessive lymphoid tissue around the eustachian tube orifice behind the pharynx that blocks the eustachian tube and interferes with proper middle ear ventilation.

Perceptive (*nerve*) deafness refers to impairment caused by disorders of the inner ear, eighth nerve, cerebral pathways, or auditory center. Other factors include infectious diseases such as meningitis, syphilis, typhoid, mumps, measles, and hemolytic streptococcal infections; tumors; trauma; injury due to toxic substances; physiological dysfunction resulting from aging or excessive noise; congenital anomalies; leukemia; anemia; and myxedema. Then too, the mother may have been exposed during the first trimester of pregnancy to German measles or ototoxic drugs, or the neonate to anoxia during delivery, to birth trauma, or to Rh incompatibility.

By use of a tuning fork, air conduction deafness can be differentiated from nerve deafness. In the Rinne test, the stem of the vibrating tuning fork is placed against the mastoid process. When the patient indicates he no longer hears the sound, the still-vibrating prongs are held opposite the auditory meatus. The result is described as "Rinne positive" if the sound is heard longer by air, "Rinne negative" if the sound is heard longer by bone, and "Rinne equal" if the sound is heard equally by air and bone. In the normal individual, sound is heard about twice as long by air conduction as by bone conduction.

Management

In treating conductive deafness, efforts are directed at removing the cause, including removal of obstructing lymphoid tissue. In the case of otosclerosis, surgical intervention is often successful. Perceptive deafness is more difficult to treat, and if the underlying cause cannot be corrected, rehabilitation measures, including audiometric studies, evaluation for a hearing aid, and, if necessary, instruction in lip reading, should be carried out.

MENIERE'S DISEASE

Ménière's disease or syndrome is a common condition of the second half of life. Although many theories have been suggested to explain the basic disturbance of the labyrinth, the cause remains unknown. Research continues in efforts to find ways of curing this distressing condition. It is also referred to as *endolymphatic hydrops*.

Pathophysiology

There are degenerative changes in the membranous labyrinth. Swelling of the canals results in paroxysms of vertigo lasting hours or all day and often accompanied by pallor, prostration, vomiting, slight mental confusion, pain behind the ear, and headache. The vertigo of Ménière's disease must be distinguished from faintness, lightheadedness, and other forms of so-called dizziness. It occurs invariably as a result of a disturbance of the equilibratory apparatus. Ringing in the ears and nerve deafness may develop in the late stages.

Management

A low-sodium diet may be advised to control edema. Vitamin therapy and antinauseant preparations may afford relief. The patient should be cautioned to avoid any sudden jarring or turning movement. In severe and intractable cases it may be necessary to destroy the inner ear.

TOPICS FOR DISCUSSION

1. From the standpoint of the evolution of man, which part of the nervous system is the more ancient, the cerebrospinal (voluntary) or the autonomic (involuntary)?

2. What special precautions does Nature take to protect nerve tracts that do not possess a neurilemma sheath and hence cannot regenerate?

3. What serious diseases and injuries could be cured if nerve tracts without neurilemma sheaths could be made to regenerate?

4. In what respects are the endocrine glands under the control of the nervous system?

5. Name some familial nervous disorders.

6. What practices would favor the development of familial nervous system disorders?

7. Which disturbances of water and electrolytes affect nerve excitability?

8. What chemical substances are involved in transmission of nerve impulses?

9. Contrast neuralgia and neuritis.

10. What is the chief general function of the sense organs? How does the sensory deprivation of aging tend to separate the elderly from the mainstream of society?

11. What nervous system disorders chiefly affect children?

12. What nervous system disorders chiefly affect adults?

16

common diseases of the circulatory system, the blood, and the blood-forming organs

The circulatory system includes the heart and blood vessels, which together are generally referred to as the *cardiovascular system*. Because this system is so intimately related to the blood and blood-forming organs, it is logical for our purposes to present all of them together. In discussing, for example, the general characteristics of anemia—a disease of the blood and blood-forming organs—we should certainly wish to note that associated with it are such *circulatory* manifestations as palpitation and shortness of breath. The circulatory system performs the essential task of delivering nutrients to the body cells, at the same time picking up waste materials to be suitably disposed of. In the presence of some malfunction in the blood-forming organs, the system is unable to deliver blood efficiently and the composition of the blood that is delivered is of suboptimal quality.

Some of the statistics on the cardiovascular system tax one's credulity. Every day the heart pumps 3,000 gallons of blood through nearly 60,000 miles of blood vessels at the rate of 4 quarts a minute. The only rest this indefatigable pump enjoys is the half second between contractions and the slightly relaxed rate permitted during sleep.

The ancients paid the great tribute to the heart of viewing it as the seat of the emotions—although it looks more like a pear or a clenched fist than like a valentine. A surprisingly large proportion of medical practice is devoted to diseases of the heart and blood vessels. The latter have been equated with one's life span in the statement, "A man is as old as his arteries." Happily, the cardiovascular system usually responds to appropriate medical treatment. When developing cardiovascular illnesses are detected early, and when one's way of life is changed appropriately, gratifying improvement is the usual reward.

PATHOPHYSIOLOGIC PROCESSES WHICH CAN BE INVOLVED
IN DISEASES OF THE CIRCULATORY SYSTEM,
THE BLOOD, AND THE BLOOD-FORMING ORGANS

	Genetics: Diseases Due to Hereditary Factors	Disease Due to Hypersensitivity and Autoimmunity	Infectious Diseases	Diseases Due to Physical Agents	Diseases Due to Chemical Agents	Neoplasia	Disturbances of Fluid and Electrolyte Balance	Diseases of Malnutrition	Endocrine Dysfunction	Stress Factors in Disease	The Aging Process	Psychosomatic Factors in Disease
Congenital Anomalies	■						■	■				
Coronary Artery Disease	■	■	■		■			■	■	■	■	■
Congestive Heart Failure		■	■		■			■	■	■	■	
Heart Block	■	■			■	■	■		■		■	■
Bacterial Endocarditis			■					■				
Primary Hypertension	■		■			■		■	■	■	■	■
Aneurysm and Aortitis	■		■								■	
Varicose Veins	■									■	■	
Peripheral Vascular Disorders	■		■	■	■						■	■
Sickle Cell Anemia	■											
Iron Deficiency Anemia			■	■				■	■			
Leukemia	■		■	■								

CONGENITAL ANOMALIES
(CONGENITAL HEART DISEASE)

An individual born with a cardiac anomaly or defect is said to have congenital heart disease. Embryonic defects in the budding circulatory system may develop during the period when the heart and great vessels are molded from the primitive blood vessel tube. One or several abnormalities may arise in a single embryo, depending on the embryonic stage at which normal development is altered. The varieties of anomalies are nearly limitless. The presence of an anomaly should be suspected when a young child has enlargement or failure of the heart, a diastolic murmur, a loud systolic murmur or thrill, or cyanosis of heart origin at any age. Careful history, physical examination, chest x-rays, and electrocardiogram facilitate accurate diagnosis. Cardiac catheterization and angiocardiograms are other diagnostic tools.

MODERN
MANAGEMENT
OF
CONGENITAL
ANOMALIES
A SIGNIFICANT
CHAPTER IN
MEDICINE

Pathophysiology of Common Congenital Anomalies

Tetralogy of Fallot   Tetralogy of Fallot refers to the presence of pulmonary stenosis associated with a defect of the interventricular septum, a shift of the aorta to the right side, and hypertrophy of the right ventricle. It causes varying degrees of cyanosis. The more severe the stenosis, the more severe the cyanosis. In moderate stenosis, pulmonary arterial flow can maintain reasonably normal arterial oxygen saturation. After a few months, however, the flow through the pulmonary artery becomes inadequate to meet the needs of the growing infant, and blood is shunted from the right side of the heart to the left, producing cyanosis.

Transposition of the great vessels   In this anomaly, which is often referred to simply as *transposition,* the pulmonary artery arises from the left ventricle and the aorta from the right ventricle. Most of the blood returned to the right atrium by the venae cavae goes directly to the aorta without passing through the lungs. The pulmonary circulation is largely a closed circuit, with blood from the lungs returning mainly to the pulmonary artery. The combination of ventricular defects, atrial defects, and a patent ductus causes shunting of blood. Transposition is the most common cause of cyanosis during infancy.

Ventricular septal defect   This defect, which is variable in size, usually appears in the membranous portion of the interventricular septum. It is the most frequent congenital circulatory anomaly, and its size largely determines the severity of illness. Oxygenated blood from the left ventricle is forced into the right ventricle in systole, with the result that pulmonary blood flow is greater than systemic blood flow. Because of secondary pulmonary changes, pressure in the right ventricle may become so high that the direction of shunt is reversed and unoxygenated blood is mixed with aortic blood.

Atrial septal defect   Atrial septal defects can occur in two places: low in the interatrial septum, or at or just below the foramen ovale. Blood pressure is far lower in the right atrium than in the left; therefore, in either atrial defect, blood flows from the left side to the right, causing overload of the pulmonary circuit. Right ventricular failure may eventually result due to the pulmonary hypertension that develops. Reversed flow through the atrial defect then causes cyanosis.

Patent ductus arteriosus   In this condition an opening persists from fetal life between the aorta and the pulmonary artery, whereas normally the ductus closes shortly after birth. Aortic blood flows throughout systole and diastole into the low-pressure pulmonary artery, flooding the lungs. The work of both ventricles is increased, particularly that of the left. Usually no symptoms occur.

Isolated pulmonic stenosis   This lesion usually involves the valve. Impairment of pulmonary flow varies. The severity of stenosis can be judged by the degree of right ventricular enlargement, pressure increase, and hypertrophy. Pressures in the pulmonary artery remain low.

Aortic stenosis   Congenital aortic stenosis usually involves the valve or the valve muscles. Heart output is limited; the left ventricle is overworked. Patients usually have no symptoms until late in the course of the disease.

Coarctation of the aorta   In this abnormality, there is a localized constriction of the aorta occurring at or below the entrance of the obliterated ductus arteriosus. The mechanics resemble those of aortic stenosis except that the stenosis is more distal. Blood pressure is increased in the upper extremities and in the cranium.

Management of Common Congenital Anomalies

Until recent years only general supportive care could be offered the unfortunate victim of congenital heart disease. A current bright chapter in medicine includes progress in understanding the basic mechanisms involved in these defects, development of specific surgical procedures, and overall management. Today, surgery combined with "total nursing care" means cure of the defect and the prospect of a normal life expectancy for large numbers of affected persons.

CORONARY ARTERY DISEASE

Although the coronary arteries are subject to a great variety of diseases, many of these processes do not affect the heart itself. In this discussion we are interested only in the processes that involve the heart and thereby cause heart disease. The term *coronary artery disease,* or *coronary heart disease,* means that the blood supply of the heart is disturbed due to disease of the coronary arteries. As a result of this interference, the heart is damaged.

Pathophysiology

The most common cause of coronary artery disease is atherosclerosis, which was described in Chapter 12. Hypertension, diabetes mellitus, hypothyroidism, hypercholesterolemic states, obesity, and old age are among the factors that contribute to its development. Ingestion

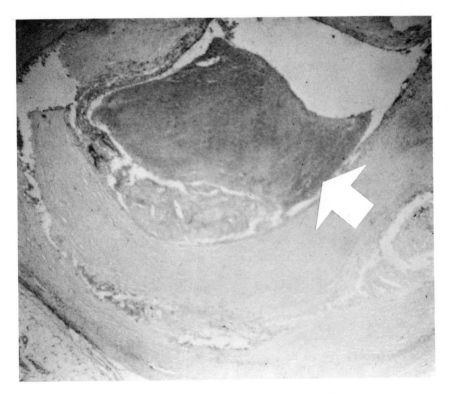

Thrombosis of coronary artery. Central portion of artery is blocked by thrombus (*arrow*) preventing normal circulation of blood to heart muscle.

CORONARY
ARTERY DISEASE
A MULTIFACTORIAL
PROCESS

of a diet high in fats, particularly saturated fats, is thought to be associated, since such a diet raises the cholesterol level and probably promotes atherosclerosis. Syphilitic or rheumatic arteritis, aortitis causing obstruction of coronary artery openings, embolism, polyarteritis, and congenital cardiovascular anomalies are additional factors that may contribute to atherosclerosis. Premenopausal women have fewer complications of atherosclerosis than men of the same age, as the secretion of estrogen acts as a protective mechanism; after menopause, however, women show a slow but steady rise in coronary artery disease.

Symptoms arise only when heart muscle damage becomes severe enough to cause a serious blood deficit. The clinical disease that develops varies according to the size and location of the damage and its consequences; that is, the severity, rate of development, and duration of the deficit. The chief diseases that are seen are angina pectoris and myocardial infarction, and our discussion will be limited to these.

Angina pectoris Angina pectoris is also called the *anginal syndrome* and *cardiac pain of effort*. There is paroxysmal pain in the anterior chest which is so severe that the patient must stop whatever he is doing. In most cases it is brought on by walking outdoors, although it may occur at rest due to emotional factors; less commonly it may be due to overeating or walking in cold, windy weather.

The pain is due to a temporary inability of the coronary arteries to supply enough oxygenated blood to the heart muscle, and is believed to be caused by stimulation of afferent nerve endings in the myocardium by the products of myocardial hypoxia. Relative myocardial ischemia may stem from increased oxygen demand, as occurs during extreme exertion, in hyperthyroidism, and in other conditions that make the heart work harder than normal.

Myocardial infarction In a sense, myocardial infarction represents a further stage of angina pectoris. It results when a sudden occlusion of a coronary artery blocks the blood supply to the heart. There is usually severe pain and a sensation of substernal oppression, which may be followed by shock, cardiac dysfunction, and sudden death. Myocardial infarction means that a part of the heart muscle (myocardium) has died because its oxygen supply is cut off. If this episode of *ischemia* is acute, the patient will probably die suddenly, and then there will be no necrosis or infarction. If, on the other hand, he survives the initial episode, the heart muscle will first become necrotic; this will be followed by some degree of healing as the body musters all its forces to repair the damage. In many instances the *collateral circulation*—consisting of new branches of arteries that form to bring the blood supply to the damaged area, and newly enlarged branches of some arteries—is sufficient to maintain a reasonably adequate supply of blood to the heart for as long as the patient lives.

In many instances of early death following infarction, an acute *arrhyth-*

mia—an abnormal rhythm of the heartbeat—develops and is the immediate cause of death.

Management of Angina Pectoris and Myocardial Infarction

The physician tries to determine just what factors or circumstances induce an attack of *angina* so that he can help the patient find ways of averting them. The health care team provides encouragement and reassurance to help the patient make the necessary adjustments to his condition. Several drugs are available for pain relief, the most widely used being nitroglycerin.

The patient who has suffered a *myocardial infarction* should, if possible, be placed in a cardiac care unit (CCU) for the first few days. Here all the necessary equipment and supplies are at hand for use by a team specially trained to deal with any emergency that may arise, as well as to provide the close and exacting care needed during the critical early period. The most important aspects of treatment are to correct shock, relieve pain, rest the heart, and prevent complications. After the patient's condition has been stabilized, efforts are made to rehabilitate him so that he can return to a productive life.

STATISTICS SHOW CCU A FACTOR IN REDUCING DEATH RATE

CONGESTIVE HEART FAILURE

Most persons with heart disease eventually manifest congestive heart failure. Certain conditions usually precede this state: (1) cardiac output is decreased to the point that vital organs no longer receive their oxygen and nutritional needs, (2) the pulmonary vessels become engorged because the vascular bed is not being emptied efficiently, and (3) blood returning to the heart is not propelled onward into the pulmonary vessels fast enough to prevent venous congestion. Every vital organ suffers as a result.

Pathophysiology

When, because of disease, the heart is no longer able to pump blood effectively to the peripheral organs, all body organs are disturbed. Systolic contraction fails to pump blood efficiently. One or more chambers dilate. The next systolic output is increased because the chambers contract more forcibly. Eventually the blood pressure in these distended chambers builds up during diastole. Blood backs up into the atria and the great veins, producing congestive failure. Systolic contractions weaken and cardiac output decreases. Thus, cardiac failure involves accumulation of an excessive amount of blood in the various organs, called *backward failure*, and diminished blood flow to the tissues, or *forward failure*. Now, with decreased cardiac output, renal blood flow is reduced, so that glomerular filtration diminishes and excretion of water and sodium decreases. This retained fluid causes an increase in tissue and blood volume and thus aggravates the circulatory congestion. Because of the increased renal venous pressure, excretion of sodium and water is reduced even further.

The patient's symptoms may be quite severe. He becomes increasingly dyspneic, even when resting in bed. Because of the congestion now present in the liver and other organs, he is unable to eat properly. He is physically exhausted and may suffer from excessive drowsiness and memory impairment.

Management

Physical and emotional rest are of prime importance. Attention to diet, body alignment, and general hygiene are beneficial. Digitalis derivatives and diuretics are generally administered. Prevention of recurrent episodes is the major goal of everyone involved in the patient's care.

HEART BLOCK

HEART BLOCK
A DANGEROUS
COMPLICATION
OF ACUTE
MYOCARDIAL
INFARCTION

A heart block is a disturbance that prevents stimuli from the atria from reaching the ventricles. The block may be *partial*—some stimuli are disrupted—or *complete*—all stimuli are disrupted.

Pathophysiology

Sinoatrial (SA) block   In this heart block, an occasional normal impulse fails to leave the region of the SA node because of a temporary block. Not being stimulated, the atria and ventricles do not contract. Following the next normal SA impulse that is not blocked, the atria and ventricles do contract. With frequent SA block, dizziness, syncope, or convulsions may occur.

Intra-atrial (IA) block   This form of heart block results from a delay in spread of the impulse through the atrial myocardium after its issue from the SA node. The condition is asymptomatic.

Atrioventricular (AV) block   In this heart block, some or all impulses from the SA node are impeded in the AV node and bundle. In incomplete AV block, there is simple prolongation of the P-R interval. As incomplete

THE VICIOUS CIRCLE
OF CONGESTIVE
HEART FAILURE

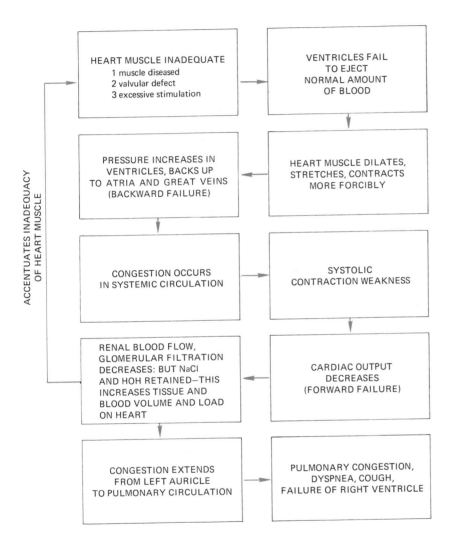

HEART MUSCLE INADEQUATE
1 muscle diseased
2 valvular defect
3 excessive stimulation

VENTRICLES FAIL
TO EJECT
NORMAL AMOUNT
OF BLOOD

PRESSURE INCREASES IN
VENTRICLES, BACKS UP
TO ATRIA AND GREAT VEINS
(BACKWARD FAILURE)

HEART MUSCLE DILATES,
STRETCHES, CONTRACTS
MORE FORCIBLY

CONGESTION OCCURS
IN SYSTEMIC CIRCULATION

SYSTOLIC
CONTRACTION WEAKNESS

RENAL BLOOD FLOW,
GLOMERULAR FILTRATION
DECREASES: BUT NaCl
AND HOH RETAINED—THIS
INCREASES TISSUE AND
BLOOD VOLUME AND LOAD
ON HEART

CARDIAC OUTPUT
DECREASES
(FORWARD FAILURE)

CONGESTION EXTENDS
FROM LEFT AURICLE
TO PULMONARY CIRCULATION

PULMONARY CONGESTION,
DYSPNEA, COUGH,
FAILURE OF RIGHT VENTRICLE

ACCENTUATES INADEQUACY
OF HEART MUSCLE

AV block progresses, the ventricular rate may become irregular. This could be misinterpreted clinically as atrial fibrillation. On the other hand, disturbances in AV conduction may progress to the point where the ventricles receive no atrial impulses. Then an independent ventricular rhythm, so-called *idioventricular rhythm,* is set up in each ventricle. Atria and ventricles beat independently of each other in complete AV block. The ventricular rate may be from 25 to 40 beats per minute slower than that of the atria.

If a patient experiences giddiness, syncope, temporary loss of con-

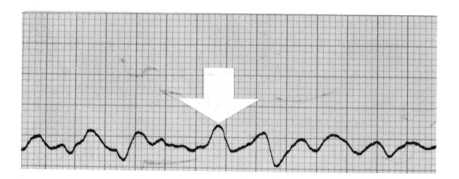

Ventricular fibrillation. High peaks represent ventricular beats (*arrow*). They occur irregularly. The tracing bears scant resemblance to a normal electrocardiogram. Ventricular fibrillation may be fatal even when vigorously treated.

sciousness, or convulsions because of complete AV block, he is suffering from the *Adams-Stokes syndrome* (often called *Stokes-Adams disease*). The symptoms result from decreased cardiac output with consequent diminished cerebral blood flow and cerebral hypoxia.

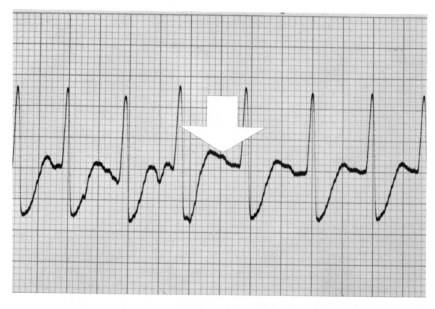

Auricular fibrillation. P waves, indicating auricular activity, occur irregularly. Arrow points to probable P wave. Tall peaks represent ventricular contractions. They occur irregularly because discharges from the auricle are irregular.

Intraventricular (IV) block   One form of IV block, bundle branch block, is characterized by a cardiac impulse that starts in the SA node and follows a normal pathway until it reaches the fork of the common bundle, beyond which point it is inhibited in one of the bundle branches. Right bundle branch block is likely to occur in elderly persons. Left bundle branch block almost always indicates heart disease. Either condition is usually asymptomatic, with diagnosis depending upon electrocardiographic findings.

Management

In many patients with heart block, an electrical pacemaker is implanted to supply the needed contraction stimulus. If Stokes-Adams disease is present external cardiac massage is performed as an emergency measure to sustain the patient until an external pacemaker is applied. Chemotherapy and complete supportive care are important aspects of treatment.

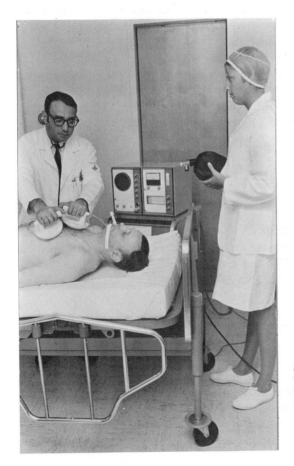

An electrical defibrillator is being applied to the patient's chest in an attempt to terminate ventricular fibrillation. The device works by sending a very short, high-voltage shock through the chest to the heart muscle. (Sharp, L. and Rabin, B.: Nursing in the Coronary Care Unit. Philadelphia, J. B. Lippincott, 1970.)

BACTERIAL ENDOCARDITIS

Bacterial endocarditis is caused by direct bacterial invasion of the endocardium—the layer of tissue that lines the cavities of the heart and covers the valve flaps. Two forms are usually described: *subacute* and *acute*. The subacute form usually results from infection of a heart valve that was damaged by rheumatic fever or is congenitally defective, although normal valves may also be attacked. The majority of cases are caused by *Streptococcus viridans,* which is of low virulence. The acute form is caused by microorganisms of greater virulence, such as *Staphylococcus aureus.*

Pathophysiology

Typically, bacterial pharyngitis, extraction of a tooth, or certain types of surgery have preceded the endocarditis. All of these cause a temporary bacteremia that is usually corrected by the body's normal protective mechanisms. But a heart valve that has been damaged becomes a lodging place where bacteria can thrive, multiply, and erode the valve leaflets. Fibrin is deposited and vegetations form. The bacteria become enmeshed in the fibrin so that the phagocytes and immune antibodies cannot destroy them, and they continue to grow. The diseased valves produce murmurs, which may change in character. As valve incompetence increases, congestive heart failure develops. There is increasing anemia and progressive loss of weight and strength. Malnutrition, cerebral or pulmonary embolism, or cardiac or renal failure may cause death.

Management

The goal of therapy is to destroy the invading microorganisms; an antibiotic specific for the organism—often penicillin—is employed for this purpose. Attention to bed rest, nutrition, and usual supportive nursing measures are essential for the patient's recovery.

PRIMARY HYPERTENSION

Primary hypertension refers to persistent abnormally high levels of blood pressure associated with arteriolar constriction. In about two thirds of all cases, the cause cannot be established on the basis of our present knowledge; such cases are referred to as *essential* or *idiopathic* hypertension, or *hypertensive vascular disease.* This type of hypertension is prevalent, and has been epidemiologically associated with the stresses of modern life and with high intakes of sodium chloride. In the remaining cases, the cause is due to an identifiable condition such as renal disease, pheochromocytoma, or adrenal tumor.

Pathophysiology

In the early stages, there are no demonstrable pathologic changes. As the disease progresses, arteriosclerosis with intimal hyalinization and medial hypertrophy occurs. Arteriolar involvement may be widespread. In many patients the kidneys are affected, and cardiac hypertrophy develops. Unfortunately, primary hypertension appears to accelerate the arteriosclerotic process, thus favoring the development of coronary artery disease, cerebrovascular accident, renal disease, and peripheral vascular changes.

There is an accelerated form of hypertension (*malignant* hypertension) that is characterized by widespread necrotizing arteriolitis with fibrinoid change and proliferative endarteritis, involving the kidneys especially.

Kidney function may be normal at first, but as the disease progresses, effective renal blood flow and maximal tubular excretory capacity diminish. Early hypertension is characterized by lability of blood pressure. In many hypertensive patients, blood pressure drops to normal with rest and removal of emotional tensions, in the presence of fever, or following myocardial infarction or cerebrovascular accident.

The course of primary hypertension is extremely variable. Eventually about 50 per cent of patients succumb to congestive failure, about 20 per cent each to myocardial infarction and cerebral hemorrhage, and about 10 per cent to uremia.

Management

The goal of treatment is to lower the blood pressure to normal levels in the hope of relieving symptoms and halting the progress of vascular disease. Since most of these patients are tense and hard-driving, they are encouraged to change their outlook on life to a more tranquil one. Diuretics and barbiturates are among the drug agents employed to achieve these ends. A low sodium diet is beneficial in many instances.

AORTIC ANEURYSM

An aortic aneurysm is a localized dilatation of the aorta due to weakness of the wall at that point. Several terms are used to describe the various types of aneurysms: a very small one due to a local infection

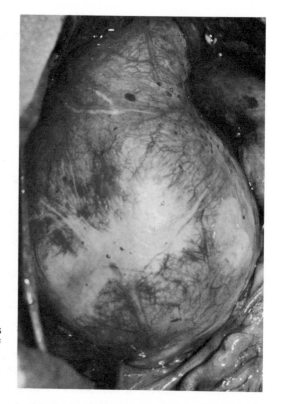

An aortic aneurysm as large as this one produces aortic insufficiency and, by its size, compression of the pulmonary artery as well. (Haimovici, H.: The Surgical Management of Vascular Diseases. Philadelphia, J. B. Lippincott, 1970.)

is a *mycotic* aneurysm; one that is larger but still limited is a *saccular* aneurysm; and one that produces dilatation of the entire artery is a *fusiform* aneurysm.

Pathophysiology

ATHEROSCLEROSIS HAS REPLACED SYPHILIS AS LEADING CAUSE OF ANEURYSM

Weakness of the arterial wall resulting in aneurysm may be caused by local trauma (as occurs in a penetrating wound), a local infection, syphilis, or arteriosclerosis. In other instances the weak spot has been present since birth. Most aortic aneurysms are situated within the thorax on the *aortic arch.* At first the symptoms are hardly noticeable, but after a time congestive heart failure develops, or there is nearly constant pain due to the pressure of the aneurysm. Dyspnea, hoarseness, cough, and dilatation of chest or arm veins are common. If the aneurysm is located in the *abdominal aorta,* there is a palpable pulsating mass that causes constant pain. Rupture of an aneurysm into the pericardium, chest, or abdomen—which becomes increasingly likely with advancing age—usually causes immediate death.

Management

The prognosis is generally poor, and without treatment the patient will die due to rupture of the aneurysm or the effects of compression. With modern surgery, however, it is now often possible to remove the aneurysm and repair the affected segment of the artery with a graft.

PERIPHERAL VASCULAR DISORDERS

The phrase *peripheral vascular disease* refers to disease of the blood vessels that supply the extremities. The veins, the arteries, the lymphatics, or all of these may be involved. In almost all patients with such disorders, the effects are those of ischemia, which, you will recall, is a deficiency of blood in a part due to impaired circulation.

ISCHEMIA THE HALLMARK OF PERIPHERAL VASCULAR DISEASES

Varicose Veins

Varicose veins are abnormally lengthened, dilated, sacculated superficial veins. Although varicosities may occur in the esophagus (esophageal varices) and the rectum (hemorrhoids), the present discussion is limited to the most common form—varicose veins of the legs.

Pathophysiology   When man assumed the upright posture, he placed an excessive burden on the veins of his legs. The venous valves and support provided veins by surrounding tissues help circulation to counteract the forces of gravity. Surrounding muscles support the deep veins, but the superficial veins have chiefly subcutaneous fat to support them. The long and short saphenous veins and their tributaries are most commonly affected by varicosities. Some veins are congenitally weak so that varicosities develop at an early age. Pregnancy, abdominal tumor, obesity, ascites, and prolonged weight bearing, all of which increase lower extremity venous pressure, are other contributing factors. If the valves are anatomically incompetent, they are unable to efficiently move blood toward the heart. Whatever the underlying cause, the venous pump—that is, the contraction of skeletal muscles against the deep veins during walking—is unable to pump blood away from the legs fast enough to reduce the high venous pressure that occurs with assumption of the upright position. In a few cases, varicose veins cause no symptoms. It is, however, more common for symptoms of muscle cramps, increased fatigability, and venous edema to appear. There may be itching and eczematoid dermatitis. Eventually there may be ulceration in the involved areas.

HEREDITY AN IMPORTANT FACTOR IN DEVELOPMENT OF VARICOSE VEINS

Management   Varicose veins are treated by bed rest, leg elevation, avoidance of prolonged standing or sitting in one position, and, whenever possible, elimination of factors that tend to increase abdominal pressure, such as tumor, ascites, obesity, and the wearing of tight girdles. If the problem arises as a result of pregnancy, debilitating disease, a postphlebitic state, or advancing age, the varicose veins should be supported by elastic bandages and stockings, pneumatic stockings, or a special type of paste boot known as Unna's boot. Ligation (tying) of these veins may be helpful. In many cases a stripping procedure in which the varicose veins are removed becomes necessary.

Thromboangiitis Obliterans

Thromboangiitis obliterans, or *Buerger's disease,* is an inflammatory occlusive vascular disease whose etiology remains in doubt. It affects men far more frequently than women, the ratio being 75 to 1, and is most likely to develop between the ages of 20 and 45. Buerger's disease is far more common among Jews than any other ethnic group. Tobacco smoking aggravates the disorder. There are structural changes in the peripheral arteries, veins, and nerves, with associated venous thrombosis, which frequently leads to gangrene.

There is a *chronic* and an *acute* stage of the disease. In the chronic form, there is widespread and serious involvement: both the arterial and venous walls are inflamed and their lumens are blocked by thrombi, with the result that there is ischemia of the distal parts of the leg and foot. Reflex vasospasm of normal arteries further reduces the blood supply. The patient may complain of sensations of coldness, numbness, tingling, and burning in the affected part. The earliest symptom is usually intermittent claudication, which means cramplike calf pains felt after walking a short distance.

As this process of *obliteration* of vessels goes on, the symptoms become so severe that gangrene sets in and amputation of the part often becomes necessary.

Management   The objectives in treatment are to increase the circulation to the legs and protect them from trauma and infection. The patient obviously must stop smoking, since nicotine causes arterial constriction. Certain exercises may be prescribed, and careful attention is given to seeing that the patient follows a program of adequate rest and scrupulous hygiene measures.

Raynaud's Disease or Syndrome

In this vascular disorder there are attacks of *cyanosis* of the fingers and toes. It occurs almost exclusively in young women. The cause may be primary vascular disease, psychic stress, an abnormal cervical rib, cold, sensitivity to certain chemical agents, or pinching of sympathetic nerves due to osteoarthritis. These stimuli can cause such severe spasm that eventually there are marked changes in the skin which may result in the development of painful, slow-healing ulcers. There is marked dilatation of the skin capillaries in involved areas. Gangrene of the fingertips is a late development.

Management The health care team endeavors to educate the patient about the need for a "therapeutic environment": she must learn to avoid cold or protect herself from it, to avoid emotionally upsetting situations, and to handle sharp objects (such as needles and knives) with great care. Drugs to dilate the peripheral vessels may be beneficial.

LEUKEMIA

Leukemia—meaning *white blood*—is a disease characterized by a marked increase in the number of white blood cells in the circulating blood. The universal feature of all leukemias is the presence of immature white cells of any type, and extensive overgrowth of the tissue producing that particular cell. These features—*abnormal cell types* that exhibit *uncontrolled and destructive growth*—would seem to place leukemia among the malignant neoplasms. There is much investigation going on today concerned with the possibility of a *viral* basis for leukemia; several leukemias of mice have been shown to be caused by viruses. Intensive research is underway to find a cure for this fatal disease.

VIRUSES, RADIATION, CHEMICALS MAY ALL BE IMPLICATED

Pathophysiology

Both *acute* and *chronic* forms of leukemia are recognized, and each of these is further classified according to the cell type that predominates; e.g., if the lymphoid cells are increased in number it is identified as *lymphatic leukemia*. The acute leukemias are seen most often in children and young adults. The chronic types in general develop at later ages and have a slower course. The patient experiences symptoms of anemia (e.g., weakness, fatigue, palpitation) and of infiltration and enlargement of the affected organs (e.g., a feeling of dragging or pressure). There is a marked tendency to abnormal bleeding, which worsens as the disease goes on.

Management

The health care personnel direct their efforts toward helping the patient live as nearly normal a life in as much comfort for as long as possible. This means, of course, that close attention must be paid to his nutritional needs, measures to relieve pain, immediate treatment of infection, and the need for psychological and emotional support. Several drugs produce a temporary remission of the disease.

SICKLE CELL ANEMIA

Sickle cell anemia is the result of a *hemoglobinopathy*—a condition in which the normal hemoglobin has been replaced, due to a genetic defect, by another type of noxious hemoglobin. It occurs exclusively in Negroes or in persons of other races who have some Negro ancestry. The disease takes its name from the sickled, or crescent, shape assumed by the red blood cells when they are exposed to low oxygen tension.

Pathophysiology

About one Negro in 600 in the United States has sickle cell anemia; some 8 to 13 per cent do not manifest anemia but have the sickling trait, known as *sicklemia,* which can readily be demonstrated by blood studies.

The usual symptoms of a severe anemia are present. The patient is moderately jaundiced, and may experience arthralgia with fever. There may be episodes of severe abdominal pain with vomiting. Hemiplegia, cranial nerve paralysis, and other neurologic disturbances may result due to cerebral thromboses. Because of the anemia, the patient is underdeveloped, with a short trunk and long extremities. The skull may be tower-shaped. The long bones show cortical thickening, irregular density, and evidence of new bone formation within the medullary canal. The heart usually is enlarged on both sides, and a murmur simulating that of rheumatic or congenital heart disease may be present. Cholelithiasis may develop.

Few patients live beyond the age of 40. They are extremely susceptible to infection, pulmonary embolism, and thrombosis, and one of these usually is the cause of death.

Management

Treatment is symptomatic, since no curative measures have been found. Cortisone may be of value in arresting painful crises. Persons with sicklemia should be cautioned against flying in unpressurized airplanes, since such reduced oxygen tension increases the sickling tendency.

IRON DEFICIENCY ANEMIA

A deficiency of iron is quite common, since less than 10 per cent of *all* iron ingested, by whatever means, is absorbed. Thus a well-balanced diet supplies only the requirements of a normal adult male in good health. One can readily see that any condition (not necessarily a disease) that imposes high iron requirements may, if not treated, result in iron deficiency anemia. A list of such conditions would include menstruation, pregnancy, inadequate diet, faulty absorption of iron, and blood loss due to illness.

IRON DEFICIENCY GREATEST CAUSE OF ANEMIA THROUGHOUT THE WORLD

Pathophysiology

Iron deficiency anemia is characterized by small red cells that are relatively lacking in pigment (hypochromia). The cause is depletion of the body's iron stores. Such digestive disorders as chronic diarrhea and hookworm infection result in decreased iron absorption. During pregnancy, iron requirements are increased because of the needs of the fetus, and immediately following childbirth, maternal iron losses are high. Infants frequently develop iron deficiency anemia during this period of rapid growth while receiving a diet consisting chiefly of milk; indeed, severe iron deficiency may develop in older babies who have been kept too long on a milk diet. In the case of adults, especially men, unless the diet is grossly abnormal, deficient iron intake is not an adequate explanation, and x-ray examinations of the gastrointestinal tract and repeated stool examinations for blood are made in order to discover the source of loss. Normal menstrual bleeding adds considerably to iron losses, and in the case of a woman whose menstrual flow is prolonged or heavy, the iron loss will be much greater.

The symptoms of iron deficiency anemia come on gradually. Weakness, fatigability, irritability, heartburn, flatulence, vague abdominal pains, and anorexia are common. The skin and mucous membranes are pale. The sclerae appear blue or pearly white. The nails become brittle. There may be papillary atrophy of the tongue, and in some patients fissures arise at the corners of the mouth. A systolic heart murmur may be heard, pointing to slight cardiac enlargement.

Management

Iron is a specific in this anemia, and is often prescribed as ferrous sulfate. This treatment is continued for at least 1 month after the hemoglobin level is stabilized in order to replace the body iron stores. A high-protein diet is recommended, as well as vitamin supplementation, particularly vitamin C. Any disorder that is contributing to the anemia should, of course, be vigorously treated.

TOPICS FOR DISCUSSION

1. At what point in the long evolution of man do you suppose that the cardiovascular system incorporated part of the extracellular fluid as plasma? (See Smith, H. W.: From Fish to Philosopher. Doubleday and Company, Inc., 1961.)

2. What effects do the following body fluid imbalances exert on heart action?
   a. sodium deficit
   b. sodium excess (distinguish between short term and long term)
   c. potassium deficit
   d. potassium excess
   e. magnesium deficit
   f. magnesium excess
   g. calcium deficit
   h. calcium excess

3. Which of the above body fluid disturbances produce characteristic electrocardiographic tracings?

4. What disorders are classified as nutritional anemias? Deficit of what specific nutrient is responsible for each nutritional anemia?

5. Which do you regard as having the brighter outlook as a replacement for a hopelessly diseased heart: a heart transplant or an artificial heart?

6. Can a heart without extrinsic nerve connections continue to beat effectively? What evidence do you have for your answer?

7. Whether a diet high in saturated fats promotes heart disease, particularly disease of the coronary arteries, has long been a subject of controversy. What is your opinion?

8. In the patient receiving adequate iron, the hemoglobin level is a good indication of the state of protein nutrition. This is not the case when the patient is iron deficient. Why?

9. In what forms of cardiovascular disease is the low-sodium diet valuable?

10. In what patients might a strict low-sodium diet (250 mg.—about 11 mEq.—or less of sodium per day) be preferable to the use of the new potent diuretics?

11. What body conservation measures go into effect after a person has been on a low-sodium diet for a few days? Is such a patient in danger of developing sodium deficit of the extracellular fluid (also called the low-sodium syndrome)?

17

common diseases of the respiratory system

The respiratory system, consisting of the lungs, the musculature required for breathing, and the air passages communicating with the outside world, quite literally provides us with the breath of life. It is within the millions of tiny air sacs, the lung alveoli, that carbon dioxide passes from blood to air, and oxygen from air to blood, through the physical process of simple diffusion. Not only is a healthy respiratory system essential for normal body metabolism, it is a necessity for a comfortable and happy life, for no one can find much satisfaction in living if every breath is a painful effort, as it is in advanced emphysema or silicosis. The dreadful and painful end result of pulmonary disorders lends emphasis to the importance of early treatment. For example, patients with early emphysema due to years of cigarette smoking have improved dramatically, approaching normality after they stopped smoking. But should emphysema progress to the sad state revealed by the development of a barrel chest, treatment can be symptomatic only.

BRONCHITIS

Bronchitis is a localized or diffuse inflammation of the bronchial tree, acute or chronic, which is caused by infection or by physical or chemical agents.

Pathophysiology

The earliest alteration in acute bronchitis is hyperemia of the mucous membrane. Desquamation, edema, leukocytic infiltration of the submucosa, and formation of sticky or mucopurulent exudate follow. The bronchial ciliated epithelium, which normally serves a self-cleansing function, is disturbed, as is the production of phagocytic cells and lymphocytes. Bacteria invade the normally sterile bronchi. Cellular debris

ALL FORMS
OF BRONCHITIS
INCREASING
IN UNITED STATES
AND GREAT BRITAIN—
POLLUTION
A PROBABLE
FACTOR

303

PATHOPHYSIOLOGIC PROCESSES WHICH CAN BE INVOLVED IN DISEASES OF THE RESPIRATORY SYSTEM

	Genetics: Diseases Due to Hereditary Factors	Disease Due to Hypersensitivity and Autoimmunity	Infectious Diseases	Diseases Due to Physical Agents	Diseases Due to Chemical Agents	Neoplasia	Disturbances of Fluid and Electrolyte Balance	Diseases of Malnutrition	Endocrine Dysfunction	Stress Factors in Disease	The Aging Process	Psychosomatic Factors in Disease
Bronchitis		■	■	■	■							
Chronic Bronchitis	■	■	■	■	■							
Common Cold	■	■						■				
Acute Laryngotracheo-bronchitis		■	■									
Pulmonary Emphysema		■	■									
Pulmonary Embolism and Pulmonary Infarction			■	■		■		■				
The Pneumoconioses												
Pneumothorax	■			■		■						
Neoplasms						■						
Pneumonia			■	■	■			■			■	
Pulmonary Tuberculosis	■	■		■	■							

and mucopurulent exudate accumulate. Cough serves the useful purpose of eliminating bronchial secretions. The inflammation is usually self-limited and normal function returns completely.

Management

Treatment is symptomatic unless a specific organism can be identified, in which case chemotherapy is employed. Postural drainage and inhalation therapy may be helpful.

CHRONIC BRONCHITIS

Chronic inflammation of the tracheobronchial tree with production of recurrent cough and sputum is designated as chronic bronchitis. It is a progressive disorder that can become seriously disabling.

Pathophysiology

In this chronic inflammation, the bronchi are thickened and inelastic. Characteristic are hypertrophy and hypersecretion of the goblet cells. Because of the chronic infection of the mucous membranes, accompanied by exudate, there may be poor bronchial drainage and obstruction of the air passages, which is aggravated by bronchospasm. Bronchial drainage depends heavily on cough production. Shortness of breath, wheezing, and cyanosis result from narrowing or obstruction of the terminal bronchioles. Pulmonary function is poor, with upper costal breathing. Vital capacity is decreased. In some patients, emphysema with alveolar dilatation and destruction of respiratory elements complicates chronic bronchitis, but in some fatal cases structural emphysema is not apparent.

Management

An intensive program of symptomatic and specific therapy is necessary. Prompt treatment of acute infection is most important. Postural drainage and inhalation therapy are employed, and tobacco smoking usually is prohibited.

ACUTE LARYNGOTRACHEOBRONCHITIS

This is an acute, often severe, respiratory infection with inflammation of the trachea and bronchi, obstruction of the larynx, severe shortness of breath, and high fever. It usually, but not always, occurs in infants and children.

Pathophysiology

In many patients, the common cold virus paves the way for secondary bacterial invasion. There is acute inflammation of the mucous membranes of the larynx, trachea, and bronchi. The combination of severe edema with constant secretion of mucus seriously obstructs the larynx, bronchi, or both. When the smaller bronchi become obstructed, the lobes may collapse. Fever is high and breathing rapid. There may be

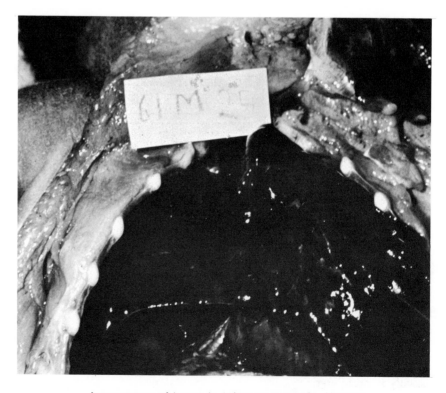

Appearance of lungs in lobar pneumonia. Normal pink, spongelike lung tissue is replaced by dark, livery consolidation.

continual unproductive cough. Considerable fluid is lost because of the hyperactive respiration, producing sodium excess of the extracellular fluid. The patient may be overwhelmed by his energetic but futile efforts to ventilate. Without treatment, pallor, cyanosis, feeble respiration, and death may follow within a few hours.

Management

An atmosphere of high humidity is essential. Symptomatic therapy includes bed rest and soothing hot drinks. Specific antibiotic therapy may be necessary if a secondary bacterial infection develops. Oxygen may be administered and tracheotomy may be necessary if respiratory obstruction is imminent.

PNEUMONIA

Pneumonia is an inflammatory consolidation of lung that may be due to certain pathogenic bacteria, to numerous viral agents, or to other causes. The major *bacterial* pneumonias are those caused by pneumococci, staphylococci, and klebsiellae. The *viral* pneumonias are caused by such agents as influenza virus, chickenpox virus, and measles virus. Other causes of pneumonia are aspiration of oil as from long-continued use of oily nose drops (*lipoid* pneumonia) and inhalation of food, gastric contents, or foreign bodies (*aspiration* or *inhalation* pneumonia); it may also be associated with another disease process, such as congestive heart failure. If a substantial part of one or more lobes is involved, the disease is called *lobar* pneumonia; if the process has a patchy distribution, it is called *bronchopneumonia*.

PNEUMONIA STILL A LEADING CAUSE OF ADULT DEATHS

Pathophysiology

The organisms are carried via the nose and throat to the lung alveoli, where they set up an acute inflammation. There is partial consolidation, or solidification, of the lung due to the filling of the alveoli with a sticky fibrinous exudate in response to the infection or irritant. The onset in bacterial pneumonias is abrupt, and is characterized by severe chills, fever, and sharp chest pain. There may be pronounced mental symptoms such as extreme restlessness or even delirium. By contrast, the onset in viral types is gradual, and the chief symptom is a hacking, nonproductive cough. Potential complications of pneumonia include septicemia, atelectasis, and shock.

Management

The physician, aided by the laboratory technicians, is careful to identify the type of pneumonia, because in some respects, especially the use of drugs, the treatment for one type may be markedly different from that for another. But regardless of the specific chemotherapy or other treatment modalities that may apply to the individual case, there are several elements in management that are important in all pneumonias. These include bed rest, oxygen if needed, communicable disease precautions, and careful attention to mouth care, nutrition, and fluid balance. With prompt treatment the infection usually is brought under control quickly, and the patient recovers completely. Since the complications of pneumonia—especially shock—may be quite serious, every effort must be made to prevent their occurrence.

PULMONARY TUBERCULOSIS

ENVIRONMENT
AND HEREDITY
IMPORTANT
FACTORS IN
ITS DEVELOPMENT

There are many strains of the tubercle bacillus, but it is believed that only the bovine and the human varieties are pathogenic for man. Infants and young children have poor resistance to the infection; at puberty there is a marked increase in the incidence of tuberculosis. Both the case rate and the mortality rate are higher in men than in women. Inborn resistance is important, i.e., some races are more susceptible than others. Socioeconomic conditions also play a part—the bacillus thrives in the crowded conditions of slums. Certain diseases also favor the development of tuberculosis, among them diabetes mellitus and the "dust" diseases.

Countries enjoying a high standard of living have a much lower incidence of pulmonary tuberculosis than underdeveloped or developing countries. Yet even today, according to Hopps, it is estimated that about 50 million of the world's inhabitants are affected, and about 5 million die from pulmonary tuberculosis every year.

Pathophysiology

The infection is in most cases acquired by inhalation. The tubercle bacilli are swept along by the lymph and the bloodstream, lodging in small clumps in the tissues. With accumulation of neighboring cells around these clumps, a protective wall forms that checks further spread and may destroy them. If this natural process is successful, the bacilli die and the tubercle becomes transformed into a small mass of fibrous tissue. But if *caseation* occurs, i.e., if the tissue becomes necrotic and changes to a cheesy mass, the bacilli are liberated and swept by the

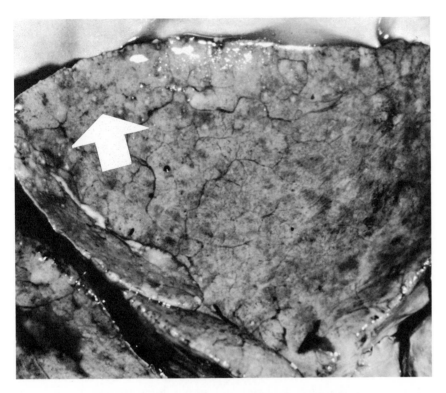

Lung in miliary tuberculosis. Tiny foci of tuberculous infection (*arrow*) are scattered throughout the lung. Many can be seen only with the aid of a magnifying glass. The descriptive name is derived from the Latin *milium* (millet seed).

lymph into the surrounding tissues, which again respond by enclosing the freed bacilli in new tubercles. Should the freed bacilli invade the bloodstream, the condition of *miliary tuberculosis* is said to exist. This is the most serious form of tuberculosis; it carries a high mortality.

Management

The patient with active tuberculosis is usually hospitalized, although complete bed rest is no longer considered necessary. Isolation techniques may be required if the tuberculosis is communicable due to production of infected sputum. A number of drugs, especially isoniazid (INH), para-aminosalicylic acid (PAS), and streptomycin, are administered to destroy the organisms. Steam inhalation to relieve cough and cool sponge baths to reduce fever are comfort measures. Surgery may be carried out in some cases to remove cavities and lesions harboring viable bacilli.

COMMON COLD

The common cold is an acute catarrhal infection of the respiratory tract. It is also referred to as an *upper respiratory infection* or *acute coryza.*

Pathophysiology

The membranes of the nose, pharynx, accessory nasal sinuses, and larynx become inflamed. These changes cause a scratchy sensation in the throat, followed by sneezing, runny nose, and general ill feeling. The senses of smell and taste are often impaired. Later the nasopharyngeal mucosa becomes engorged and the nose obstructed. A profuse serous discharge appears. If the larynx and trachea become involved, there is a hacking cough. Quite frequently the initial infection caused by a virus is followed by bacterial infection, with sinusitis, otitis, and bronchitis.

Management

Treatment is largely symptomatic unless a specific infectious agent can be identified. Bed rest and ample fluids are recommended. If a bacterial infection is superimposed (as so frequently happens), antibiotic therapy may well be indicated.

PULMONARY EMPHYSEMA

INCIDENCE RISING
SHARPLY IN
URBAN
AREAS

Pulmonary emphysema is the most common chronic lung disorder, as well as the most disabling. At present it ranks second only to heart disease as a cause of disability, and it is among the leading causes of death due to lung diseases. It is characterized by enlargement and distention of the alveoli, leading finally to their breakdown and destruction.

Pathophysiology

The patient has a chronic obstruction, or increase in airway resistance, to inflow and outflow of air. The alveoli become chronically distended. The bronchi may be chronically infected, with peribronchial fibrosis. The tracheobronchial airways are widened in inspiration as compared with expiration. The persistent hyperinflation leads to stretching and narrowing of the alveolar capillaries, which contributes to loss of elastic tissue and destruction of alveolar walls. The lungs slowly increase in size, giving the name "barrel chest" to the patient's appearance. Vital capacity is diminished. The volume of each breath decreases but much air remains in the lungs in the extreme expiratory position. Arterial oxygen saturation decreases and arterial carbon dioxide tension increases. Finally normal ventilation becomes impossible.

Management

Pulmonary emphysema is a serious disorder requiring careful medical and nursing attention. The patient must give up cigarette smoking, since cigarette smoke disrupts the ciliary cleansing mechanism of the respiratory tract. Proper environmental temperature and humidity are essential. A program of prescribed activity and exercise is undertaken. Particular attention is given to infection, bronchospasm, and increased bronchial secretion. Heart failure may be a complication, and every possible step is taken to prevent its occurrence. Various drugs, including adrenocortical steroids, may be administered.

PULMONARY EMBOLISM AND PULMONARY INFARCTION

A pulmonary embolism is an embolus, or clot, lodged in a pulmonary artery. It commonly produces pulmonary infarction, a hemorrhagic consolidation which causes necrosis due to occlusion of the blood supply.

Pathophysiology

With occlusion of a pulmonary artery, resulting in obstruction of blood flow through a portion of the pulmonary circuit, nervous reflexes come into play causing narrowing of the pulmonary arteries. As a result of this decreased pulmonary arterial capacity, the right side of the heart becomes overloaded and dilated. Poor filling of the left ventricle results in decreased cardiac output. Right-sided congestion, peripheral circulatory collapse, and even congestive heart failure may result. A large embolus can cause death within a few minutes or hours—so rapidly that infarction does not occur. A smaller embolus causes infarction. Eventually it heals, with recanalization of the occluded vessel through the collateral circulation (the communication between two sets of arteries) and restoration of pulmonary tissues.

Management

The most important part of treatment is to combat shock, hypoxia, and heart failure. Efforts are also made to prevent further immediate embolization. Oxygen, digitalis, and anticoagulants are usually administered. Some cases can be successfully treated through surgical means.

THE PNEUMOCONIOSES

THE DUST
DISEASES
CONSTITUTE
A LEADING
INDUSTRIAL
HAZARD

The group of disorders known as the pneumoconioses—often called the *dust diseases*—all have the same basis, i.e., long-standing lung irritation due to inhalation of certain dusts containing mineral substances such as asbestos and coal. Particles reaching the lung alveoli are engulfed by phagocytes and carried into the lung lymphatics. The dust-loaded phagocytes then are deposited in foci of lymphoid tissue scattered throughout the framework of the lungs and in the regional lymph nodes, causing fibrosis and destruction of lung structure.

Pathophysiology of Common Pneumoconioses

Siderosis   Siderosis is a benign, or harmless, pneumoconiosis that results from inhalation of fumes or dust containing iron particles. It develops only after 5 to 30 years of heavy exposure in occupations involving the burning, cutting, welding, or grinding of heavy steel. There are no symptoms, nor is lung function impaired. Pulmonary fibrosis is absent. There are no abnormal physical findings, and the condition does not predispose to tuberculosis. Collections of iron particles in the perivascular lymphatics appear as small, discrete, rounded shadows throughout the lung fields. No treatment is necessary.

Anthracosis   Anthracosis, which is usually not clinically significant, results from inhalation of soot or carbon smoke having no free silica content. Black carbonaceous particles, which cannot be seen on x-ray film, are deposited in the pulmonary lymphatics. The condition is not associated with disease and is commonly seen at autopsy in the lungs of city dwellers. No treatment is necessary.

Coal miners' pneumoconiosis   This term refers to retention of coal dust in focal areas of the lungs in such concentration that it can be seen on x-ray study either as fine, discrete nodules or as dense conglomerate shadows. Unsettled is the question whether the silica content of the coal dust is significant. With prolonged coal dust retention there may be shortness of breath and cough due to the progressive massive fibrosis.

The consensus is that this finding may be associated with infection by the tubercle bacillus.

Silicosis   Silicosis is the most widespread and the most serious occupational disease. It is caused by long-continued inhalation of crystalline-free silica dust. The free silica particles act as an irritant, and this stimulates fibrosis and nodule formation. At first the nodules of fibrous tissue are discrete, but later they form large fibrous areas, interfering with normal respiratory function. The condition is progressive, and eventually heart failure develops because the right ventricle must work harder to pump blood to the fibrosed lungs. Tuberculosis or bronchopneumonia is the usual cause of death.

Asbestosis   As the name suggests, asbestosis is caused by inhalation of asbestos, or magnesium silicate. The asbestos fibers are inhaled and trapped in respiratory bronchioles, where they react with body substances and become covered by a dense coating containing iron. These asbestos bodies, as they are called, cause diffuse lung fibrosis and impaired respiratory function.

Byssinosis   This pneumoconiosis is caused by inhalation of an unidentified sensitizing protein found in cotton fibers. At first there is wheezing and shortness of breath, and chronic bronchitis or emphysema may develop if exposure is prolonged. There is no characteristic x-ray finding.

Bagassosis   Bagasse is the fibrous material in sugar cane that remains after the sugar has been extracted. It is used in various manufacturing processes. Inhalation of the bagasse dust leads to bagassosis. Shortness of breath is the most common symptom, but cough, bloody sputum, fever, weakness, and weight loss are often present. Complete recovery is the rule, although chronic bronchitis and emphysema may develop in some cases.

Berylliosis   Compounds of beryllium, a metal used widely in industry, may cause berylliosis. There may be an acute lung inflammation, or formation of granulomatous nodules in the lungs. The alveolar walls are thickened. Cough, shortness of breath, and weight loss may occur, leading to progressive loss of respiratory function.

Management of the Pneumoconioses

Since success in treatment of these disorders is presently limited, prevention is the most important measure. Various dust suppression devices have been installed in "dusty" industries, and their use is increasing. Efficient ventilation is also necessary. Once clinical disease is present it is treated symptomatically for the most part, through such measures as chemotherapy and prescribed exercises.

PNEUMOTHORAX

Pneumothorax is air in the pleural cavity, the area between the parietal pleura, which lines the chest cavity, and the visceral pleura, which covers the lung. The accumulated air compresses the lung, causing collapse. Pneumothorax may result from injury or illness, or it may be induced deliberately to collapse the cavity and set the lung at rest.

Pathophysiology

A penetrating injury to the chest wall, as by gunshot, stab wounds, auto accidents, falls, crushing injuries, or blasts, allows air to enter the pleural cavity. Several lung disorders, including tuberculosis,

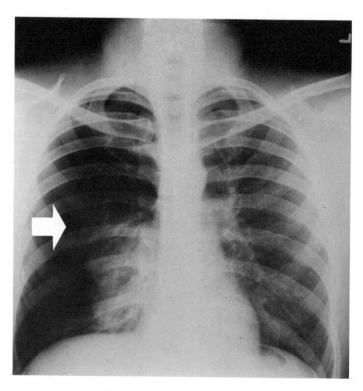

Right spontaneous pneumothorax. Lobes of right lung have collapsed due to entrance of air into right pleural cavity, probably through rupture of a congenital blister on lung surface. Arrow points to border. Lung normally fills the chest cavity. Contrast right side of chest with normal left side, in which lung fills the cavity.

lung abscess, emphysema, bronchiectasis, silicosis, and tumor, may result in pneumothorax.

Sometimes, for unknown reasons, pneumothorax occurs spontaneously in apparently healthy persons between the ages of 20 and 40. The probable cause of many such instances is the rupture of a congenital bleb on the visceral pleura. Other causes may include protracted violent coughing and diaphragmatic hernia. Usually at onset there is a sudden sharp pain in the chest, difficulty in breathing, and a dry, hacking cough. Limitation of motion and hyperinflation on the affected side are revealed by physical examination. Unilateral pneumothorax is tolerated fairly well, but bilateral pneumothorax, such as can occur following tracheotomy, may be fatal.

Management

Obviously, treatment of the underlying cause is of primary importance. In many cases bed rest is sufficient. The air is absorbed over a period of 10 to 20 days. If, however, the pneumothorax is sudden and massive, the trachea and mediastinum will shift to the opposite side due to air pressure, causing respiratory distress. Intubation is necessary to remove the air and allow the lung to reexpand.

NEOPLASMS

Lung neoplasms may be *primary,* arising within the lung or mediastinum, or *secondary,* metastasizing from a primary tumor site elsewhere. A primary tumor may be benign (known as bronchial adenoma) or malignant (known as bronchogenic carcinoma). Over the years the bronchogenic carcinoma, or simply lung cancer as it is often called, has become increasingly common, and at present it is a leading cause of death in adult males. Air pollution, cigarette smoking, and exposure to certain radioactive substances are believed to be important causative factors in its development.

LUNG NEOPLASIA CLEARLY ASSOCIATED WITH INCREASED POLLUTION AND CIGARETTE SMOKING

Pathophysiology

A *benign adenoma* is likely to bleed, causing bloody expectoration. If it obstructs a bronchus it may cause emphysema or atelectasis, and with continued growth, it may cause pain and cough. In *lung cancer,* cough is usually the first symptom, due to pathologic changes in the bronchi or the lung parenchyma. Next comes shortness of breath, because of a decrease in the pulmonary aerating surface. About 50 percent of patients experience chest pain, because of the involvement of sensory nerves in the disease process. This pain may be deep-seated or referred to the shoulder or the back. About half the patients have bloody sputum. Should a large bronchus be occluded, there may be shrinking of the chest, poor expansion, and diminished breath sounds. Localized wheezing, indicative of partial obstruction, may develop. Secondary infection often occurs. X-ray is helpful but not entirely reliable in diagnosis.

Management

In malignant lung tumors, surgical removal of the involved lobe offers the only hope of cure. Radiation may be used before or after surgery or when surgical removal of the tumor is not possible. Unfortunately, however, in the majority of cases the cancer has already spread to other sites, so that only one patient in 15 actually is cured. Surgery and radiation are also utilized in benign lung tumors, and here the results are, naturally, far more satisfactory. Whatever the type of tumor, the care of the patient is similar, with attention being given to positioning of the patient, suctioning and drainage, fluids, nutrition, and prescribed exercise and activity.

TOPICS FOR DISCUSSION

1. Trace the evolutionary predecessors of the human lung.
2. What organs and structures are included in the respiratory system?
3. What forms of pollution represent respiratory hazards?
4. Do you believe that smoking cigarettes can cause cancer? Give reasons for your belief.
5. Why does the right lung have three lobes, the left lung only two?
6. Why does stimulation of the sympathetic division of the autonomic nervous system, reacting to a threat to survival, cause dilatation of the bronchioles?
7. What are the means available for the early diagnosis of lung tumors?
8. How could a hiatus hernia produce a pneumothorax?
9. Do you anticipate an early remedy for the common cold?
10. What lung location makes for early diagnosis of lung carcinoma?
11. What lung tumor may secrete hormones usually released only by endocrine glands elsewhere in the body?

18

common diseases of the digestive system

The digestive system includes a most important tube (the alimentary canal) extending all the way from mouth to anus, and auxiliary organs and glands. Its role can scarcely be overestimated, for it converts the raw materials that enter the mouth into fairly simple chemicals suitable for use by the metabolic processes of the body. The digestive system is responsible not only for the digestion of food, but for its subsequent absorption and utilization as well.

From the evolutionary standpoint, the digestive tract is particularly fascinating, because it is homologous with (corresponds to) the invagination or inpouching of the external body surface of primitive creatures. Thus, its surface is an extension of the external body surface. Indeed, the formula used for determining intestinal surface area applies equally to estimating the external body surface area.

In view of the critical functions of this system, it should not surprise us to learn that it is subject to an enormous number of diseases. Many of them respond readily to medical treatment, whereas others can be as intractable as any ailment in the compendium of diseases.

PEPTIC ULCER

Peptic ulcer is a limited erosion of the mucous membrane of the lower end of the esophagus, stomach, or duodenum. The word *peptic* is used because peptic juice (pepsin, a protein-digesting enzyme) along with hydrochloric acid is secreted by the stomach in order to bring about the digestion of meat and other proteins reaching the stomach.

Pathophysiology

Hypersecretion of acid gastric juice (hydrochloric acid) and pepsin is responsible for ulcer production. Peptic ulcer occurs only in the presence of this free gastric acid. Psychic stress is thought to con-

PATHOPHYSIOLOGIC PROCESSES WHICH CAN BE INVOLVED IN DISEASES OF THE DIGESTIVE SYSTEM

	Genetics; Diseases Due to Hereditary Factors	Disease Due to Hypersensitivity and Autoimmunity	Infectious Diseases	Diseases Due to Physical Agents	Diseases Due to Chemical Agents	Neoplasia	Disturbances of Fluid and Electrolyte Balance	Diseases of Malnutrition	Endocrine Dysfunction	Stress Factors in Disease	The Aging Process	Psychosomatic Factors in Disease
Peptic Ulcer									■	■		■
Pancreatitis			■		■				■			
Gastroenteritis and Food Poisoning			■				■	■				
Regional Enteritis			■			■						■
Appendicitis			■	■								
Peritonitis			■	■	■	■						
Diverticulosis and Diverticulitis	■						■				■	
Malabsorption Syndrome	■		■	■				■				
Parasitic Infections			■									
Neoplasms	■					■	■					
Viral Hepatitis			■									
Ulcerative Colitis		■	■									■
Cystic Fibrosis of the Pancreas	■		■				■	■				

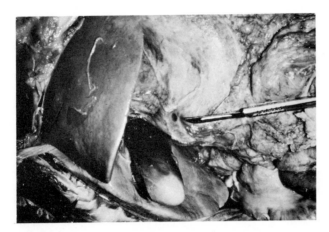

Perforated stomach ulcer; tip of scalpel points to perforation in stomach wall.

tribute to this hyperacidity. Although peptic ulcer may develop at the lower end of the esophagus, it is most likely to occur on the lesser curvature of the stomach or in the first portion of the duodenum. The ulcer margins are sharply defined; the surrounding mucosa may be normal or inflamed. The crater floor is usually clean, consisting of a thick layer of exudate overlying a deeper layer of granulation and fibrous tissue. In chronic ulcer, however, the muscular layer may be replaced by fibrous tissue and the surrounding tissues distorted by scarring. About 50 per cent of patients with duodenal ulcer secrete excessive amounts of hydrochloric acid in response to maximal histamine stimulation. The most prominent symptom is abdominal pain, which may range from mild discomfort to excruciating distress. Ingestion of food usually provides relief for an hour or two, after which the pain tends to recur. This pattern apparently occurs because food neutralizes the irritating action of the hydrochloric acid on the raw surface of the ulcer. Vomiting is a common symptom, usually following an episode of severe pain.

The presence of an ulcerating lesion of the stomach suggests the possibility of carcinoma, whereas carcinoma of the first part of the duodenum is almost unknown. Duodenal ulcer is far more frequent in men than in women, in a ratio of 10 to 1; gastric ulcer also predominates in men, the ratio being 4 to 1.

Management

Since the person with peptic ulcer is likely to be high-strung, anxious, easily upset, and given to worrying, the most important aspect of treatment is provision of mental, physical, and gastric rest. Medication

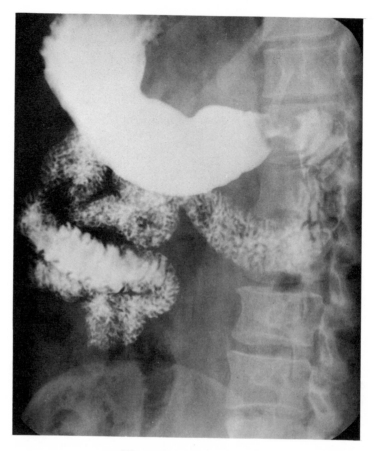

Ulcer of the duodenum.

to minimize the hyperacidity and intestinal spasm may be of help. A diet appropriate to the patient's individual needs and preferences is usually prescribed, and the value of regular rest periods is stressed.

Acute *perforation* may occur; it constitutes a major medical emergency. In this situation a hole develops through the wall of the stomach or duodenum and the gastric contents pour out into the abdominal cavity. The opening must be closed by immediate surgery.

ACUTE PANCREATITIS

As the name suggests, pancreatitis is an inflammation of the pancreas. It is due to actual digestion of the organ by an enzyme, trypsin, which the pancreas itself produces. All goes well as long as this trypsin stays in the pancreatic duct, but should the duct become blocked, as happens when gallstones form, the dammed-up secretion will rupture the smaller branches, leak into the pancreatic tissue, and digest it. Should the attacks recur, due to continued alcohol ingestion, for example, the condition is referred to as *chronic relapsing pancreatitis*.

Pathophysiology

Trauma, penetrating peptic ulcer, infectious disease, diffuse vascular disease, disorders associated with pregnancy, alcohol ingestion, overeating, and the use of certain drugs may contribute to or precipitate an attack of acute pancreatitis.

With escape of pancreatic digestive enzymes there is a severe tissue reaction, which includes edema and engorgement of blood vessels in the affected area. As the pancreatic capsule becomes distended by the dammed-up trypsin, there is intense and constant pain throughout the affected area. Then, as the enzyme is absorbed by the bloodstream, there are such systemic effects as fever, jaundice, abdominal tenderness, and, in severe cases, shock. In some instances the edema is so pronounced, because of the continued enlargement of the pancreas, that hemorrhage and necrosis follow. If the disease progresses, a bacterial infection develops to further complicate matters.

Management

In mild cases, with edema as the chief symptom, the patient improves with use of a pain-relieving drug. In more severe forms, several measures are necessary, including pain relief, treatment of shock, reduction of pancreatic secretions, prevention of infection, and maintenance of fluid and electrolyte balance.

GASTROENTERITIS; FOOD POISONING

The pathophysiology of the group of *inflammatory disorders of the stomach and intestine* falling under the general heading of gastroenteritis and food poisoning varies greatly, depending upon the cause. Over the centuries, these diseases have vied with typhus and bubonic plague as leading killers of mankind. Asiatic cholera, for example, which in times past swept throughout the world periodically, sometimes caused death within hours by producing a severe deficit in extracellular fluid. Although cholera is still prevalent in many parts of the world, it is not currently of primary concern in developed countries; but it does provide an example of the potential lethality of gastroenteric disease. The gastrointestinal tract may be exposed to toxins introduced in food or produced by bacteria growing within the intestine; the pathogen is often *Staphylo-*

coccus aureus. In either case, an infectious enterocolitis is produced, with intestinal symptoms varying from mild hypermotility to severe inflammation.

Pathophysiology of Gastroenteritis and Food Poisoning

Acute gastroenteritis   Among the causes of acute gastroenteritis are excessive drinking of alcohol; virus infection; food allergy; overuse of cathartics; absorption of metals such as arsenic, lead, mercury, and cadmium; and specific infectious diseases, including typhoid fever, bacillary or acute amebic dysentery, and cholera. Local irritation due to the causative agent gives rise to malaise, loss of appetite, nausea, vomiting, abdominal cramps, hyperactivity of the intestinal tract, and diarrhea. When vomiting is excessive, base bicarbonate excess (metabolic alkalosis) may occur; when diarrhea predominates, metabolic acidosis (base bicarbonate deficit) is more likely. Potassium deficit occurs in virtually all cases in which diarrhea is protracted and sodium excess may be present when there is pronounced watery diarrhea.

Chronic noninflammatory diarrhea   Diarrhea unassociated with gastric inflammation may develop during periods of emotional strain, or may be due to allergy to milk, wheat, rye, or egg protein, to mention just a few "triggering" substances. Loss of appetite, epigastric fullness, mild abdominal pain, and diarrhea are frequent symptoms. The loose stools are free of pus or blood but may contain undigested food residues. Cramping is usually absent.

Salmonella gastroenteritis   This type of gastroenteritis follows eating of food contaminated with bacteria of the genus Salmonella. It is often referred to as *salmonellosis*. Following an incubation period of about 8 to 48 hours after ingestion of the contaminated food, symptoms appear abruptly and may include headache, chills, fever, muscular aching, nausea, vomiting, abdominal cramps, severe diarrhea, and prostration. Rarely, death may follow within 24 hours.

Staphylococcal gastroenteritis   Staphylococcal gastroenteritis results from eating of food contaminated with staphylococcus enterotoxin. The food usually becomes contaminated through being prepared by persons whose hands harbor the pathogenic staphylococci, or who are carriers of these microorganisms. Custards, cream-filled pastry, milk, ham, and processed meat and fish are the foods most often involved. This gastroenteritis probably is the most common type of food poisoning, and is a rather frequent follow-up to summer picnics. The patient becomes violently ill within 2 to 4 hours after eating the contaminated food, and has symptoms of nausea, vomiting, abdominal cramps, diarrhea, headache, and fever. In a severe case, the patient may go into shock. The attack is usually of short duration.

SEQUENCE OF EVENTS
IN UNTREATED GASTROENTERITIS

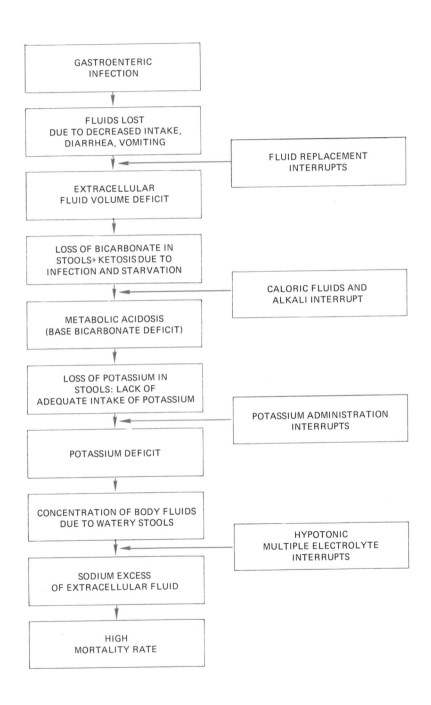

Botulism   This disease is an acute intoxication due to eating of food containing a toxin produced by *Clostridium botulinum*. The toxin is a protein that resists digestion by gastrointestinal enzymes and is the most potent poison known. The microorganism itself is not pathogenic; it liberates its toxin while growing under anaerobic (lacking in oxygen) conditions. The toxin is mainly absorbed from the upper gastrointestinal tract. It blocks the transmission of impulses from certain nerve fibers, thereby causing numerous nervous and muscular symptoms. Malaise, headache, and dizziness are followed quickly by serious visual disturbances, sometimes blindness. Then there is progressive muscular weakness until finally the victim is unable to swallow or to breathe. The mind remains clear until the end. Although individual cases of botulism may be mild, the overall mortality is high. The usual source of botulism is improperly preserved food, almost always home-preserved, for the reason that the spores of *clostridium botulinum* are not killed by the usual methods of home-canning. Exposure to moist heat at 120° C. for 30 minutes—the method used by commercial canners—kills all the spores.

Nonbacterial food poisoning   This type of food poisoning is caused by eating of plants and animals which are themselves poisonous or which contain a poison. Certain species of mushrooms, toadstools, immature or sprouting potatoes, certain fish including trigger fish, barracuda, and balloon fish, and mussels are examples of the former. Ergot poisoning (ergotism) due to eating of bread made from rye or wheat infected with ergot fungus is an example of the latter, as is poisoning due to ingestion of unwashed and uncooked foods that have been sprayed with insecticides containing toxic chemicals or that have been cooked or stored in vessels —usually very old ones—lined with antimony or cadmium. A third example, which probably came to the reader's mind immediately, is of recent origin—the contamination of many species of fish and shellfish by chemical wastes dumped into the world's waters. The symptoms in all these forms of poisoning obviously will vary with the toxic agent. In general, there is evidence of local irritation as well as neurologic disturbances.

Management of Gastroenteritis and Food Poisoning

One takes a "food history" to determine which food was responsible for the illness, and management then can be suitably planned. At the same time, secondary neurologic or fluid balance disturbances are given adequate attention. The health care team can do much to educate the patient about the importance of such rudimentary sanitary measures as proper cooking and storage of food, which go a long way toward preventing outbreaks of food poisoning and gastroenteritis.

REGIONAL ENTERITIS

Regional enteritis, also known as *Crohn's disease* for the man who first described it, is a disease of the small intestine that affects mainly young adults. Although the incidence of this disorder is much lower than that of many other inflammatory diseases of the intestine, it deserves mention in our discussion because it tends to become chronic or to recur, and because it may have serious consequences, including invalidism.

Pathophysiology

Emotional stress, which often causes bowel dysfunction, is thought to be an important contributing factor in the development of regional enteritis. The intestinal wall, especially the terminal ileum, becomes greatly thickened and rigid, and large edematous nodes develop in the adjacent mesentery. The result is pronounced narrowing of the lumen, which leads to chronic obstruction. The outcome of all this is severe symptoms of midabdominal cramps with passage of several loose bloody stools daily, and fever. These symptoms in turn result in loss of appetite, so the patient suffers considerable weight loss. In about 10 per cent of cases there is an *acute ileitis*, or inflammation of the ileum. In all other cases another distinctive feature, such as intestinal *ulcers*, perianal or perirectal *abscesses*, or *fistulas*, is present and may be the cause of serious complications.

REGIONAL ENTERITIS MARKED BY CHRONICITY, RECURRENCE, MORBIDITY, AND INVALIDISM

Management

If there are no complications, the treatment centers around relief of pain, attention to nutritional and fluid needs, relief of diarrhea, and treatment of infection. Surgery to remove the involved segment of intestine may be undertaken in the presence of such factors as perforation and hemorrhage. Regional enteritis tends to recur, whether or not surgery is performed, which suggests that a great deal remains to be learned about the disease.

ULCERATIVE COLITIS

Ulcerative colitis is another in the rather long list of illnesses about which there is much information but little definitive knowledge. Physicians understand a great deal about the lesions produced in the colon and the course and treatment of the disease—yet the underlying cause or defect remains unknown. It has been attributed to specific bacterial or viral infection; to psychic factors of stress, hostility, and anxiety; to food allergy; and to an autoimmune process.

Pathophysiology

The process apparently begins as an inflammatory infiltration of the mucosa and submucosa of the colon in which abscesses form. The overlying mucosa becomes separated from its blood supply, leading to ulceration. The mucosa is now a red, spongy surface covered with a myriad of ulcers oozing blood and pus. Even in a mild case, in which considerable healing follows the attack, the mucosal structure rarely returns to normal; in a severe case, the mucosa and musculature are destroyed and replaced by fibrous tissue. With fibrosis, crevices and pseudopolyps arise that give a rough, cobblestone appearance to the involved segment of the colon. In the majority of cases, the rectosigmoid is the first area to be affected, and finally the entire colon, even the terminal ileum, may be involved.

The onset may be acute, but usually it is insidious; the patient notices an increased urgency to defecate, and experiences mild lower abdominal cramps. There is bloody mucus in the stools. If the process extends upward, the stools become looser until eventually the patient may pass 10 to 20 or even more stools daily, associated with severe cramps—there is no respite even at night. These watery feces are mixed with pus, blood, and mucus, or may consist entirely of blood and pus.

In the fulminant form, the patient is suddenly seized with an attack of violent diarrhea, severe cramps, and high fever, which is followed by profound toxemia. He may succumb to the initial attack, with the cause of death usually attributed to hemorrhage. Perhaps one in every four patients recovers completely after a single attack. But far more often, ulcerative colitis is a disease of remission and exacerbation.

Management

The goal of therapy is to provide the necessary physical and psychological support so that the patient's own defenses can combat the disease. Strict bed rest and unrestricted fluid intake are indicated, but if the patient cannot eat or drink, water, electrolytes, nutrients, and vitamins are given parenterally. As far as possible, emotional problems should be solved and difficult environmental factors eliminated; the health care team, by being alert to the patient's overall needs and conditions, can contribute greatly to his comfort.

Should colonic obstruction or neoplasm develop, as not infrequently happens, surgical intervention may be necessary. In this operation, the colon is removed from cecum to sigmoid, with establishment of a permanent ileostomy. The rectum may be resected at the same time or at a later date.

APPENDICITIS

The vermiform appendix serves no function that is known, yet it is the source of the most common surgical lesion of the abdomen—appendicitis. This inflammatory disease may occur at any age but is most common in young adults.

Pathophysiology

The appendix is, you will recall, an offshoot of the cecum, sharing with the cecal lumen the fecal contents of the colon. The lumen of the appendix ends blindly so that when obstruction and inflammation are absent—the normal condition—its fecal contents are evacuated back into the cecum. But when an obstruction, such as is caused by a fecalith (a hardened mass formed around fecal matter) or earlier fibrosis, develops, the lumen becomes distended and venous return is disrupted. This leads, in turn, to poor oxygenation of the area, permitting bacteria to invade and multiply. If the process goes on, the appendix will fill with pus and finally rupture, and this will result in peritonitis—inflammation of the peritoneum. The peritonitis may remain *localized* if, as frequently happens, it is walled off by formation of abscesses around the appendix. If this walling-off is inadequate, *generalized* peritonitis follows, in which the intestinal contents pour out into the abdominal cavity.

The usual symptoms include fever, loss of appetite, nausea, vomiting, and pain and tenderness in the lower right part of the abdomen. The pain increases in severity until rupture occurs, when the pain stops suddenly and dramatically—but only because the outpouring of pus has relieved the local tension, not because the patient's condition has improved.

Management

An acutely inflamed appendix should be removed surgically as soon as possible after diagnosis. By contrast with the postoperative course of just 30 or so years ago, when the patient was kept in bed for a number of days—and thereby became weaker rather than stronger—today's patient usually is permitted to be out of bed within a few hours after surgery, and goes home within 3 or 4 days for a brief recuperative period.

When surgery is not promptly performed, the appendix may rupture.

In some instances the body defenses form a protective wall around the ruptured appendix. The result is an appendiceal abscess. In other cases, successful walling off does not occur. Then peritonitis develops.

PERITONITIS

Peritonitis is a condition in which the peritoneal cavity—the area between the two layers of peritoneum that, respectively, line the abdominal cavity and cover the viscera—becomes inflamed due to infection. The infection is usually bacterial in nature, but it may be due to the presence of blood, urine, bile, or pancreatic juice in the abdominal cavity.

Pathophysiology

Among the numerous underlying causes of peritonitis are *inflammation* or *perforation* of the gastrointestinal tract resulting from appendicitis, peptic ulcer, diverticulitis, and ulcerative colitis; in the female, *infection* of the genital tract; *trauma* to the abdominal wall; *dissemination* of tubercle bacilli, streptococci, and pneumococci; and accidental *soiling* at operation. Because of the ensuing severe irritation, the normally clear and glistening membrane turns dull and opaque. A serofibrinous exudate forms, which later becomes purulent.

Decreased motor activity causes severe abdominal distention, with associated vomiting and sometimes diarrhea. The temperature rises, the pulse quickens, and the white blood count increases. Extracellular fluid volume deficit and other fluid imbalances complicate the picture. The overwhelming illness imparts a pinched, drawn appearance to the patient's face—the "hippocratic" facies. Finally, as the intestinal wall becomes inflamed, peristalsis disappears, and the condition becomes one of acute obstruction.

Management

The first step in treatment is to remove the cause, e.g., in appendicitis, to remove the inflamed appendix if peritonitis is early, in ruptured duodenal ulcer, to close the duodenal opening. If the peritonitis is localized, the inflammation will subside, and the patient recovers. If, however, the peritonitis is generalized, the patient will remain extremely ill due to the widespread infection, and will require close medical and nursing care. This involves, in addition to measures to combat the infection, attention to fluid and electrolyte balance, nose and mouth care, and adequate drainage of the gastrointestinal tract and of the wound itself.

DIVERTICULOSIS AND DIVERTICULITIS

A diverticulum (plural, diverticula) is a protrusion of the mucosa and submucosa at a weak point along the muscular coat of the intestine. *Diverticulosis* refers merely to the existence of diverticula. When a diverticulum becomes obstructed and thus leads to infection and inflammation, the condition is known as *diverticulitis*.

Pathophysiology

Diverticula arise at points of increased pressure along the intestinal wall, by the entrance of blood vessels and the bile and pancreatic ducts. Fully developed diverticula are spherical sacs connected with the intestinal lumen by a narrow neck. They are most likely to develop in the fifth decade or later, especially in the obese. Diverticulosis of the colon is asymptomatic. When the neck of the diverticulum becomes obstructed, as by a fecalith, the stasis thus produced promotes inflammation and infection—diverticulitis. The process may remain localized and subside, or with continued obstruction, may spread and produce abscess formation. Intestinal obstruction may result. The diverticulum may perforate, leading to peritonitis or fistula formation. Eventually, the bowel wall may become thickened and even stenosed.

With acute diverticulitis, the patient experiences left lower quadrant pain, nausea, vomiting, abdominal distention, and colic. Obstinate constipation (obstipation), diarrhea, or both may occur. Infection causes chills and fever and the white blood count may be normal or elevated.

DIVERTICULAR DISEASE THE MOST COMMON PATHOLOGIC PROCESS IN THE COLON

Management

Diverticulosis requires no treatment other than a bland, non-irritating diet. The treatment of diverticulitis is, of course, more complicated. Bed rest, antibiotic therapy, and careful management of body fluid disturbances are necessary. A low-residue diet is followed. Heat is applied to the abdomen, and warm saline enemas are given. Chronic diverticulitis may improve with use of a low-residue diet. Complications such as abscess, perforation, massive hemorrhage, or fistula necessitate immediate surgery with removal of the involved segment.

THE MALABSORPTION SYNDROME

This term refers to deficiency in the absorption of food. The word "syndrome" is used because any one of a number of diseases may be responsible. Whatever the underlying cause, the hallmark of all the diseases of malabsorption is a deficiency in fat absorption, causing the frequent passage of unformed, bulky, foul-smelling stools.

Pathophysiology

Any of several disease categories may be responsible for malabsorption, among them impaired digestion, as occurs in cirrhosis, and lymphatic obstruction, as occurs in lymphoma. For purposes of our discussion, however, the most important cause is a biochemical abnormality, and in this group of disorders are included tropical sprue and non-tropical sprue (also known as idiopathic steatorrhea), and celiac disease. The first two are diseases of adults, the last is a disease of children. The defect is similar in all of them: the villi of the intestinal mucosa are blunted or atrophied to the point of being lost altogether. The result is that there is a loss of absorptive surface within the intestine, and consequent reduced food absorption. Symptoms of diarrhea, steatorrhea, weight loss, weakness, vitamin deficiency, and microcytic anemia appear.

Infection, malnutrition, dietary protein deficiency, folic acid deficiency, a genetic metabolic abnormality, and an enzyme deficiency have all been suggested as contributing factors.

Then, too, a host of other disorders may be precipitating factors. A list of these would have to include extensive bowel resection, intestinal fistulas, bile duct obstruction (as occurs in pancreatitis), lymphomatosis, regional enteritis, intestinal tuberculosis, intestinal diverticula, diabetes, and radiation injury. We might say that the digestive system's ability to convert food into substances that can be utilized by the various tissues accurately reflects the body's overall state of health.

Management

In general, therapy centers around replacement of the deficient substance, which might be, for example, a digestive enzyme, insulin, ox bile, vitamin B_{12}, or folic acid; or removal from the diet of the offending substance, for example, gluten in tropical sprue and adult celiac disease. Corticosteroids, antibiotics, and other drugs are administered selectively, and, when appropriate—as when fistulas are present—surgery to correct the condition may be undertaken.

PARASITIC INFECTIONS

The list of parasites that may infest the gastrointestinal tract of man and thus cause intestinal infection is of a bewildering variety and length. Diseases caused by parasites are more common and widespread than bacterial and viral diseases, in both man and animals, although—in the highly developed countries—they give less cause for concern. It would be impossible, in a book such as this, to list and describe all the parasitic infections to which man is susceptible. The following table is offered as a *representative* list of a few parasitic diseases that afflict many millions of persons every year and cause millions of deaths.

Many of the parasitic diseases (e.g., schistosomiasis) are extremely prevalent in certain areas of the world, particularly the tropics, and a few

A LARGE FRACTION OF THE WORLD'S POPULATION IS AFFLICTED WITH PARASITIC DISEASE AT ALL TIMES

REPRESENTATIVE DISEASES CAUSED BY ANIMAL PARASITES

Phylum	Organism	Disease	Pathophysiology
Protozoa	*Entamoeba histolytica*	Amebiasis	Parasitic cysts ingested by man in food or drink contaminated by fecal matter; symptoms of cramps, diarrhea, fatigue, fever; complications include liver abscess, hepatitis, pulmonary abscess.
Arthropoda	Plasmodium species	Malaria	Transmitted by bite of mosquitoes of genus *Anopheles* or in transfusion of infected blood; symptoms of paroxysms of fever accompanied by shivering, pallor, cyanosis, followed by profuse sweating; an important cause of death and, despite heroic efforts at eradication, the most serious parasitic infection of man.
Protozoa	Trypanosoma species	African trypanosomiasis (sleeping sickness)	Transmitted by tsetse fly, which injects trypanosomes into bloodstream; symptoms of severe headache, feeling of great oppression, loss of nocturnal sleep.

REPRESENTATIVE DISEASES CAUSED BY ANIMAL PARASITES (Cont.)

Phylum	Organism	Disease	Pathophysiology
Platyhel-minths (flatworms)	Schistosoma species	Schisto-somiasis	Eggs and adult worms deposited in small venules of intestine and migrate through intestine and urinary bladder to accumulate in liver, lungs, and central nervous system; symptoms of hepatitis, fever, weight loss, diarrhea; if disease becomes chronic there is severe liver and intestinal damage; next to malaria, it is the most serious parasitic infection of man.
Nematoda (round-worms)	*Trichinella spiralis*	Trichinosis	Hogs infected by eating uncooked meat scraps and garbage or infected rats; man acquires infection by ingesting partially cooked pork products; larvae then deposited in striated muscles and vital organs; symptoms of muscle inflammation, muscle stiffness and weakness, edema, and pain.

(e.g., trichinosis) are fairly frequent in North America. With ever-increasing world travel, the possibility that individuals may return home having acquired an intestinal parasite increases.

Management

Specific drugs are available for treatment of many intestinal parasitic infections of man, and in some infections surgical measures may be employed. Probably, however, the most essential aspects of treatment are preventive in nature: educating the public about the importance of scrupulous attention to personal hygiene, proper cooking of all pork products, and avoiding water and food substances that may be contaminated; and carrying out, on a mass scale, various programs aimed at controlling or eradicating the parasites and their vectors.

NEOPLASMS

Both benign and malignant neoplasms occur in all parts of the alimentary tract; unfortunately, however, benign growths are relatively rare; malignant tumors of the gastrointestinal tract on the other hand, account for 25 per cent of all deaths from neoplasms.

Pathophysiology

Benign neoplasms of the gastrointestinal tract include fibromas, neurofibromas, myomas, adenomas, lipomas, hemangiomas, and papillomas. They give rise to symptoms of bleeding, nausea, anorexia, and epigastric pain—which are also early symptoms of gastric carcinoma. Polyps larger than 2 cm. in diameter are often malignant; in familial polyposis of the colon, carcinoma of the large intestine is almost certain to develop unless the polyposis is treated by removal of the colon.

Carcinoma of the gastrointestinal tract is mainly seen in persons older than 40 years. Size, location, and nature of the tumor, whether ulcerating, infiltrating, or polypoid, dictate the course and symptoms in the individual case; in more than half of these tumors symptoms arise sufficiently early to permit accurate diagnosis.

GREAT MAJORITY OF CARCINOMAS ARISE FROM MUCOSA

In the *esophagus,* an important symptom is the inability to swallow a bolus of food, along with the sensation that the bolus is stuck at a point somewhere behind the sternum. Later the patient is unable to swallow even liquids. Pain with efforts to swallow or a sensation of persistent boring pain will develop.

Carcinoma of the *stomach* causes symptoms of upper abdominal distress (which may or may not be more severe after eating), epigastric pain similar to that due to ulcer, poor appetite, vomiting, weight loss, anemia, and gastrointestinal bleeding.

Intermittent midabdominal cramps, evidence of bleeding, and anemia not due to an identified disease of the stomach or colon suggests the presence of a carcinoma of the *small intestine.*

A marked change in bowel habit, usually in the form of diarrhea, suggests the possibility of carcinoma of the *colon.* In addition, there is weight loss, abdominal pain, and vomiting, and blood may be passed by rectum. The symptoms of *rectal* carcinoma are quite similar to those just mentioned.

Management

Surgical removal of both benign and malignant tumors offers the greatest possibility of cure. This is not always possible, however, since many gastrointestinal cancers are inoperable because of extension or metastasis by the time symptoms are noted. Radiation therapy and chemotherapy are adjunctive modalities that provide relief of symptoms or bring about temporary remission in numerous cases, particularly those in which surgery is not possible. In operable cancer of the colon, the surgical procedure is an ostomy—the creation of a new opening of the bowel onto the skin. There are two main types: in *ileostomy* the ileum is opened onto the skin, and in *colostomy* the colon is opened onto the skin.

VIRAL HEPATITIS

At the present time the two most frequent types of viral hepatitis are infectious hepatitis and serum hepatitis, and our discussion will be confined to these. *Infectious* hepatitis is usually transmitted through fecally contaminated food or water (the *fecal-oral route*). Its occurrence may be sporadic or epidemic, depending upon the distribution of the infected material and the susceptibility of the population exposed; conditions of crowding and poor sanitation favor an epidemic outbreak. *Serum* hepatitis is transmitted mainly via virus-infected blood used for transfusion, although lately there has been a rising frequency of serum hepatitis due to sharing of infected needles by "mainlining" narcotic addicts. Occasionally it is transmitted through inadequately sterilized dental and surgical instruments.

Pathophysiology

The course is similar in both types. There is an abrupt onset, with anorexia, nausea, fever, and malaise. The liver is enlarged and tender, and there is pain in the right upper quadrant. About 5 days later jaundice appears in many patients and the fever begins to subside. The jaundice is due to the backing up of bilirubin in the liver resulting from impaired liver function. In some patients the spleen becomes enlarged. Other symptoms, seen in some cases, include severe generalized pruritus, urticaria, and intermittent diarrhea.

Most patients recover uneventfully within 6 to 8 weeks, although they may continue to note mild residual symptoms of right quadrant pain and tenderness and intolerance of fatty foods. Liver function may continue to be slightly depressed for as long as a year or more.

This is the usual picture of viral hepatitis, which applies especially to young adults. In a few patients, however, especially elderly ones, the illness takes an acute course, marked by symptoms of vomiting, extreme jaundice, bile in the urine, delirium, coma, and finally death. This is the picture of *acute hepatic necrosis,* or *acute yellow atrophy.*

Management

The physician may order that strict isolation technique be maintained during the active phase of the disease. The patient should remain in bed as long as jaundice, abdominal pain, and liver tenderness are present and until liver function tests approach normal; usually a minimum of 3 weeks is desirable. Health care personnel should encourage the patient to eat foods that appeal to him; foods high in protein and carbohydrate are most desirable. A satisfactory diet contains about 125 grams of protein, 350 grams of carbohydrate, and 100 grams of fat per day. Adrenocortical steroids and antibiotics may be prescribed according to individual need.

CYSTIC FIBROSIS OF THE PANCREAS

This condition is also known as *mucoviscidosis, fibrocystic disease of the pancreas,* and *pancreatic cystic fibrosis.* It is an inherited disease of the exocrine glands which affects the pancreas, respiratory system, and sweat glands. Cystic fibrosis usually appears in infancy and is characterized by chronic respiratory infection, insufficiency of the pancreas, and susceptibility to heat prostration.

CYSTIC FIBROSIS TRANSMITTED AS AN AUTOSOMAL RECESSIVE TRAIT

Pathophysiology

The significant feature is the changes produced in the secretions of the pancreas, the intestinal glands, and the bronchial mucus-secreting glands, the change being one of much increased viscidity, or stickiness.

The mucous glands of the *trachea and bronchi* are filled with mucus, so that segments of lung become blocked off, leading to chronic infection and fibrosis. Areas of atelectasis and emphysema develop, and eventually, the larger bronchi fill with a purulent secretion from which *Staphylococcus aureus* or *Pseudomonas aeruginosa* can be cultured. Death may result from occlusion of the tracheobronchial tree by these purulent secretions or from cor pulmonale.

In the *pancreas* the ducts are dilated and filled with viscid mucus, which prevents important digestive enzymes from entering the duodenum. The intestine is blocked by viscid (inspissated) meconium, leading to obstruction, a condition known as *meconium ileus.*

These infants fail to gain weight, in spite of good appetite and vigor, and have a chronic cough, with a rapid respiratory rate. They pass large, frequent, foul-smelling stools. Rectal prolapse is a fairly frequent occurrence. Cough is the most troublesome complaint, and it may be associated with vomiting. The baby becomes barrel-chested. In almost every case the sweat glands are involved; during periods of hot weather or fever, there may be great losses of sodium, chloride, and potassium.

Although the outlook has improved considerably, thanks to antibiotic therapy, the prognosis remains poor. Less than 10 per cent of these children reach adulthood.

Management

Dietary measures are of prime importance. Common considerations are pancreatic enzyme replacement, sufficient calories, adequate protein intake, low fat intake, and multivitamins.

At night and during daytime rest periods the child may stay in a mist tent in which fine droplets of water are carried to the deep portions of the respiratory passages. A program of physical therapy, including breathing exercises and postural drainage, is prescribed. Antibiotics are administered to combat acute or chronic pulmonary infection. Surgical intervention may be necessary should intestinal obstruction or intussusception (prolapse of one part of the intestine into the lumen of the adjoining part) develop.

TOPICS FOR DISCUSSION

1. Why is the digestive tract said to be an extension of the external body surface?

2. What are the protective functions of the digestive tract?

3. What segment of the digestive tract is chiefly responsible for absorption?

4. Would you agree that diseases of the digestive tract have been one of the chief causes of death throughout history?

5. Why is carcinoma one of the most frequent neoplasms of the digestive tract?

6. What digestive illnesses may, on occasion, be psychosomatic in origin?

7. What digestive diseases are familial?

8. In what respects is the anal sphincter a most remarkable structure? (Read: Bornemeier, W.: Sphincter protecting hemorrhoidectomy. The American Journal of Proctology, *11*:48–52, 1960.)

9. How would you define constipation? (Most persons do not define it correctly!)

10. What are the cardinal functions of the large intestine?

11. What digestive tract disorders are most remediable? Which are extremely difficult to treat successfully?

12. What digestive disorders arise from vestigial structures inherited through the ages from primitive ancestors?

19

common diseases of the urinary system

The urinary system consists of the urinary tract (male or female) and the male genital organs. The system is also known as the *genitourinary system*. The kidneys are the most important part of the urinary system, and we shall discuss these organs and their disorders first.

It would be a mistake to regard the kidneys as designed primarily for waste disposal, for they have a major regulatory function. The urinary tract aids in maintaining the proper environment for the normal functioning of the body cells. The composition of our body fluid depends not so much on what we eat as on what our kidneys keep—in fact, according to the great physiologist Homer Smith, the tubule cells of the kidneys exceed in importance any other cells of the body. Certainly they are the master chemists of the tight little pond we call body fluid.

When, because of intrinsic kidney disease or disease of other parts of the urinary system, the kidneys cannot function normally, illness follows. Such illness will have widespread effects on all body systems, including the cardiovascular and musculoskeletal. Fortunately, disorders of the kidney and its auxiliary structures usually respond well to treatment, particularly when that treatment is started in the early stages of disease.

In *From Fish to Philosopher*, Homer Smith has provided us with some striking statistics concerning the kidneys: Their 2 million tubules would stretch almost 50 miles if joined end to end. The filtering surface of our 2 million glomeruli is equal to nearly half the body surface area. The liquid filtered through the glomeruli amounts to about 125 ml. per minute, or 180 liters (about 190 quarts) daily; this filtrate contains 1,100 gm. of sodium chloride, 425 gm. of sodium bicarbonate, and 145 gm. of glucose. Almost all the sodium chloride and sodium bicarbonate is reabsorbed, as are important amounts of potassium, calcium, magnesium, phosphate, sulfate, amino acids, vitamins, and other essential substances. The filtrate is reduced to an average of 1.5 liters of urine *daily*; the kidneys require 1,200 ml. (1.2 liters) of blood *per minute* to produce this filtrate. Although the kidneys account for only 0.5 per cent of body weight, they receive 40 times as much blood as any other organ.

PATHOPHYSIOLOGIC PROCESSES WHICH CAN BE INVOLVED IN DISEASES OF THE UROLOGIC SYSTEM

	Genetics: Diseases Due to Hereditary Factors	Disease Due to Hypersensitivity and Autoimmunity	Infectious Diseases	Diseases Due to Physical Agents	Diseases Due to Chemical Agents	Neoplasia	Disturbances of Fluid and Electrolyte Balance	Diseases of Malnutrition	Endocrine Dysfunction	Stress Factors in Disease	The Aging Process	Psychosomatic Factors in Disease
Congenital Anomalies	■		■	■			■					
Acute Renal Failure		■	■	■	■							
Renal Tuberculosis	■		■									
Acute Glomerulonephritis		■					■					
Nephrotic Syndrome		■	■						■		■	
Arteriolar Nephrosclerosis	■						■		■		■	■
Acute Pyelonephritis			■									
Neoplasms				■		■						
Calculi			■		■		■		■		■	
Perinephritic Abscess			■									
Cystitis			■	■		■		■	■			
Ureteritis												
Prostatism						■					■	
Benign Prostatic Hypertrophy											■	
Fibrosis			■									
Gonorrhea			■									
Epididymitis			■	■								
Urethritis			■	■								
Prostatitis			■								■	

Up to now, the only vital organ that has been transplanted successfully in a significant number of cases is the kidney. Moreover, the artificial kidney can maintain a patient in reasonably good health for some years; as yet, similar feats involving other major body organs have not been accomplished.

In times past, the kidneys were regarded as among the lowliest of organs. But in 1804, the French chemist Fourceroy revealed a dawning understanding of the importance of these organs when he said, "The urine of man . . . which commonly inspires men only with contempt and disgust . . . has become, in the hands of the chemists, a source of important discoveries." Indeed, as Fourceroy so well emphasized, examination of the urine can be of enormous help in diagnosis not only of diseases that primarily affect the kidneys but of those that involve other organs and tissues as well. The odor, color, specific gravity, and reaction of the urine give the physician some helpful information about his patient's general state of health; when to this is added such information as the presence or absence of glucose, ketone bodies, albumin, blood, pus, and casts, the physician has a useful picture of the specific state of one body system.

EXAMINATION OF URINE; ABNORMAL FINDINGS

Odor

Urine that smells strongly of ammonia has merely been standing —it does not provide any significant information. On the other hand, certain illnesses produce definite urinary odors. The urine of a patient with phenylketonuria, for example, is distinctive and unforgettable.

Color

Normally urine is yellow or amber, depending largely on the volume of water drunk. Urine darkens with inadequate water intake or heavy water losses, as may occur during fever, periods of hot weather, or profuse sweating from any cause. In diabetes mellitus, the urine is pale even though it contains sugar, and in a severe untreated case, it may resemble a mixture of honey and water. When kidney concentrating ability (ability to produce urine of high specific gravity) is impaired, the urine is pale. The color may be smoky if a few red cells are present and bright red or brown if much blood is present.

Specific Gravity

The specific gravity of pure water is 1.000; that of normal urine is from 1.010 to 1.025. Normally the specific gravity varies about 10 points during the course of a day, so that variations lower or higher often point to the existence of renal disease.

Reaction

The pH of normal urine is slightly acid (recall that the symbol pH refers to the hydrogen ion concentration, the measure of alkalinity and acidity). Urine may become alkaline in the presence of certain bladder infections or some cases of alkalosis. It will become alkaline if it is allowed to stand for several hours in a warm atmosphere. This alkalinity gives urine the characteristic pungent odor of ammonia. Obviously, urine to be tested should be fresh.

URINALYSIS AN
ELEMENT OF
EVERY PHYSICAL
EXAMINATION

Glucose

The finding of glucose in the urine (glycosuria) usually means that diabetes mellitus is present. However, one positive specimen does not make the diagnosis. Urine should be checked repeatedly, and further tests, including blood studies, should be performed.

Ketone Bodies

Ketone bodies—acetone and diacetic acid—in the urine indicate the presence of ketoacidosis, or base bicarbonate deficit. Ketoacidosis is usually a serious complication of diabetes mellitus. Ketone bodies may also be found in the urine (ketonuria) in persons who are severely dehydrated or starved.

Albumin

Normally a trace of albumin passes into the urine but this trace is so small that it is not detected by usual methods. The presence of detectable albumin in the urine (albuminuria) in most cases indicates that nephritis or nephrosis is present.

Blood

Blood in the urine (hematuria) is generally ominous. An infection, calculus, or neoplasm of the urinary tract is the usual cause.

Other causes include toxicity due to drugs, and hemorrhagic diseases. When the quantity of red cells is sufficient to color the urine red, *gross hematuria* exists; in many instances, however, the hematuria is *occult,* i.e., detectable only on microscopic examination of the urine sediment.

Pus

Pus in the urine (pyuria), as evidenced by numerous polymorphonuclear cells seen microscopically, is due to an infection of the urologic tract; the infection might be pyelitis, pyelonephritis, tuberculosis of the kidney, cystitis, or urethritis.

Casts

Casts are elements formed in the renal tubules. The lumen becomes partially filled with a substance consisting of albumin, red blood cells, white blood cells, and epithelial cells, which hardens and forms a cast—hence the term. When found in the urine (cylindruria) they denote the presence of nephritis. Usually cylindruria and albuminuria occur together. The casts disappear when urine is left standing, so only fresh urine specimens should be examined.

Crystals

Crystals are generally found in concentrated urine specimens (crystalluria) but, with few exceptions, they are of no pathological significance.

ACUTE RENAL FAILURE

Acute renal failure refers to sudden and complete failure of excretory function.

Pathophysiology

Acute renal failure develops over a period of days to weeks. It may follow *necrosis of renal tubules,* as occurs, for example, in severe and prolonged shock and in poisoning due to certain heavy metals or drugs. Severe *infection,* as may occur as a complication of diabetes mellitus, is another cause. A third important factor is *vascular injury,* which is an ever-present threat during cardiac surgery and in sickle cell anemia. Severe *hypersensitivity states* (described in Chap. 3) may produce acute failure; the collagen diseases are in this category. Finally, *obstruction* due to calculi, tumors, or other cause may result in acute renal failure.

In the early stage, the only symptom suggesting kidney damage may be failure to void normally. Lumbar pain and tenderness may develop. In this stage of *oliguria,* or marked reduction in urinary excretion, less than 400 ml. of urine per day is excreted, and it is loaded with albumin and casts. If oliguria persists for more than 10 days, the patient is not likely to survive.

Management

DIALYSIS MAY
SPELL DIFFERENCE
BETWEEN SURVIVAL
AND DEATH

Acute renal failure is a critical event. Since, as has been described, it follows other disorders, the first objective of treatment is to bring the underlying disease under control insofar as possible. The artificial kidney (dialyzer) plays an important role in this phase of treatment and has saved the lives of numerous patients. The next step, also of great importance, is to institute fluid balance measures. Prompt and vigorous treatment of infection with antibiotics, blood transfusion if indicated, and close attention to diet are also necessary. In fact, the overall management of the patient in acute renal failure brings into play all the skills of every member of the health care team, from physician to orderly. Catheterization is avoided whenever possible in order to reduce the possibility of sepsis, which is the largest single cause of death in these patients.

NEPHRITIS

Nephritis means inflammation of the kidney, specifically a diffuse, progressive, degenerative, or proliferative lesion involving the parenchyma, the interstitial tissue, or the vascular system of the kidneys. This inclusive term thus refers to glomerulonephritis, the nephroses, nephrosclerosis, and pyelonephritis.

GLOMERULONEPHRITIS

Glomerulonephritis, still often called *Bright's disease* for the man who first described it more than 100 years ago, is characterized pathologically by diffuse inflammatory changes in the glomeruli. (Actually, the eponym has come to designate several renal diseases having similar characteristics of albuminuria, hypoproteinemia, and renal failure.)

Acute, subacute, and chronic forms are recognized. *Acute* glomerulonephritis is characterized by acute inflammation, acute renal insufficiency, edema, and, in many cases, hypertension. Albuminuria and edema are the cardinal findings in the *subacute* phase, often called the *nephrotic* phase. In the *chronic* form there is hypertension and renal failure. Recovery usually follows episodes of acute glomerulonephritis; but with repeated infections, the subacute phase, and finally the chronic—and lethal—phase follow.

Pathophysiology

Acute glomerulonephritis is an acute, nonsuppurative, inflammatory and proliferative disease in which no bacteria are demonstrable. It affects children and adolescents much more frequently than adults. It follows streptococcal infection—sometimes nonstreptococcal infection—in any part of the body. There is an interval of approximately 2 weeks between infection and onset of glomerulonephritis.

SEQUENCE OF EVENTS:
ACUTE GLOMERULONEPHRITIS

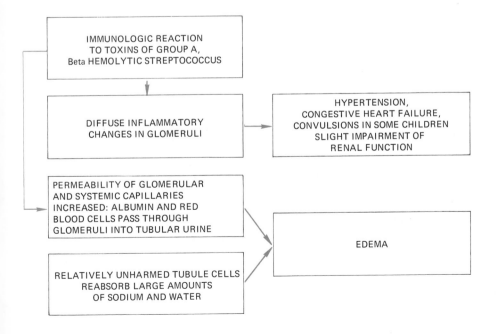

EVIDENCE
MOUNTS FOR
AUTOIMMUNE
BASIS

There is compelling evidence pointing to an *autoimmune* (autoclastic) basis for glomerulonephritis (see Chap. 3). The latent period between streptococcal infection and renal disease, the absence of bacterial invasion, and the proliferative nature of the renal lesions all suggest that an antigen-antibody reaction involving the glomeruli is at work.

The onset is usually abrupt, with symptoms of headache, fever up to 101° F., poor appetite, nausea, and vomiting. Oliguria is usual; anuria is rare. Edema develops in many patients due to loss of plasma from the abnormally permeable capillaries, not only in the glomeruli but throughout the body. Convulsions may occur, in children especially, as a result of cerebral edema. There may be back pain. Mild to moderate hypertension is common as a result of cardiac effort to force blood through the jammed glomeruli. In some cases, congestive heart failure develops.

In many instances casts are seen after a few days. Those formed from red blood cells are a pathognomonic (specific) sign of acute glomerulonephritis; others consist of protein from the glomerulus and epithelium, granules, and fatty substance from the tubules.

At this stage the kidneys are swollen and congested due to inflammation. With adequate treatment, however, the acute attack usually clears completely (especially in children) and is unlikely to be followed by a second attack. Complete healing takes place in upward of 85 per cent of cases.

Should urinary abnormalities continue, however, along with further decreasing renal function and hypertension, the *subacute* stage is considered to be present.

Should proteinuria persist for more than 1 year after the initial episode, the patient has entered the *latent chronic phase.* Yet he may experience few or no symptoms and renal function may be normal or nearly normal. This stage may go on for as long as 20 or 30 years. During this phase the chief symptom is edema, due to loss of albumin both from capillaries of the glomeruli and from those of the subcutaneous tissues. Albuminuria due to glomerular damage is pronounced, and diverse types of casts appear. Kidney function is, nevertheless, only slightly impaired in this stage.

Finally the stage of chronic glomerulonephritis is reached. In this phase, the kidney is scarred. Its size is below normal, and its surface is dotted with fine granules. When examined under the microscope, the diseased kidney bears scant resemblance to a normal kidney. The tubules have been replaced by scar tissue; large numbers of hyalinized cells can be seen under low power. Some are shrunken, but others have hypertrophied to carry on the essential work of the kidney and keep the patient alive. The convoluted tubules have disappeared for the most part; those leading from the overworked glomeruli are hypertrophied. Islands of these tubules project above the surface of the kidney, contributing to the granular appearance.

STEPWISE
PROGRESSION
OF
GLOMERULO-
NEPHRITIS

Now renal failure comes on rapidly. Only small amounts of albumin

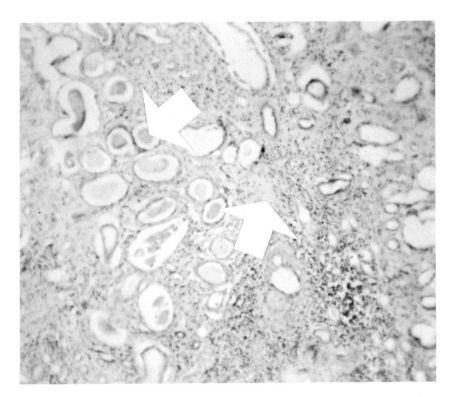

Chronic glomerulonephritis. Normal glomeruli are largely replaced by hyaline material (*upper arrow*). In many areas, tubules are replaced by fibrosis (*lower arrow*).

and casts are likely to be found in the urine; the concentrating power of the kidney has largely been lost because the atrophied convoluted tubules can no longer absorb water normally. The specific gravity is usually fixed at around 1.010; nitrogen retention increases, and azotemia (the presence of urea and other nitrogenous bodies in the blood) follows. Edema disappears but the blood pressure climbs. The left side of the heart enlarges. Hypertension may cause brain and retinal hemorrhages; indeed, hypertension dominates this phase.

Polyuria represents the efforts of the failing kidney to excrete waste products. Since the kidney can no longer concentrate urine, it must pour out great quantities of fluid to carry the solids.

Management

The treatment of acute glomerulonephritis is obviously a major undertaking that requires a full team effort. It centers around management of the individual problems. An antibiotic is administered to bring infection under control. The patient is kept at bed rest until the hematuria, edema, and hypertension have cleared. Constant monitoring of fluid and electrolyte balance is carried out. Meticulous dietary measures are essential.

Antihypertensive therapy may be needed. Dialysis may be effective in severe edema. If the disease progresses to the stage of latent chronic glomerulonephritis, no active treatment is necessary, since there are no symptoms or abnormal physical findings and the patient can anticipate a state of good health lasting many years. But, once renal function decreases to below 10 to 20 per cent of normal—the stage of advanced chronic disease —the course is steadily downhill. Although the patient may still have months or even a few years left to him, the disease will eventually be fatal.

NEPHROTIC SYNDROME

Nephrotic syndrome refers to the concurrent occurrence of marked proteinuria, hypoalbuminemia, and generalized edema. The causes of nephrotic syndrome are many. *All involve the glomeruli*, and all result in tubular degeneration. A list of causes would include inflammatory renal diseases (e.g., acute glomerulonephritis), glomerular disease associated with another systemic disease (e.g., secondary syphilis), mechanical disorders (e.g., thrombosis of a renal vein), poisons (e.g., mercury), and miscellaneous causes (e.g., renal transplant).

Pathophysiology

CONSEQUENCES
OF SEVERE
PROTEIN LOSS

The massive urinary losses of albumin—the protein that maintains the osmotic pressure of the blood—effect a plasma-to-interstitial fluid shift of water and electrolytes. This causes edema, which develops first in dependent parts and later is generalized. Protein losses in the urine may amount to from 7 to 20 gm. per day. Hypertension is present in some cases, based on the type of glomerular disease. The high protein losses result in malnutrition, and this, in turn, is responsible for muscle wasting. Hyperlipemia (abnormally high blood lipids) is also present.

Management

The first need in treatment is to treat the underlying disease as vigorously as possible, and then to treat the syndrome itself. This is accomplished through dietary sodium restriction and administration of diuretics. As the nephrotic syndrome is chronic in most cases, the patient is encouraged to follow his customary routine as far as possible.

ARTERIOLAR NEPHROSCLEROSIS

The kidney is always involved in all forms of hypertension, although it is not always clear whether the kidney damage is a cause or an effect of the hypertension. The term *arteriolar nephrosclerosis* refers to thickening of the afferent renal arterioles—the minute arterial branches that convey blood to the glomeruli. As a consequence of this sclerosis, there is fibrosis, ischemic necrosis, and destruction of glomeruli (described earlier in this chapter; the general effects of hypertension were mentioned in Chap. 16). To take that discussion a step further, one can see that hypertension, rather than renal disease per se, may cause a patient's death by placing an enormous workload on the heart and thus leading to heart failure, or by placing an enormous workload on the arteries to the brain and thus leading to cerebral hemorrhage.

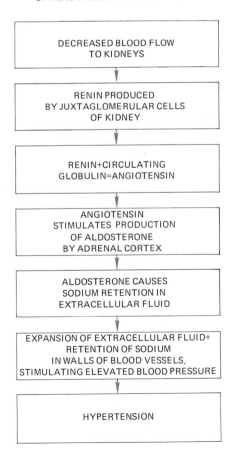

SEQUENCE IN DEVELOPMENT
OF RENOVASCULAR HYPERTENSION

DECREASED BLOOD FLOW
TO KIDNEYS

RENIN PRODUCED
BY JUXTAGLOMERULAR CELLS
OF KIDNEY

RENIN+CIRCULATING
GLOBULIN=ANGIOTENSIN

ANGIOTENSIN
STIMULATES PRODUCTION
OF ALDOSTERONE
BY ADRENAL CORTEX

ALDOSTERONE CAUSES
SODIUM RETENTION IN
EXTRACELLULAR FLUID

EXPANSION OF EXTRACELLULAR FLUID+
RETENTION OF SODIUM
IN WALLS OF BLOOD VESSELS,
STIMULATING ELEVATED BLOOD PRESSURE

HYPERTENSION

Pathophysiology

Arteriolar nephrosclerosis may run a *benign* or a *malignant* course. The benign form is most likely to be found in persons above 35 years of age. There are few symptoms, and renal insufficiency does not appear until late in the course. The disease pattern in this type is patchy, with areas where glomeruli and tubules have disappeared alternating with areas where they are intact. The malignant form actually represents the end stage of chronic glomerulonephritis. This is the situation referred to as *malignant nephrosclerosis* or *malignant hypertension*. The course is far more rapid than the benign form, with the stages of albuminuria, hypertension, failing renal function, and eye changes proceeding rapidly. These patients are usually in younger age groups.

VICIOUS CIRCLE OF HYPERTENSION AND RENAL SCLEROSIS

Management

The overall management of glomerulonephritis and hypertension has been described earlier. We would emphasize here the importance of helping the patient to find ways to deal more effectively with stressful situations, if he cannot avoid them. Use of diuretics and other therapeutic modalities is described elsewhere in this book.

PYELONEPHRITIS

Pyelonephritis is an acute diffuse infection of the kidney pelvis and underlying kidney tissues caused by pyogenic (pus-forming) bacteria. Pyelitis and pyelonephritis may be considered a single disease, since there is always involvement of the substance of the kidney in infections of the kidney pelvis. The disease primarily involves the interstitial tissue of the kidney, although eventually the nephrons become involved. *Acute* and *chronic* forms are recognized, although there is some uncertainty regarding their relationship since many patients who have had several attacks of acute pyelonephritis never progress to the chronic stage. One or both kidneys may be involved and the infection may be primary or secondary to another disorder. Pyelonephritis is the most common type of renal disease.

Pathophysiology

Acute pyelonephritis affects both the kidney pelvis and the interstitial tissue. Infection occurs by way of the bloodstream or lymphatics from foci of infection elsewhere in the body, by direct spread from adjacent structures, or by ascending infection from the bladder. The most common causative organism is *E. coli,* which is found in about half the cases. Other causative bacteria include the colon bacillus, staphylococcus, streptococcus, *Proteus vulgaris, Pseudomonas aeruginosa,* and *Aerobacter aerogenes.* Mixed infections are common.

Among the important predisposing factors the following should be mentioned: (1) obstruction—flow of urine is impeded, which favors bacterial infection; (2) age and sex—incidence is high during the first 18 months of life and in women of childbearing age; (3) urinary tract instrumentation—bacteria are carried into the tract during catheterization, cystoscopy, and similar procedures; (4) diabetes mellitus—renal papillary necrosis, a severe form of acute pyelonephritis, is frequently found in diabetics.

BACTERIAL BASIS OF PYELONEPHRITIS

The kidney is swollen, soft, and congested and the lining of the pelvis is diffusely inflamed. Many small abscesses are seen in this area of inflammation; they bulge under the kidney capsule or protrude from the surface as small pustules.

Usually the onset is sudden with symptoms of chills, fever, abdominal pain, backache, general toxicity, nausea, and vomiting. Urinary output may be decreased, although frequency and urgency are noted. Pus cells and bacteria are found in the urine.

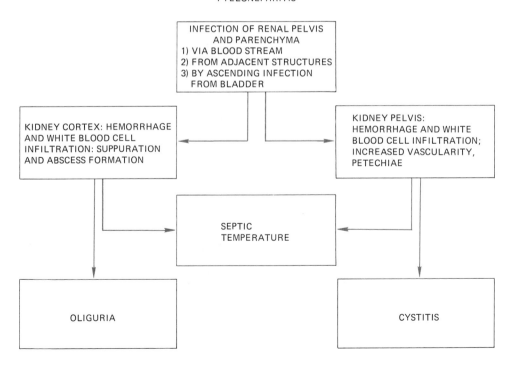

SEQUENCE OF EVENTS:
PYELONEPHRITIS

INFECTION OF RENAL PELVIS AND PARENCHYMA
1) VIA BLOOD STREAM
2) FROM ADJACENT STRUCTURES
3) BY ASCENDING INFECTION FROM BLADDER

KIDNEY CORTEX: HEMORRHAGE AND WHITE BLOOD CELL INFILTRATION: SUPPURATION AND ABSCESS FORMATION

KIDNEY PELVIS: HEMORRHAGE AND WHITE BLOOD CELL INFILTRATION; INCREASED VASCULARITY, PETECHIAE

SEPTIC TEMPERATURE

OLIGURIA

CYSTITIS

Chronic pyelonephritis is the name given to the condition resulting from injury due to previous bacterial infections, as well as the progressive stage due to recurring bacterial infection. There are now irreversible degenerative changes in the kidney due to extensive scarring. The kidney is small and atrophic, the pelvic mucosa is pale and fibrotic, and many nephrons are destroyed. In addition, areas of acute infection may be noted, which could account for the continued presence of urinary pus and bactria. Hypertension develops in some cases, bringing with it the complications of coronary and cerebrovascular disease.

The patient with acute pyelonephritis is acutely ill. His symptoms include flank pain, chills, fever, and nausea, and he may note frequency and burning on urination. Any obstruction to urinary flow must be corrected. The physician prescribes an antibiotic after sensitivity testing of the urine has identified the responsible organism. Bed rest and adequate fluid intake are important factors in care. In the absence of complications the prognosis for complete cure is excellent. Should the disease enter the chronic stage, as may occur with recurrence of infection or continued obstruction, the patient may appear to be asymptomatic except for slight fever, anemia, and gastrointestinal discomfort. Here the goal is to prevent further damage, for which intensive antibiotic therapy is employed. The patient may be able to continue his customary routine for months or even many years, until uremia, intercurrent infection, or coronary or cerebrovascular complications develop in the terminal stage.

DIALYSIS AND TRANSPLANTATION

Two therapeutic modalities have been developed in recent years that are significantly changing the picture in renal disease. These are renal dialysis and renal transplantation.

Dialysis

Renal dialysis removes harmful substances in the patient who is seriously ill due to acute or chronic renal failure or exogenous poisoning, or who has generalized edema. The methods of dialysis utilized at present are hemodialysis (also referred to as *extracorporeal dialysis*) and peritoneal dialysis. The basic principle of both methods is diffusion of substances through a semipermeable membrane in response to a concentration gradient from the plasma to a dialysate. The choice of method is based on the patient's clinical condition and the facilities available.

Hemodialysis   The semipermeable membrane used in hemodialysis is cellophane. This membrane has pores similar to those of the glomerular capillaries. As blood is removed from the patient's radial or brachial artery, it is pumped through the cellophane tube, which is immersed in the dialysate, or electrolyte solution. In this way water, exogenous poison, plus urea and other end-products of protein catabolism are removed from the blood. Blood continuously recirculates between the patient and dialysate for a period of 4 to 7 hours. The dialysate is changed at intervals to prevent accumulation of toxins. The procedure is complicated, requiring a knowledgeable team, precise technique, and extensive equipment. It is also expensive.

Peritoneal dialysis   In contrast to hemodialysis, which is considerably more effective, peritoneal dialysis is both less expensive and simpler, since neither a specially equipped hospital nor highly trained personnel is required. Nevertheless, competent nursing personnel and supervision by a physician are certainly necessary. In this method, the dialysate is introduced at intervals into the peritoneal cavity, the surface of the peritoneum acting as the semipermeable membrane. Thus toxins and wastes are removed from the patient's body.

A new chapter in medical history   The invention, development, and refinement of renal dialysis, or the artificial kidney, as it was called in the early 1900's when the work was begun, is surely one of medicine's exciting chapters. Without any doubt, renal dialysis has been the means of sustaining large numbers of patients who would otherwise have succumbed to acute or chronic renal failure or to certain types of poisoning. Survival rates range from a few months to many years. With further improvements in technique and equipment, still higher survival rates may be anticipated. Patients have been enabled to return to their customary occupations and to resume productive living. And today, thanks to the availability of home dialysis units, many patients enjoy considerable independence, since they can arrange their dialysis procedures in the manner best suited to their particular needs.

Transplantation

The advent of renal transplantation has brought the hope of leading a nearly normal life to the patient dying of end-stage renal disease. Although transplantation is still considered an experimental procedure, a successful "take" offers the recipient a better quality of life than the best hemodialysis program. Many of the techniques in use today were developed by Alexis Carrel at the turn of the century. His subjects were dogs, and although the transplants were initially functional they quickly underwent a destructive process. Then in 1944 Peter Medawar (later Sir Peter Medawar) worked out the genetic basis and described this process of rejection. The first human kidney transplantation was accomplished in Boston in 1954 by Dr. Joseph Murray and colleagues.

Any patient with end-stage chronic renal disease who can no longer

PRINCIPLE OF SELF—NOT SELF BASIS FOR TRANSPLANT REJECTION

be managed satisfactorily on a conservative outpatient basis may be considered for renal transplantation. Both donor and recipient require expert evaluation, which is carried out in a hospital. The donor's examination consists of tissue typing, physical examination, electrocardiogram, evaluation of kidney function, and other measures. The recipient, while awaiting the transplant operation, is maintained by means of dialysis, physical therapy, and additional measures designed to put him in optimal condition for surgery. The operation consists of transplanting the donor kidney retroperitoneally into either iliac fossa of the recipient. The ureter of the new kidney is transplanted into the bladder or anastomosed to the recipient's ureter. Infection is a critical postoperative complication, because the immunosuppressive drugs administered to reduce or overcome the patient's natural defenses that would otherwise cause rejection of the graft as a foreign substance also increase his susceptibility to infection.

The factor of *histocompatibility* (acceptance or rejection of grafted tissue) is all-important. The closer the relationship between donor and recipient, the more likely is the transplant to be accepted by the body tissue (recall the self-not self concept described in Chap. 3). The seventh report of the Human Kidney Transplant Registry covers 2,321 transplants performed up to January, 1969. The 1-year recipient survival rate was 91 per cent where the donor was a twin or other sibling; 83 per cent where the donor was a parent; and only 42 per cent where a cadaver kidney was used.

The chief areas of research are, in addition to histocompatibility, organ storage and preservation, and immunology. Then there is the urgent problem of expense, since the total cost of transplantation and the lifelong care that is thereafter necessary is astronomical. Despite the formidable problems remaining to be solved, it appears that transplantation is on the way to becoming an acceptable method of treating otherwise incurable renal disease.

NEOPLASMS

The urologic system is the site of about one-fifth of all tumors in adults and about one-fourth of all tumors in children.

Pathophysiology

Kidney   Tumors may arise in the renal parenchyma, pelvis, or capsule, and well over 70 per cent of these are carcinomas. Males 45 to 60 years of age are mainly affected. Although spontaneous regression of renal carcinoma has been documented, the overall prognosis is poor. Hematuria, weight loss, flank pain, fever, and abdominal pain are the prominent symptoms, resulting from tumor engorgement on kidney tissues and blood vessels. The most common renal tumor of childhood is Wilms' tumor, which usually develops before the child is 5 years old, with the chief finding being an abdominal mass.

Bladder   Tumors of the bladder epithelium may at first appear to be benign, only to become invasive or recur following removal. Industrial exposure to aniline dyes is the most frequent contributing factor; excessive cigarette smoking has also been implicated. Hematuria is the chief symptom. If the tumor obstructs the ureteral opening or the bladder neck, azotemia may develop, and with infection of the tumor surface, there is painful urination, pus in the urine, burning, and frequency. Hemorrhage may occur. Tumor enlargement causes pelvic and leg pain due to pressure on nerves.

Urethra   These tumors are rare in both men and women, which is fortunate, since the prognosis is always poor. Most are of the squamous cell type and arise from the distal urethra. Bleeding from the urethra and difficulty in voiding are the usual symptoms.

UROLOGIC
NEOPLASMS
HEAVILY
INFLUENCED
BY INDUSTRIAL
EXPOSURE

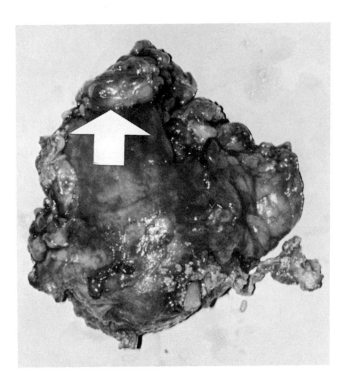

Carcinoma of the bladder showing numerous raised overgrowths. Arrow points to one such overgrowth.

Management

As in all other types of cancer, time is of the essence. In many instances early diagnosis makes the difference between a long and comfortable survival period and rapid metastasis and death. Surgery for operable neoplasms is frequently followed by radiotherapy and chemotherapy. In inoperable cases, relief of pain and other symptoms can usually be provided by drugs.

CALCULI

Urinary calculi (singular, calculus), or stones, may form in the kidney, ureter, bladder, or urethra. They result from the deposit of crystalline substances (calcium oxalate, calcium phosphate, uric acid, and cystine) that are normally excreted in urine. These *concretions* vary in size from granular deposits (sand or gravel) to stones as large as an orange.

Pathophysiology

The cause of calculi is not known, although it appears that infection, urinary stasis, high urinary concentration, sulfonamide therapy, long periods of immobilization, and excessive excretion of phosphorus are predisposing factors.

Excessive ingestion of calcium leading to hypervitaminosis D is a possible factor; so is abnormal excretion of uric acid, such as occurs in gout. Hyperparathyroidism due to a tumor may cause too much calcium phosphate to be removed from bone and deposited in the kidneys. There may be multiple calculi, and both kidneys may be affected. The stones may cause obstruction leading to urinary stasis; this favors infection. Many patients are asymptomatic until the stones enter and obstruct the ureter, when *renal colic* occurs. This excruciating pain originates in the renal area and radiates down the thigh; the patient writhes in agony. The attack may last for several hours. The little urine that is passed is bloody because of the abrasive action of the stone.

EFFECT OF
CALCIUM
METABOLISM

Management

Since in some cases calculi are passed spontaneously, the physician usually delays instrumental intervention until it is certain that the calculi will not be passed. The patient who passes calculi is instructed to drink liquids copiously. Antispasmodics and certain phosphate salts may be prescribed, the latter in the hope of preventing further calculus formation. Stones that are not passed spontaneously must be removed. As they tend to recur, the patient must follow a prophylactic program including high fluid intake, avoidance of all factors that might predispose to infection, and adherence to the prescribed diet.

RENAL TUBERCULOSIS

Although renal tuberculosis is uncommon, it merits a place in this book because it is always secondary to tuberculosis elsewhere in the body, developing from foci carried by the bloodstream to the kidney at the time of the primary infection.

Pathophysiology

The infectious process generally begins in one of the renal pyramids. Tuberculous ulceration into the renal pelvis follows as the bacilli are carried down with the urine into the bladder. The wall of the ureter becomes thickened and its lumen narrowed; the lumen may be completely blocked, effectively cutting off the kidney from the bladder. Bladder infection and destruction of the ureterovesical valve follow, favoring an ascending infection of the remaining healthy kidney. Suggestive early symptoms are pus in the urine and renal hemorrhage, causing hematuria. Later on there is urinary pain and frequency.

Management

Medical treatment is nearly always effective. A two-drug program consisting of streptomycin and isoniazid or para-aminosalicylic acid is effective in the majority of patients. Nephrectomy or another surgical procedure may on occasion be necessary if there is obstruction with a complicating pyogenic infection. The potential danger is, of course, a serious involvement of the second kidney, and therefore every effort is made to prevent this development.

CYSTITIS

Cystitis is an acute or chronic inflammation of the urinary bladder. It is fairly common and would be even more frequent were it not for the natural resistance of the bladder lining, which tends to prevent an inflammatory process from becoming established following the occasional invasion of the bladder by bacteria.

Pathophysiology

Cystitis has many causes, of which the most common will be mentioned. Normally, the contents of the bladder are sterile; bacteria are carried there via infection of the kidney, prostate, or urethra. Any condition that prevents normal adequate emptying of the bladder will contribute to cystitis; this category includes irritation due to foreign bodies or calculi, enlargement of the prostate, urethral stricture, unsterile catheterization, major surgical procedures, difficult childbirth, and prolonged immobilization. Patients with poorly controlled diabetes mellitus often are affected. In women, cystitis may develop following urethral irritation after sexual intercourse ("honeymoon cystitis").

The bladder trigone may show increased vascularity or even generalized edema and ulceration. In cystitis of long duration, the bladder may become thick-walled and contracted, so that its capacity is reduced. Frequency, burning, and hematuria result from the irritation; if bacteremia is present there will be chills and fever.

Management

Any obstruction to urinary drainage must be removed. Antibacterial therapy and ample fluid intake are prescribed. Symptomatic therapy, including bed rest and sitz baths, helps to relieve the pain and discomfort. In chronic cystitis, repeated bladder irrigation with a saline solution may be necessary. Alcohol and highly seasoned foods must be eliminated from the diet.

CONGENITAL ANOMALIES OF THE URINARY SYSTEM

Congenital anomalies are found more often in the urinary system than in any other, probably because of the complex development during embryonic life of the specialized structures of this system. Some of these defects, such as absence of both kidneys, are incompatible with life. Several cause mechanical difficulties contributing to urinary stasis, infection, formation of calculi, renal insufficiency, and hypertension. Anomalous structures may be mistaken for cysts or tumors. Finally, certain anomalies of the system are frequently seen in association with disorders of other systems or organs.

Pathophysiology

Kidney   Renal anomalies include abnormalities of number, size, structure, form, and location. Clinical symptoms become apparent if the defect interferes with the transport of urine. One or both kidneys may be absent (renal agenesis), or there may be an extra kidney (supernumerary kidney). The kidneys may be fused in a horseshoe shape (horseshoe kidney) or abnormal in location (ectopic kidney). Abnormal (aberrant) arteries may obstruct the ureter. In polycystic disease, a rare familial condition, the kidneys are converted into masses of cysts. Congenital kidney anomalies may be associated with congenital heart disease or cerebral aneurysm.

Ureters   The incidence of ureteral anomalies is high; like those of the kidney, such defects become evident when transport of urine is disrupted. The ureter may drain abnormally, so that urine passes into the urethra, prostate, vagina, uterus, seminal vesicle, or bowel (ureteral reflux). Ureteral obstruction may cause distention of the renal pelvis and calyx with urine—a condition called *hydronephrosis*.

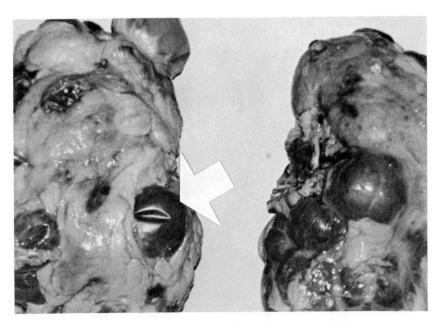

Cystic disease of the kidneys. Normally smooth kidney surface is interrupted by many swellings, or cysts (*arrow*). The cysts have largely replaced functional renal tissue, making normal function impossible.

Bladder   Among the bladder anomalies that should be noted, two—absence of the bladder (agenesis) and dwarf bladder (hypoplasia)—are extremely rare. Diverticula, which we discussed in relation to the digestive system (Chap. 18) are also seen in the bladder; occasionally they are congenital, but more often are acquired in adulthood as a result of an obstruction. Bladder reduplication, or bladder division, means that the bladder is divided by a septum into two more or less distinct parts. Bladder exstrophy is a congenital malformation in which the bladder appears to be turned inside out, i.e., the internal surface of the posterior wall shows through the opening in the anterior wall.

Urethra   Numerous congenital malformations can involve the urethra; only the most common ones will be mentioned here. Congenital urethral *valves* are deep mucosal folds situated in the posterior urethra which may cause urethral obstruction. A urethral *stricture* is a pathologic narrowing of the lumen. As with the bladder, urethral duplication is possible.

Management

Many congenital urologic anomalies can be treated by surgical means. In some instances an anomalous malpositioned structure can be transposed to the normal position.

THE MALE GENITAL TRACT

DISEASES OF
MALE GENITAL
TRACT CAUSE
FUNCTIONAL
ABNORMALITIES
OF BOTH
SYSTEMS

Although several organs of the male genital tract really belong to the reproductive system, their diseases cause changes in the urologic system, so it is logical to include them here. Furthermore, it is the urologist who treats these diseases.

Prostatism

It will be recalled that the prostate is an accessory sex organ located just below the urinary bladder; it produces seminal fluid containing substances needed for sperm nutrition. The urinary stream travels in the urethra through the center of the gland. Prostatism refers to any prostate disease that causes obstruction of the bladder outlet. The most common causes are benign prostatic hypertrophy, fibrosis, and carcinoma. Prostatism is extremely common in men above 60 years of age.

Benign prostatic hypertrophy   Under the influence of male hormones (or perhaps another factor not recognized at present) the periurethral glandular tissue undergoes hyperplasia and the gland enlarges. This expansion is not in itself critical; what is of concern is the inward encroachment of this tissue, which causes a marked decrease in the diameter of the prostatic urethra.

Multiple nodules develop under the epithelium of the posterior urethra. As they enlarge they compress the prostatic tissue laterally. The bladder becomes increasingly irritable and urgency, frequency, and smarting are noted, even though the urinary stream is normal. Then partial urinary obstruction develops along with nocturia, increased frequency, incomplete emptying of the bladder, a small feeble stream, and straining on urination. The congestion may cause hematuria; eventually there may be overflow, dribbling, and a developing uremia. The stagnant urine easily becomes infected, giving rise to symptoms of chills, fever, nausea, and vomiting. Palliative treatment, such as avoidance of highly seasoned foods, cold, dampness, and alcohol, may be sufficient in mild cases. The patient is also advised to avoid sexual excesses. When these measures prove insufficient, a prostatectomy (removal of the gland) is performed.

Carcinoma   Prostatic carcinoma occurs in 15 to 30 per cent of males above the age of 60. The usual site of origin is the posterior lobe of the prostate, whence the tumor spreads by local infiltration into the remainder of the gland, the seminal vesicles, and the bladder. The symptoms generally are similar to those of benign prostatic hypertrophy. Unfortunately, this carcinoma is highly malignant and metastasizes to bone, brain, and lungs; hormonal therapy, however, usually affords a long period of comfort, even though it may increase the chances for cerebrovascular accidents. Once this therapy is no longer effective—in most cases after several years—a prostatectomy is carried out.

Fibrosis   This disorder is often associated with urethral strictures because the inflammatory process may involve both organs. Fibrosis may also cause increased rigidity of the urethrovesical junction. Prostatectomy is undertaken in most cases.

Carcinoma

Prostatic carcinoma has already been mentioned. The penis and the testes are also sites of malignant neoplasms.

Penis   Carcinoma of the penis is relatively common among uncircumcised men and extremely rare among circumcised men. These neoplasms are of the squamous cell type and are, fortunately, relatively slow-growing. They account for about 3 per cent of all skin cancers. They are treated by local measures or, if necessary, by amputation.

Testis   Tumors of the testis may develop in adults between the ages of 20 and 35 years; they are, in fact, the most common type of neoplasm in this age group. These tumors are usually highly malignant, and tend to metastasize via the bloodstream and the lymphatics. Orchiectomy (removal of a testis) followed by irradiation is carried out. In some instances, the involved lymph glands are surgically removed.

Gonorrhea

A sharp increase in the incidence of this disease over the past several years has made everyone concerned with public health aware that enormous efforts must be made to bring this plague under control. Several days after sexual exposure in which gonococcal infection has occurred, there is a purulent and painful urethral discharge. The infection spreads to the seminal vesicles and the epididymis, causing urethritis, prostatitis, and seminal vesiculitis, and thence to sites outside the genital tract where it results in such infections as arthritis, endocarditis, and meningitis. Penicillin is still the drug of choice for treatment of gonorrhea, although the emergence of resistant gonococcal strains now makes it necessary to employ a much larger dose than in the past.

Epididymitis

The epididymis is the excretory duct of the testis. Any urinary tract infection may produce epididymitis, since the organisms pass upward through the urethra, the ejaculatory duct, the vas deferens, and the epididymis. Epididymitis is, therefore, a secondary infection. The epididymis becomes enlarged and hard, and the groin area becomes very painful. Bed rest, scrotal support, and heat applications are effective measures. Antibiotic therapy may be indicated.

Urethritis

Neisseria gonorrhoeae, the causative organism of gonorrhea, can attack the mucous membrane of the urethra, causing increased vascularity and other signs of inflammation along with symptoms of urinary pain and discomfort and a thick purulent discharge from the meatus. This type of urethritis is referred to as *gonococcal urethritis.* When urethritis is caused by organisms other than *N. gonorrhoeae,* it is designated *nonspecific* urethritis. Bacteria normally present in the distal urethra cause no difficulty unless the tissue is traumatized, as may occur with catheterization or vigorous sexual intercourse. Then these bacteria are carried along the urethra to cause inflammation and other symptoms just mentioned. Penicillin is prescribed if the urethritis is gonococcal in nature. Avoidance of catheterization, intake of copious amounts of fluids, and such comfort measures as frequent sitz baths are recommended.

USUAL URINE ABNORMALITIES IN RENAL DISEASE

Disease	Appearance	Volume	Specific Gravity	Protein	Deposit
Acute glomerulonephritis	Smoky or red	Decreased	High	Present	Red cells and casts
Nephrotic syndrome	Normal or pale	Normal	Normal range at first, low and fixed later	Present in large amounts	Casts
Chronic renal disease	Pale	Increased	Low and fixed	Trace	Casts and few red cells
Acute pyelonephritis	Cloudy; "fishy" odor	Often decreased	Normal range unless previous renal damage	Present	Pus cells and bacteria

Prostatitis

Like urethritis, prostatitis may also follow gonococcal infection. The *chronic* form is quite common during the middle years. Although there may be no symptoms, the prostate is enlarged and soft, with areas of induration. Usually the seminal vesicles are involved in the inflammatory process. In the *acute* form the patient notes chills and fever, and may have urinary symptoms. The prostate is swollen and tender, and abscesses may be noted. Bed rest, heat, high liquid intake, and other general comfort measures are carried out.

TOPICS FOR DISCUSSION

1. What essential regulatory functions does the urinary system exercise?

2. Why may the cells of the renal tubules be more important than brain cells?

3. Would you accept dialysis by the artificial kidney and all the discomfort and trouble it entails? Temporarily? Permanently?

4. What psychological traits are desirable in the patient who must undergo hemodialysis for a prolonged period?

5. For what organs other than the kidney are there replacements?

6. In what types of poisoning is the artificial kidney useful? If an artificial kidney was unavailable, what other form of dialysis could be used?

7. How does the urologic system interrelate with the reproductive system?

8. What changes can occur in the kidney as a result of psychic tension? What disease might result?

9. How do males and females differ in their susceptibility to infection of the urogenital tract? Why?

10. How can a thorough understanding of the nephron facilitate understanding of diseases of the kidney?

11. What might be the ethical, financial, and legal implications associated with a community-wide renal dialysis program?

12. What moral and ethical problems are involved in considering renal transplantation?

20

common diseases of the reproductive system

Among all the manifestations of human existence, probably none has stirred man's imagination as powerfully as has the idea of reproduction of his own kind. One group of writers put it this way: "In all Nature's wide universe of miracles there is no process more wondrous, no mechanism more incredibly fantastic, than the one by which a tiny speck of tissue, the human egg, develops into a 7-pound baby. So miraculous did primitive peoples consider this phenomenon that they frequently ascribed it all to superhuman intervention and even overlooked the fact that sexual intercourse was a necessary precursor." * One might add that although volumes have been written on ovulation, gestation, infant and maternal care, and growth and development, no one yet knows what causes the "alarm" to ring after a period of almost exactly 9 months, thereby setting in motion the chain of events that culminates in the birth of a human being.

The reproductive system is the only one not intimately involved in homeostasis. It has, nevertheless, an obvious close relationship to the endocrine system, since reproductive system function is under hormonal control, which itself is under pituitary regulation. This relationship suggests the important part played by both psychic and somatic factors in reproductive system physiology and pathophysiology.

THE MENSTRUAL CYCLE

It will be recalled that the normal mentrual cycle consists of three phases. During the *proliferative* phase (fifth to fourteenth day of the cycle) the anterior pituitary gland stimulates secretion of follicle-stimulating hormone (FSH), causing a rise in estrogen level and proliferation of endometrial tissue. This phase is followed by the *secretory* phase

* Fitzpatrick, E., Reeder, S. R., and Mastroianni, L., Jr.: Maternity Nursing. ed. 12. Philadelphia, J. B. Lippincott Co., 1971.

PATHOPHYSIOLOGIC PROCESSES WHICH CAN BE INVOLVED
IN DISEASES OF THE REPRODUCTIVE SYSTEM

	Genetics: Diseases Due to Hereditary Factors	Disease Due to Hypersensitivity and Autoimmunity	Infectious Diseases	Diseases Due to Physical Agents	Diseases Due to Chemical Agents	Neoplasia	Disturbances of Fluid and Electrolyte Balance	Diseases of Malnutrition	Endocrine Dysfunction	Stress Factors in Disease	The Aging Process	Psychosomatic Factors in Disease
Dysmenorrhea			■			■			■			■
Premenstrual Tension							■		■			■
Menopausal Syndrome	■			■	■				■	■	■	■
Abortion			■	■	■				■			■
Toxemia of Pregnancy					■		■	■	■			
Neoplasms (Female)						■						
Endocervicitis			■									
Pelvic Inflammatory Disease			■									
Neoplasms (Male)						■						

(fourteenth to twenty-fifth days) when the endometrial glands lengthen and endometrial hyperplasia and vascularization occur in preparation for the fertilized ovum. In the absence of fertilization, the corpus luteum atrophies and the endometrium desquamates, thereby bringing about the *menstrual* phase (after the twenty-eighth day), when the necrotic endometrial tissue, consisting of blood, endometrial fragments, and mucin from the endometrial glands, is discharged. The first day of menstruation is counted as the first day of the menstrual cycle.

MENSTRUAL DISORDERS

Dysmenorrhea, or painful menstruation, may be *primary* (unassociated with known pathology) or *secondary* (associated with a frank physical disorder). Emotional and psychologic factors are thought to contribute prominently to the primary type.

PSYCHIC FACTORS MAY PLAY PROMINENT ROLE

Pathophysiology

Cramping pain, which may be mild or severe, is felt in the lower abdomen. It may be associated with expulsion of casts or clots. Pain may start just before menstruation, or it may appear during the period; its duration may be from a few hours to several days.

In primary dysmenorrhea the pain may be due to an increase in uterine irritability leading to intense uterine contractions. In the secondary type the list of possibilities includes endometriosis (in which tissue resembling endometrium proliferates aberrantly in the pelvic cavity), pelvic tumors, stenosis of the uterine cervix, uterine displacement, and pelvic inflammatory disease. Poor postural habits or constipation may contribute to both forms. The birth of a child usually brings an abrupt and dramatic end to primary dysmenorrhea; surgical or medical treatment is required to correct the secondary type.

Management

Heat, in the form of a hot water bottle or an electric pad, and mild analgesics usually ease the crampy pain. The patient is encouraged to get sufficient rest and to correct or avoid "tension" factors in her daily activities. If an underlying physical disorder is the cause of the discomfort, it should, of course, be corrected if possible. Many "old wives' tales" continue to be passed along by persons who are ignorant of facts relating to female physiology. In such instances, it may be that explanation and reassurance by the physician and the health care team are all the treatment that is needed.

PREMENSTRUAL TENSION

Premenstrual tension develops in many women 5 to 10 days preceding the menstrual period. This clinical syndrome is characterized by symptoms of edginess, irritability, pronounced emotional swings, feelings of intolerable tension, insomnia, headache, vertigo, nausea, depression, edema, and sore breasts—all of which disappear shortly after menstruation begins.

Pathophysiology

The theories suggested to explain premenstrual tension almost equal the potential symptoms in number. Certainly psychosomatic factors are sometimes contributory; conversely, premenstrual tension may cause psychologic disturbances, as evidenced by the fact that many of the crimes committed by women are carried out during this unsettling time. Other factors cited include an increase in antidiuretic hormone (ADH), causing abnormal retention of water; undesignated "menstrual toxins"; disturbances of the autonomic nervous system (virtually the same as psychosomatic factors); hypoglycemia; allergy to ovarian hormones; and temporary endocrine imbalance.

Management

A low-salt diet and diuretics relieve the edema that is usually associated with premenstrual tension. It is, of course, to the patient's benefit to make efforts aimed at correcting the emotional "trigger" factors in her life. If these efforts are not sufficient, psychiatric treatment may be sought.

ABORTION

Abortion, often called miscarriage by the layman, is the termination of pregnancy before the fetus is viable. Abortion may be *spontaneous,* that is, one in which the process starts of its own accord, or *induced,* that is, one that is accomplished through artificial means, whether for therapeutic or other reasons.

Pathophysiology

SPONTANEOUS
ABORTION A
USEFUL
PHENOMENON

Spontaneous abortion   About 75 per cent of *spontaneous abortions* occur during the second and third months of pregnancy; about one pregnancy in every ten terminates in this way. The commonest cause is an inherent defect in the product of conception, either an abnormal embryo or an abnormal trophoblast (the layer of cells that secures food for the embryo). Abortion from this cause really serves a useful purpose, for it is Nature's way of extinguishing embryos that are imperfect. Severe infection, heart failure, endocrine dysfunction, trauma, and reproductive tract abnormalities are other causes.

The first symptom is bleeding, due to separation of the fertilized ovum from its uterine attachment. The bleeding may be slight at first and may continue for several days until uterine cramps appear, or it may be profuse and followed immediately by cramps. Contractions of the uterus cause the cervix to soften and dilate so that finally the embryo is expelled either partially or completely.

DEVELOPMENT OF ABORTION

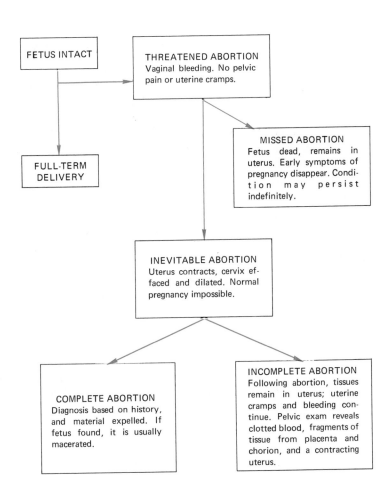

In *threatened* abortion, a patient in early pregnancy has vaginal bleeding and may have mild cramps. The cervix is closed. With adequate treatment the pregnancy may proceed normally. *Inevitable* abortion means that the process has gone so far that it is impossible to prevent termination of the pregnancy. Bleeding is profuse, and the cervical canal is dilating. An *incomplete* abortion is one in which part of the product of conception has been passed but part is retained in the uterus, so that bleeding continues until the retained part (referred to as the *secundine*) has been expelled. In *complete* abortion the entire product of conception is expelled. A *missed* abortion is the situation in which the fetus dies in the uterus but is retained there for 2 months or longer before being expelled. The term *habitual* abortion refers to the occurrence of spontaneous abortion in three or more successive pregnancies.

Induced abortion: therapeutic type   In therapeutic, or medical, abortion, the physician terminates the pregnancy after it has been determined that the pregnancy poses a threat to the physical or mental health of the mother or because it involves a high risk of fetal malformation. The number of such abortions has increased in recent years as a result of liberalization of abortion laws in many states. Several induction techniques are available; whichever one is employed, the procedure is always carried out under surgical asepsis in a hospital setting.

Induced abortion: criminal type   Criminal abortion is the termination of pregnancy accomplished outside of appropriate medical facilities. It is usually done by nonphysicians. Ingestion of strong cathartic drugs, and the insertion of a foreign body into the uterus, are among the methods employed. These crude efforts carried out in a septic environment often end not in successful abortion, but in puerperal sepsis, a severe infection that is frequently associated with shock and generalized peritonitis; it is often fatal. Thus criminal abortion is the direct cause of the majority of maternal deaths in the United States.

Management

Treatment is planned on the basis of symptoms. Conservative measures, such as light diet, bed rest, and avoidance of straining, may be sufficient in threatened abortion. Incomplete abortion is treated by curettage (gentle surgical scraping) and drugs that stimulate uterine contractions. In most cases of missed abortion the uterus is permitted to empty itself. Since for many women the experience of an abortion is a cause of deep grief, health care personnel should be especially attentive to the psychologic state and needs of these patients.

TOXEMIA OF PREGNANCY

Toxemia of pregnancy ranks with hemorrhage and puerperal sepsis as one of the three major complications responsible for the largest number of maternal deaths in the United States. These disorders of gestation and early puerperium are characterized by one or more of the following signs: hypertension, edema, albuminuria, and in severe cases convulsions and coma. Despite intensive research, the cause remains unknown; toxemia represents one of the most important unsolved problems in the entire field of human reproduction.

Numerous factors, including endocrine dysfunction, metabolic disorders, body fluid disturbances, production of toxins, uterine ischemia, and malnutrition (especially protein deficit), are under investigation. Multiple pregnancies, hydatidiform mole, and diabetes more than double the likelihood of toxemia.

Toxemia of pregnancy is divided into two stages: the nonconvulsive stage, *preeclampsia,* and the convulsive stage, *eclampsia.* Preeclampsia is, as the term suggests, the forerunner of eclampsia; unless the preeclamptic stage is interrupted by either treatment or delivery, the eclamptic stage is almost certain to follow.

MOST CASES OF TOXEMIA ARE PREVENTABLE

The pathologic mechanism is generalized arteriolar spasm resulting in tissue hypoxia. Portal vein thrombosis may occur; brain and kidney edema is common. Sodium and water are retained. Increased blood pressure, excessive weight gain, edema, and albuminuria are manifested in headache, drowsiness, visual disturbances, dizziness, forgetfulness, nausea and vomiting, and respiratory changes. If the eclamptic stage supervenes, the jaws and then the eyelids begin to open and close violently. The other facial muscles and then all the body muscles alternately contract and relax rapidly. These movements are so forceful that the patient may throw herself out of bed and bite her tongue unless protective measures are taken. Foam, often tinged with blood, appears about the mouth and nostrils. The face is purple and congested, and the eyes are bloodshot—altogether a horrible and unforgettable picture. Coma or further convulsions may follow. In the terminal stage, the convulsions stop entirely; vascular collapse, falling blood pressure, and overwhelming pulmonary edema bring about death.

Management

Prophylaxis is obviously the most important factor in controlling toxemia, since preeclampsia is almost alway preventable. At the earliest sign of difficulty the physician will instruct the patient regarding reduced sodium intake, bed rest, and restriction of activity, and will measure blood pressure, weight, and urinary output frequently. If these steps are not corrective, the patient will be hospitalized and placed under vigilant care; sedatives, diuretics, strict dietary control, and supportive measures often suffice. If, however, eclampsia develops, delivery will be undertaken as soon as sedation and diuresis have been accomplished.

MENOPAUSAL SYNDROME

The *climacteric* is the long period during which ovarian activity gradually ceases. The term is often used interchangeably with *menopause,* the cessation of menses. The popular phrase for both of these is "change of life." Menopause is a normal physiologic process that usually takes place between the ages of 40 and 50. It is the result of ovarian atrophy, which converts the ovary to a small, pale, wrinkled structure one third the size of the active organ.

Pathophysiology

Many, probably most, women experience little or no discomfort during this time, whereas others suffer distressing (although essentially harmless) symptoms of increased nervousness, fatigability, sweating, and palpitations; perhaps the most annoying symptom is hot flashes, which may be mild and transitory or may last as long as 2 minutes and occur every 10 to 30 minutes throughout the day and night.

The cause of all these disturbances is estrogen deficiency, which appears when the ovary ceases to respond to gonadotropic stimulation by hormones of the anterior pituitary. Estrogen induces a positive calcium balance and continued osteoblastic activity; hence the lack of it is believed to account for postmenopausal osteoporosis. Skin thickness gradually decreases, as do muscle size and tension. The vagina, endometrium, and breasts atrophy. In some women—perhaps those whose diet has long been deficient in calcium or who have been relatively inactive—osteoporosis may become so pronounced several years after menopause that they suffer vertebral collapse and kidney stones due to excessive calcium excretion.

DOES DRUG-INDUCED OVARIAN STIMULATION INCREASE LIKELIHOOD OF CANCER?

Management

Estrogen therapy has proved useful in ameliorating or, in some cases, preventing the postmenopausal syndrome. The most important question relating to such therapy is whether or not endogenous estrogen induces neoplastic changes in estrogen-sensitive tissues. The consensus appears to be that, while such therapy should not be prescribed in the presence of malignant disease, it is both safe and beneficial in women who are free of malignant disease. If osteoporosis is part of the picture, increased dietary calcium, attention to adequate physical activity and exercise, and administration of steroids may be needed in addition.

ENDOCERVICITIS

Endocervicitis is, as the term suggests, an inflammation of the cervical mucosa and glands. It is a common infection; since the lining of the cervix is not swept away every month, an infection may remain there for some time, and may easily extend into the uterus, tubes, and pelvic cavity.

Pathophysiology

Endocervicitis is caused by either of two types of organisms: ordinary pyogenic bacteria such as staphylococci and streptococci, or gonococci (during an attack of gonorrhea). Inflammation may cause cervical erosion, with symptoms of spotting or bleeding, a thick purulent leukorrhea (white discharge), backache, low abdominal pain, and menstrual disturbances. Cervical erosion and infection seem to play a significant part in the development of cervical cancer.

Management

Douches and antiseptics are palliative measures, but in many cases destruction of cervical glands with a cautery or excision of the diseased tissue is the only means of cure. If the cervicitis is severe and chronic, the diseased portion of the cervical mucosa is removed (conization), thereby eliminating the constant irritation and the leukorrhea.

PELVIC INFLAMMATORY DISEASE

Pelvic inflammatory disease, or P.I.D. as it is often abbreviated, refers to an inflammatory disorder of the pelvic cavity. The inflammation may involve the ovaries (*oophoritis*), the fallopian tubes (*salpingitis*), the pelvic peritoneum, or the pelvic vascular system.

Pathophysiology

The infective microorganisms—usually gonococci, less often streptococci or staphylococci—easily gain access to the pelvic structures via the vagina, lymphatic channels, uterine veins, or fallopian tubes. When the tubercle bacillus is the responsible organism it is spread via the bloodstream, and the pelvic disease may not be manifest until many years after the primary lesion in the lungs has become inactive. The infection gives rise to a malodorous discharge, along with symptoms of backache, abdominal and pelvic pain, fever, nausea and vomiting, and menstrual disturbances.

Management

The main objective of patient care is to prevent extension of the infection within the patient and its transmission to attendants and others; isolation may be necessary if there is an associated gonorrhea. Antibiotic therapy is usually prescribed. Heat in the form of warm sitz baths and abdominal applications improves circulation to the area. Untreated P.I.D. may have serious consequences: scar tissue may close the fallopian tubes, resulting in sterility; an ectopic pregnancy can occur if the fertilized ovum is unable to pass the stricture; or the formation of adhesions may necessitate removal of the uterus, tubes, and ovaries.

NEOPLASMS OF THE FEMALE REPRODUCTIVE TRACT AND THE FEMALE BREAST

Carcinoma of the Breast

Although most disorders of the female breast are of a benign nature, one highly malignant disease—carcinoma—strikes at least 65,000 women annually. Unlike certain other types of cancer, such as gastric cancer, which are definitely declining in incidence, carcinoma of the female breast has maintained a leading place as a cause of death due to malignancy for at least 50 years, with about 28,000 deaths every year; this unhappy statistic makes it one of the most critical problems facing cancer research today.

Pathophysiology In the majority of cases, the carcinoma begins in the upper outer segment of the breast, forming a hard nodule that can be felt by the palm. Tumor spread is by infiltration (tumor cells spreading throughout the breast, overlying skin, and underlying muscle), the lymphatics (tumor cells carried to the axillary lymph nodes and to the lymph nodes in the chest and the neck), and by the bloodstream (tumor cells carried to distant organs). A movable nontender lump may be the earliest symptom; later there may be skin dimpling and nipple retraction, followed finally by fixation of the breast to the chest wall, the appearance of nodules in the axilla, and ulceration.

Management   Approved treatment includes removal of the breast and muscles of the chest wall. If the tumor has spread to the axilla, the lymphatic glands are excised as well. If the carcinoma is deemed to be inoperable because of metastasis, hormonal therapy, radiotherapy, and chemotherapy will usually be employed for palliation. The woman who has undergone radical breast surgery must have a gynecologic examination regularly for the rest of her life.

Benign Tumors of the Breast

Cystic disease (cystic hyperplasia); fibroadenoma   Cystic disease of the breast is common in women between 30 and 50 years of age. In this disease normal breast tissue proliferates and forms masses throughout the breasts; these small nodules may feel like lead shot. As the nodules become fibrotic, they block the ducts and cause cysts to form. Although cystic disease is innocuous, its manifestations may cause the physician to suspect malignancy; he may, therefore, perform a biopsy. If there are multiple cysts, especially if the woman is beyond childbearing age, a mastectomy, or removal of the breast, may be undertaken.

A fibroadenoma is a benign tumor formed by overgrowth of both fibrous and glandular tissue. As a rule it appears in the breasts of girls in their teens and twenties. The tumor is firm, round, and movable. It is easily removed through a small incision and has no malignant potential.

Malignant Tumors of the Uterus and Cervix

If one studies United States cancer mortality tables covering the past 40 years, he will be impressed by the steady decline shown in the death rate from uterine cancer. This decline is almost certainly due to educating women to have annual or semiannual gynecologic examinations, including a "Pap" smear (so called for Dr. George Papanicolaou, who developed the technique). In this test a sample of vaginal secretion is examined and interpreted by the pathologist; he then grades the smear, using Papanicolaou's classification, from Class 1 (absence of atypical or abnormal cells) to Class 5 (cytology conclusive of malignancy). The test thus makes possible *early* detection of cancer of the *cervix*, the neck of the uterus. Since cancer of the *corpus,* the body of the uterus, grows from the cervix in about 90 per cent of cases, it is easy to appreciate the

EDUCATION OF PUBLIC VITAL ASPECT OF CANCER CONTROL

tremendous significance of the "Pap" smear in reducing the uterine cancer death rate.

The early symptoms of cervical carcinoma are leukorrhea and irregular vaginal spotting or bleeding. As the cancer advances, tissues outside the cervix are invaded; next the corpus of the uterus is involved; and finally the cancer spreads to the bladder, the rectum, and distant organs such as the lung—a distressing picture, and one that all health practitioners should endeavor to prevent.

Benign Tumors of the Cervix and Uterus

A polyp is a protruding growth on a mucous membrane. When arising on the cervical or uterine mucous membrane, it may cause sudden bleeding or irregular spotting, especially following physical exertion or sexual intercourse. There may be an associated leukorrhea. While cervical polyps can often be seen by inspection, curettage is necessary for diagnosis of intrauterine polyps. A polyp that has been removed is carefully examined by the pathologist to detect malignant change. Uterine fibroids, or benign tumors of muscle, are found in about a third of all women over 40 years of age. The patient may experience no symptoms at all, or may have menstrual disturbances and pressure symptoms on adjacent structures. A purulent discharge may be seen. The patient may have experienced repeated spontaneous abortions.

Management

The medical and surgical management of tumors of the female reproductive tract is so complex that only the briefest outline can be sketched here. It may range from the relatively simple dilatation and curettage ("D and C") in the case of certain menstrual disturbances, to the drastic type of surgery known as pelvic exenteration, in which several or all of the pelvic organs are removed. A benign uterine fibroid may never cause symptoms and may be safely left alone; but should it cause severe symptoms, such as heavy bleeding, it must be removed. A malignant tumor should always be removed, if this is possible; such surgery is usually followed by radiation or deep x-ray therapy, with the goal of destroying any remaining cancer cells. Chemotherapy is almost always employed in these cases. Even when the tumor is deemed to be inoperable because of extensive metastases, medical measures may ensure the patient many months of fairly comfortable existence.

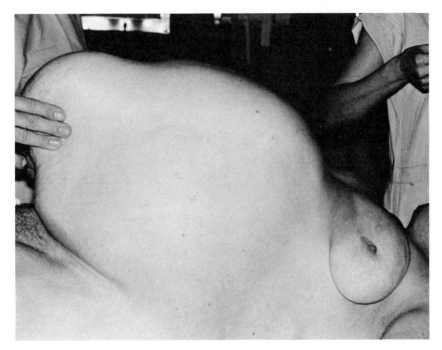

Ovarian tumor. These tumors may weigh in excess of 25 pounds. At one time, such a tumor caused death because of complications due to its sheer size. Today these tumors can be removed surgically.

NEOPLASMS OF THE MALE GENITAL TRACT

These disorders are described in Chap. 19, to which the reader is referred.

TOPICS FOR DISCUSSION

1. What disorders of the reproductive system are potentially psychosomatic?

2. Which endocrine organ largely controls the activity of both male and female sexual glands?

3. Name an endocrine gland (not a sex gland) that produces a male sex hormone in both males and females.

4. What is the purpose of the menstrual cycle?

5. How can genetic disease sometimes be predicted by examination of the amniotic fluid?

6. Discuss the significance of Papanicolaou's smear or stain.

7. What self-examination should women carry out periodically?

8. What self-examination should men do periodically?

9. What are some of the hazards of oral contraceptives?

10. Does the reproductive system participate importantly in body homeostasis? Explain.

21

common diseases of the skin

The skin, sometimes called the common integument, which is the body's largest organ, performs several essential functions. It serves as a protective barrier for the entire body, shielding it from invasion by bacteria and other foreign materials and defending the underlying tissues from physical and chemical assaults. Being waterproof, it helps the body maintain its moist interior. The skin plays an essential role in temperature regulation: its sweat glands help cool the body, as does dilation of its blood vessels; and it conserves body heat by vascular constriction. The skin is a sense organ, having receptors for touch, pain, heat, and pressure. Sodium, chloride, potassium, and magnesium are excreted in perspiration. When the kidneys fail, the integument excretes nitrogenous waste products such as urea; the body surface becomes covered with "uremic frost." Vitamin D forms when the skin is exposed to ultraviolet rays from the sun. Skin area, usually referred to as body surface area (BSA), probably represents the best available gauge for drug dosage.

The skin often mirrors the state of health of the body. Facial pallor is universally regarded as a sign of disease, while rosy cheeks convey the impression of buoyant health. Many infectious disorders, such as chickenpox, measles, and scarlet fever, lend a distinctive appearance to the skin, as do chronic infections such as syphilis and leprosy. Metabolic and endocrine disorders have their dermatologic accompaniments: there is the pigmentation of adrenal insufficiency, and the striae of adrenal overactivity; the jaundice of liver disorders, and the yellow pigmentation of carotinemia. The skin reflects occupations (e.g., the leathery wrinkled skin of the cowboy, or the pallor of the prisoner or indoor worker), as well as age (e.g., the smooth skin of the baby, or the wrinkled visage of the aged).

With a few exceptions, the same toxic, infectious, degenerative, and metabolic processes that affect the internal organs may involve the skin. It is said that as a result of disturbances of normal skin function due to various intrinsic or extrinsic harmful influences, over 300 patterns of skin disease may be produced.

THE SKIN A
BAROMETER
OF HEALTH

PATHOPHYSIOLOGIC PROCESSES WHICH CAN BE INVOLVED
IN DISEASES OF THE INTEGUMENT

	Genetics: Diseases Due to Hereditary Factors	Disease Due to Hypersensitivity and Autoimmunity	Infectious Diseases	Diseases Due to Physical Agents	Diseases Due to Chemical Agents	Neoplasia	Disturbances of Fluid and Electrolyte Balance	Diseases of Malnutrition	Endocrine Dysfunction	Stress Factors in Disease	The Aging Process	Psychosomatic Factors in Disease
Acne Vulgaris			■						■			
Impetigo			■									
Erysipelas			■									
Herpesvirus Infections			■									■
Dermatophytes		■	■									
Pemphigus			■					■				
Epithelioma						■						
Systemic Lupus Erythematosus		■	■									
Keratosis	■		■	■		■					■	■
Psoriasis	■		■	■						■		

ACNE VULGARIS

Acne vulgaris, or common acne, is an inflammatory disease occurring in areas where the sebaceous glands are largest, most numerous, and most active. It is most frequently seen during puberty, and affects both sexes equally.

Pathophysiology

Acne results from overactivity of the hair follicles and sebaceous glands. This causes oversecretion of oil and thickening of the pores. The primary lesion of acne is the comedone, or blackhead (exposure to air causes the black color). The disorder is characterized by blackheads and pimples, oily scalp, and dandruff.

ACNE A DISEASE OF YOUTH

The natural history of acne vulgaris varies greatly from individual to individual. It may be transient, leaving only a few dilated pores; in advanced cases, superficial pustules are found about the excretory ducts of the sebaceous glands, and superficial or deep noninflammatory cysts may develop. With prompt and adequate treatment, little, if any, scarring is seen. In persistent cases, bacterial and chemical by-products cause irritation and destruction of epidermal cells, so that the skin remains pitted and scarred once the inflammatory process has subsided. In extreme cases, the unsightly lesions cover not only the face, but the back, chest, shoulders, and upper arms as well. The psychosomatic "scars" may, in fact, be more serious and long-lasting than the physical ones.

Management

Numerous types of treatments, involving x-rays, stringent diet, or hormones, have been advocated, but none has proved especially successful. Perhaps the most effective treatment is scrupulous attention to cleanliness of skin and clothing, and patience—many cases clear spontaneously within a year or two of onset. A useful method for removing acne scars is dermabrasion. In this procedure, the skin is first frozen with a topical spray anesthetic. This makes possible mechanical removal of the epidermis and superficial dermis by means of a high-speed rotary steel brush.

IMPETIGO

Impetigo, or *impetigo contagiosa*, is a primary superficial skin infection caused by strains of staphylococci and streptococci. It is primarily a childhood disorder, and is most common during warm weather. It is highly contagious—the main reason it is of interest to us.

Pathophysiology

Impetigo involves the superficial layers of the epidermis. It is commonly spread by the hands and by contaminated towels. The bacteria enter the stratum corneum, or horny layer of the skin. A vesicle, or tiny blister, develops, followed by a pustule, a pus-filled sac, which may be larger than 1 cm. in diameter. White blood cells rush in from the underlying corium to combat the infection. Edema and inflammation develop. The pustule ruptures within hours to 2 days, and a crust forms. When this crust is removed, the pustule oozes. The entire face and body may be affected. A fatal systemic infection may occur in infants, but this is not likely.

Management

A highly important part of treatment is to remove the crusts so that the medication can penetrate. The medication usually used is neomycin and bacitracin ointment; in extensive involvement systemic penicillin may be required. Because of the contagiousness of impetigo, the patient should be instructed to follow such measures as use of paper tissues instead of handkerchiefs, careful washing of affected parts, and daily changing of linens.

ERYSIPELAS

ANTIBIOTICS
A CORNERSTONE
OF TREATMENT

Erysipelas is an acute streptococcal infection of the lymphatics of the skin. Except in infants and aged or debilitated persons, the disease is no longer a major problem since the advent of penicillin and other antibiotics.

Pathophysiology

Erysipelas usually involves the face. Just how the organisms are introduced into the skin is not clearly understood; it is possible that the primary infection is a nasopharyngitis, from which the streptococci are transferred to the skin. Thus the organisms may gain entrance through minute abrasions. Erysipelas of the trunk or extremities is sometimes seen in infants and following surgery or wounding in older persons. In these cases the streptococci probably are carried from external sources; without treatment, this type is commonly fatal.

Affected areas are pink to red and have a hard shiny surface. The infection spreads peripherally from its site of appearance. The advancing edge is sharply defined and slightly elevated. Mononuclear leukocytes and lymphocytes crowd into the lymphatics to destroy the streptococci swarming in the lymph space. When deep tissues are involved there is suppuration. Malaise, fever, and elevated systemic white blood count result from the presence of toxins in the lesion. The disease is contagious only when there is exudation from the lesions.

Management

Penicillin or another broad-spectrum antibiotic usually brings about a rapid response. Local cool or cold packs are applied for comfort.

HERPESVIRUS INFECTIONS

Among the group of disorders designated *herpesvirus infections,* which includes herpes zoster, herpes simplex, cytomegalovirus infections, and some others with exotic names, we are concerned mainly with those most likely to be seen by the reader, i.e., herpes zoster and herpes simplex. Despite many similarities in the clinical manifestations of these two infections, there seems to be no such similarity in their causative viruses.

Pathophysiology

Herpes zoster   Herpes zoster, popularly known as *shingles,* and varicella, popularly known as *chickenpox,* are now thought to be caused by a single virus. The reason for the differences in their clinical appearances goes back to the phenomenon that was discussed in Chapter 3, i.e., host response, or host immunity.

SINGLE VIRUS CONCEPT NOW GENERALLY ACCEPTED

There is inflammation of the posterior root ganglion of the spinal cord. The distribution follows the ganglion nerve. Aching pain is followed by an eruption that circles the trunk as far as, but not beyond, the linea alba, or middle line. In this *eruptive* stage there are papules (small circumscribed elevations), followed by vesicles (small sacs containing liquid). Scarring may result. The ganglia show evidence of severe inflammation; as the process advances there is degeneration of ganglion cells and posterior root, peripheral nerve, and posterior column nerve fibers. In some cases lesions are found in the esophagus, stomach, pancreas, adrenals, and ovaries.

Herpes simplex   Herpes simplex, also called *fever blister* and *cold sore,* is a recurrent infection due to a virus that remains dormant in the skin until activated by exposure to sunlight, an upper respiratory infection, a febrile illness, or physical or emotional stress. Single or multiple clusters of small vesicles filled with clear fluid are followed by herpetic eruptions on the lips, cornea, or external genital organs. Herpes simplex is a frequent complication of febrile disease. It is a rare cause of fatal encephalitis. In contrast to herpes zoster, herpes simplex does not affect the spinal fluid or follow the nerve distribution.

Management

Treatment of both types of herpesvirus is largely symptomatic since no specific therapy exists. Soothing dressings and topical anesthetics may be needed to relieve pain and itching. Most cases resolve spontaneously within a few days to several weeks.

DERMATOPHYTOSES

The group of disorders known as the *dermatophytoses* includes all superficial fungus infections of the skin and its appendages. They are manifested in an allergic skin rash that results from absorption of the fungus or its toxic products. Fungi of the genera Trichophyton, Microsporum, and Epidermophyton are the responsible organisms. They are classified as ringworm fungi.

Pathophysiology

The ringworm fungi have a distinctive property in that they possess an enzyme that enables them to digest keratin, the protein that is the main constituent of hair, nails, epidermis, and horny tissues. Thus these fungi are capable of disintegrating the nails, dissolving the hair, and destroying the keratinized cells of the stratum corneum. They rarely, however, invade living tissue; but sensitization to them may be induced. This is what occurs in inflammatory reactions occurring during the course of ringworm of the scalp and in acute inflammatory reactions of the feet.

These fungi provide some interesting and important information about the host-parasite relationship in ringworm infections. When the infection is highly inflammatory, spontaneous cure is likely. This is either because the fungus is unable to continue to proliferate, being desquamated along with other products of inflammation, or because the environment is no longer hospitable, owing to disruption of normal keratin synthesis. Hence, in order to entrench itself successfully, the organism must provoke only moderate or minimal reaction. For example, in the common ringworm infection of the feet caused by *T. rubrum,* the inflammatory changes are slight but the infection may persist for years.

Management

Griseofulvin is effective in many types of fungus infection, such as tinea capitis (of scalp), tinea barbae (of bearded area of face and neck), and recurrent tinea pedis (of feet). Various lotions, medicinal paints, wet packs, and baths are usually prescribed, with the specific measures planned according to the patient's needs.

PEMPHIGUS

Pemphigus is an uncommon disease of unknown etiology. It affects both sexes, and usually begins between the ages of 40 and 60 years. Since pemphigus has just been described as an uncommon disease, the reader may well ask why it is listed among the common diseases of the skin. It is a serious, often fatal, disease, and this feature itself sets it off from the many skin disorders that are not dangerous. Beyond this fact, pemphigus is of interest because it is one of the diseases on which extensive research has been carried out in an effort to discover the causative factors—whether toxic, viral, metabolic, enzymatic, or other—without success. Thus, to the dermatologist, the internist, and the neurologist—to say nothing of the patient and his family—pemphigus remains a challenge.

Pathophysiology

The distinctive feature of pemphigus is the formation of bullae, which are large blisters filled with serous fluid, on the skin and mucous membranes. It is characterized histologically by acantholysis, i.e., atrophy and detachment of the prickle cells of the skin. These cells, it will be recalled, are provided with delicate radiating processes that connect with similar cells. In pemphigus these cells become separated from each other, and lie singly or in clumps in the blister fluid. As the fluid contains water, electrolytes, and protein, loss of these substances causes blood changes.

The course of pemphigus is marked by anemia, inflammation, and infection. The bullae spread at the edges, show little tendency to heal, and rupture easily. They follow a random distribution but are most frequent on the scalp, groin, hands, feet, and, in fact, any area exposed to friction and pressure. The oral mucosa is severely affected, as is the mucosa of the pharynx, larynx, nose, conjunctiva, genitalia, and anus. As these destructive processes advance, the patient becomes increasingly weaker and toxic, and finally is unable to eat or drink.

Management

The mortality in untreated pemphigus is above 90 per cent. With the availability of adrenal steroids and ACTH (corticotropin), this rate has been sharply reduced. As is the situation in many other diseases marked by inflammation, the steroids control the disease but do not cure it. Prednisone is usually prescribed. The supportive care is fairly complicated, involving such measures as attention to fluids and electrolytes, transfusions, and prescribed baths; in addition, psychotic disturbances due to steroid therapy must be treated when they occur.

KERATOSIS

A keratosis is a horny growth, such as a wart or callus, characteristically arising from the stratum corneum of the epidermis. Two types of keratosis are recognized, one innocuous and the other potentially lethal; we shall describe an example of each.

Pathophysiology

SIMILARITY OF
BENIGN AND
MALIGNANT TYPES

Seborrheic keratosis   This form of hypertrophic growth is also called *senile wart* (verruca senilis), and *basal cell papilloma.* Although benign, seborrheic keratosis can readily be confused with pigmented mole, or melanoma, and with basal cell carcinoma, both potentially deadly. Seborrheic keratosis consists of numerous soft moles. It is usually found on exposed areas, and most often develops in middle-aged persons. The moles, or "soft warts," are raised and often hyperpigmented. Their surface is soft and greasy (seborrhea means *tallow flow*). They appear to be glued to the skin. Beneath the horny overgrowth, plugs of laminated keratin, the chief epidermal protein, may be found at various levels of the stratum germinativum. These plugs may look like an inverted papilloma; they should not be confused with epidermoid carcinoma.

Senile keratosis   Unlike the harmless seborrheic keratosis, senile keratosis flies a red flag: it is a precancerous disorder. It is characterized by the presence of small firm lesions on the face and back of the hand. Older persons, young ones accustomed to long periods of exposure to the sun, and fair-skinned persons of northern European ancestry are especially susceptible. Just as in seborrheic keratosis, hyperkeratosis is present; but in senile keratosis, epidermal cells show irregular multiplication with highly pigmented nuclei and loss of cellular polarity. Numerous mitoses crowd the nuclei. The microscopic picture of senile keratosis may strongly resemble carcinoma in situ (see Chap. 7).

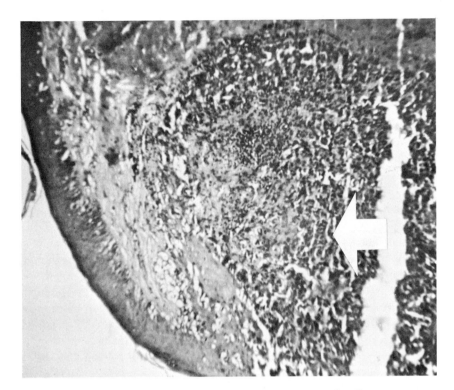

Malignant melanoma—one of the most deadly forms of neoplasia. Although this section is from the skin, the melanoma cells (*arrow*) bear no resemblance to normal skin cells. These cells are highly undifferentiated (anaplastic) in contrast to normal cells, which are differentiated according to function.

Management

When bothersome to the patient, the lesions of seborrheic keratosis can be removed by chemical or surgical means. Preferably, senile keratoses should be removed. Electrocautery or surgery is the preferred method. The physician may prescribe a sun-screening lotion to prevent further lesions in young patients.

PSORIASIS

Psoriasis is a rather common disorder classified as a papulosquamous dermatosis. It accounts for approximately 4 per cent of all the cases seen by dermatologists; certain authorities have estimated that 0.5

to 1 per cent of the total population of the United States has had psoriasis at some time. Oddly enough, the afflicted person is likely to be in robust health in all other respects. The average age of onset is 20 years.

Pathophysiology

Psoriasis is characterized by the presence of reddish-brown raised areas and tiny patches covered by sheaths of silvery scales. Removal of the scales reveals fine bleeding points, which correspond to the tops of the papillae of the corium. The significant lesions are found in the epidermis; its stratum corneum is thickened. Edema fluid between the cells of the stratum germinativum prevents formation of keratin, the chief epidermal protein. This state, known as *parakeratosis,* is pronounced. Air spaces give the psoriatic scales their silvery appearance. An inflammatory exudate bathes the upper portion of the corium; white blood cells infiltrate the epidermis, forming microabscesses in or under the stratum corneum. Following injury, lesions may appear in previously uninvolved areas. This may account for the prevalence of lesions at points exposed to injury, such as the elbows, knees, and buttocks.

In some patients, a destructive form of arthritis involving the distal interphalangeal joints is associated. Commonly a psoriatic attack coincides with flare-ups of the joint disease.

Management

PSORIASIS IS
A DISEASE OF
HEALTHY PEOPLE

There is neither remedy nor cure for psoriasis. It often happens that a type of treatment will be effective when first tried, but becomes less so with continued use. Various local therapies, such as applications of crude coal tar in conjunction with ultraviolet radiation (the Goeckerman treatment), may prove helpful. Systemic administration of adrenocortical steroids may be tried in rapidly spreading cases, but this is not without risk. Reassurance about the benign nature of psoriasis, and optimism about the patient's general health status, are probably as beneficial as any form of treatment.

EPITHELIOMA

An epithelioma is a malignant tumor consisting mainly of epithelial cells and primarily derived from the skin or a mucous surface. The *basal cell* epithelioma is relatively benign, whereas the *squamous cell* type is highly malignant.

Pathophysiology

Overexposure to sunlight over many years produces a suitable "soil" for epithelioma; the incidence in farmers, sailors, fishermen, outdoor sportsmen, and sunbathers is directly related to the amount of exposure. Light-skinned persons are most sensitive to sunlight. Skin burned by x-ray and radium may show malignant degeneration many years after exposure.

Basal cell epithelioma usually develops in persons over 40 years of age. It arises from the basal cells of the epidermis or the skin appendages, i.e., glands and hair follicles. Almost all basal cell epitheliomas develop on the head and neck areas; they are rarely found on the palms or soles. The initial lesion is typically a small papule, which enlarges slowly. Within a few months, the border becomes shiny and translucent, and a central ulcer appears. These tumors are slow-growing and do not metastasize; destructive forms may, however, invade cartilage, bone, blood vessels, or large areas of skin surface, and thereby cause death.

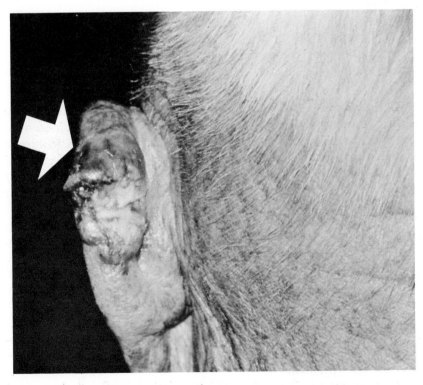

Neglected fungating carcinoma of the left ear (*arrow*). Note the ulceration of the left side of the tumor.

Squamous cell, or prickle cell, epithelioma is rare in women—possibly because they customarily give their skin more attention than do men—being seen most frequently in men of the 50-to-70-year age group. The tumor arises from the prickle cell layer of the epidermis and is characterized by rapid growth, atypical forms, and metastases. It may be primary or may arise from a senile keratosis or leukoplakia. Chronic occupational trauma may contribute to formation of the initial tumor. Although squamous cell carcinoma may develop on any area of skin or mucous membrane, it is most common on the lower lip, ears, tongue, and dorsum of the hands.

Management

SKIN CANCER
HAS
HIGHEST CURE
RATE OF
ANY
CANCER

The cure rate in basal cell epithelioma is 100 per cent, provided it is treated early and adequately. Surgical excision, curettement, chemocautery, radiation, electrosurgery, or a combination of these methods is carried out, and, as in any type of cancer, faithful follow-up is necessary. Squamous cell carcinoma, being an invasive tumor, requires intensive surgical or radiation therapy or both, as well as thorough follow-up.

SYSTEMIC LUPUS ERYTHEMATOSUS

Systemic lupus erythematosus is of great interest to medical science. It can affect many organ systems; its course may be fulminant or indolent; it is five to ten times more frequent in women than in men; it may occur at any age, including early youth and extreme old age. And although the disease has been recognized by physicians since at least the thirteenth century, its cause remains unknown—surely a disease that defies definition. Is SLE, as it is usually called, an autoimmune disease? There is considerable evidence, including the finding of LE (lupus erythemotosus) cells in the blood of patients, to strongly support this idea.

Pathophysiology

The clinical picture varies. The disease may have an acute onset, with high fever suggesting acute infection, or it may develop insidiously over months or years marked by periodic fever and vague constitutional symptoms.

The characteristic "butterfly rash" (red lesions on the flush areas of the face) is present in many, but certainly not all, patients. Ears, neck, upper back, and arms may be similarly affected. Later, these eruptions may become purpuric or bullous. There may be edema of the face and ankles, and erosion of the lips and mouth. Joint symptoms range from moderate pain to acute inflammation. With advancing visceral involvement, pneumonitis and pleurisy are likely to develop. X-ray studies reveal asymptomatic foci of atelectasis. A diffuse myocarditis may develop, resulting in congestive heart failure. Splenomegaly with lymph node enlargement and renal lesions may appear.

The subacute form clears spontaneously in the majority of cases. The acute form may remit spontaneously, but if severe renal or visceral changes are present, death occurs within weeks or months.

Management

The goal in managing the subacute form is to prevent an acute attack, and to this end, rest, nutritional therapy, and vitamin supplementation are utilized in conjunction with systemic drugs. In the acute form, hospitalization is necessary. Systemic steroids, antimalarial drugs, and corticosteroid creams may be beneficial, along with the measures mentioned above. Although there is no cure available at present, prolonged remission is possible with adequate treatment.

TOPICS FOR DISCUSSION

1. How does the integument adapt through the processes of evolution to varying conditions of temperature and sunlight?

2. Summarize the functions of the skin.

3. How does the skin mirror the state of the body circulation?

4. What skin disorders may be psychic in origin?

5. What internal tumors may be reflected by skin tumors?

6. To what skin disorders are fair-skinned individuals especially susceptible?

7. What internal diseases (exclusive of neoplasms) may be indicated by specific skin lesions?

8. What is the physiological significance of the body surface area?

9. What methods can be used to determine body surface area? (Read. Snively, W., Montenegro, J., and Dick, R.: Quick Method for Estimating Body Surface Area. JAMA, *197*:208 (July 18), 1966.)

10. What skin diseases may be familial?

11. How do skin areas vary in their susceptibility to various skin disorders?

bibliography

General

Major, R.: Classic Descriptions of Disease. Springfield, Illinois, Charles C Thomas, 1945.

Geschickter, C., and Cannon, A.: Color Atlas of Pathology. vol. 1. Philadelphia, J. B. Lippincott, 1950.

Apperly, F.: Patterns of Disease. Philadelphia, J. B. Lippincott, 1951.

Grant, J.: An Atlas of Anatomy. Baltimore, Williams & Wilkins, 1962.

Geschickter, C., and Cannon, A.: Color Atlas of Pathology. vol. 3. Philadelphia, J. B. Lippincott, 1963.

Guyton, A.: Function of the Human Body. Philadelphia, W. B. Saunders, 1964.

Hopps, H.: Principles of Pathology. eds. 1, 2. New York, Appleton-Century-Crofts, 1964.

Lyght, C., et al.: The Merck Manual of Diagnosis and Therapy. Rahway, N.J., Merck & Co., Inc., 1966.

Beeson, P., and McDermott, W.: Cecil-Loeb Textbook of Medicine. vols. I and II. eds. 12, 13. Philadelphia, W. B. Saunders, 1967, 1971.

Douthwaite, A.: French's Index of Differential Diagnosis. Baltimore, Williams & Wilkins, 1967.

Sodeman, W., and Sodeman, W.: Pathologic Physiology. Philadelphia, W. B. Saunders, 1967.

Passmore, R., and Robson, J.: A Companion to Medical Studies. vol. I. Philadelphia, F. A. Davis, 1968.

Talso, P., and Remenchik, A.: Internal Medicine. St. Louis, C. V. Mosby Co., 1968.

Chaffee, E., and Greisheimer, E.: Basic Physiology and Anatomy. Philadelphia, J. B. Lippincott, 1969.

Boyd, W.: A Textbook of Pathology. Philadelphia, Lea & Febiger, 1970.

Brunner, L., et al.: Textbook of Medical-Surgical Nursing. Philadelphia, J. B. Lippincott, 1970.

Passmore, R., and Robson, J.: A Companion to Medical Studies. vol. II. Philadelphia, F. A. Davis, 1970.

Smith, D. W., Germain, C. P. H., and Gips, C. D.: Care of the Adult Patient. Philadelphia, J. B. Lippincott, 1971.

Boyd, W.: An Introduction to the Study of Disease. eds. 5, 6. Philadelphia, Lea & Febiger, 1971.

Fluid Balance

Moyer, C.: Fluid Balance. Chicago, Year Book Publishers, 1952.
Snively, W., and Sweeney, M.: Fluid Balance Handbook for Practitioners. Springfield, Illinois, Charles C Thomas, 1956.
Weisberg, H.: Water, Electrolyte, and Acid-Base Balance. Baltimore, Williams & Wilkins, 1962.
Leithead, C., and Lind, A.: Heat Stress and Heat Disorders. Philadelphia, F. A. Davis, 1964.
Metheny, N., and Snively, W.: Nurses' Handbook of Fluid Balance. Philadelphia, J. B. Lippincott, 1967.
Garrett, T.: Baxter Guide to Fluid Therapy. Morton Grove, Illinois, Baxter Laboratories, 1969.
Snively, W., and Thuerbach, J.: Sea of Life. New York, David McKay, 1969.
Goldberger, E.: A Primer of Water, Electrolyte and Acid-Base Syndromes. Philadelphia, Lea & Febiger, 1970.

Endocrinology

Selye, H.: The Stress of Life. New York, McGraw-Hill Book Co., 1956.
Netter, F.: Endocrine System and Selected Metabolic Diseases. New York, Ciba Pharmaceutical Co., 1965.
Schmitt, G.: Diabetes for Diabetics. Miami, Diabetes Press of America, 1968.
Williams, R.: Textbook of Endocrinology. Philadelphia, W. B. Saunders, 1968.

Genitourinary Disease

Kintzel, K. C. (ed.): Advanced Concepts in Clinical Nursing. Philadelphia, J. B. Lippincott, 1971.

Pediatrics

Shirkey, H.: Pediatric Therapy. St. Louis, C. V. Mosby Co., 1968.
Krugman, S., and Ward, R.: Infectious Diseases of Children. St. Louis, C. V. Mosby Co., 1968.
Blake, F. G., Wright, H., and Waechter, E. H.: Nursing Care of Children. Philadelphia, J. B. Lippincott, 1970.

Psychosomatic Disease

Freedman, A., and Kaplan, H.: Comprehensive Textbook of Psychiatry. Baltimore, Williams & Wilkins, 1967.

Aging

Veterans Administration: Research in Aging. Washington, D.C., Veterans Administration, 1959.

Clinical Chemistry

Tietz, N.: Fundamentals of Clinical Chemistry. Philadelphia, W. B. Saunders, 1970.

Therapy

Garb, S., Crim, B., and Thomas, G.: Pharmacology and Patient Care. New York, Springer, 1970.
Goth, A.: Medical Pharmacology. St. Louis, C. V. Mosby, 1970.
AMA Drug Evaluations. Chicago, American Medical Association, 1971.

Microbiology

Pelczar, M. J., Jr., and Reid, R. D.: Microbiology. New York, McGraw-Hill, 1965.
Carpenter, P.: Microbiology. Philadelphia, W. B. Saunders, 1967.
Wheeler, M., and Volk, W.: Basic Microbiology. Philadelphia, J. B. Lippincott, 1969.
Brock, T. D.: Biology of Microorganisms. Englewood Cliffs, Prentice-Hall, 1970.

Nutrition

Wohl, M., and Goodhart, R.: Modern Nutrition in Health and Disease. Philadelphia, Lea & Febiger, 1960.
Mitchell, H. S., Rynbergen, H. J., Anderson, L., and Dibble, M.: Cooper's Nutrition in Health and Disease. Philadelphia, J. B. Lippincott, 1968.

Dermatology

Tobias, N.: Essentials of Dermatology. Philadelphia, J. B. Lippincott, 1963.

index